Routledge Revivals

Fifty Years in Public Health

First published in 1935, this book provides a valuable contribution to the history of Public Health and Preventive Medicine. Written as a recollection of the experiences and knowledge of Sir Arthur Newsholme, the book covers a period in which phenomenal progress was made.

Fifty Years in Public Health

A Personal Narrative with Comments

Sir Arthur Newsholme

Routledge
Taylor & Francis Group

First published in 1935
by George Allen & Unwin

This edition first published in 2015 by Routledge
2 Park Square, Milton Park, Abingdon, Oxon, OX14 4RN
and by Routledge
711 Third Avenue, New York, NY 10017

Routledge is an imprint of the Taylor & Francis Group, an informa business

Publisher's Note
The publisher has gone to great lengths to ensure the quality of this reprint but points out that some imperfections in the original copies may be apparent.

Disclaimer
The publisher has made every effort to trace copyright holders and welcomes correspondence from those they have been unable to contact.

A Library of Congress record exists under LC control number: 35014104

ISBN 13: 978-1-138-90645-7 (hbk)
ISBN 13: 978-1-315-69548-8 (ebk)
ISBN 13: 978-1-138-90647-1 (pbk)

Fifty Years in Public Health

A Personal Narrative With Comments

by

Sir Arthur Newsholme

K.C.B., M.D., F.R.C.P.

Sometime Chief Medical Officer of Health
to the Local Government Board
Sometime Lecturer in Public Health
Johns Hopkins University

LONDON

George Allen & Unwin Ltd

MUSEUM STREET

FIRST PUBLISHED IN 1935

PRINTED IN GREAT BRITAIN BY
UNWIN BROTHERS LTD., WOKING

To the Memory of

My Wife

whose uninterrupted comradeship during fifty-two years ensured my happiness, my capacity for work, and its measure of success

PREFACE

I HAVE often been urged to write Recollections of my long life, which has been chiefly engaged in that rapidly growing branch of applied Preventive Medicine known as Public Health and in its associated epidemiological problems.

The difficulties of the task have led to prolonged hesitation; and had it not been that the writing of this volume was enjoined on me by one who for fifty-two years shared much of my work, it might have remained unwritten.

Among the difficulties I foresaw was the impracticability of doing justice in a personal narrative to the work of many who have been engaged in work like my own, some of them known, some unknown to me.

When my memory has served, aided by re-perusal of reports and journals, I have mentioned or outlined work collateral to my own; but I must here and there have overlooked some work of others, mention of which would have been made in a complete record. But I remind myself and my readers that a complete record is beyond my powers, and that this volume, as it is entitled, is in the main a personal narrative, concerning itself with events in my own life. I ask that it be read with that in mind.

As, except in its two first chapters, my Recollections have been intentionally limited to occurrences bearing on Public Health, I am hopeful that, even with the above-stated limitation, this volume may prove not only interesting but also valuable as a contribution to the history of Public Health and Preventive Medicine during a period in which phenomenal progress has been made.

This hope is confirmed by my conviction that only after studying how Public Health—or any other science, theoretical or applied—has come to be what it is can one fully understand its present position, and prepare for further advance with a minimum risk of mistakes.

In the present volume I have dealt chiefly with Public Health first as seen from the viewpoint of private medical practice, and then as seen—steadily increasing in scope—in my experience as a medical officer of health up to the year 1908.

In a second volume—if it is ever written—I hope to give an account of Public Health progress as seen from a personal angle in more recent years, first in England and afterwards in other countries.

I have said above that this is mainly a volume of personal recollections, but I have not hesitated to give my later thoughts on the subjects discussed, while placing on record past imperfections of theories and work.

I am able to place on record in these pages contemporaneous statements, which is perhaps the least unsatisfactory way of writing history, when these contemporaneous facts and conclusions are checked in the light of the fuller knowledge of 1934. This is possible because for five years I was Editor of *Public Health*, the journal of the Society of Medical Officers of Health, because of contributions to medical journals and to the Proceedings of different Societies, and lastly because in my annual reports for Brighton current Public Health problems were discussed year by year.

My apologia for devoting so much space to my predecessors in Public Health work is given on page 72.

ARTHUR NEWSHOLME

February
1935

CONTENTS

Part Three

MEDICAL PRACTICE AND PUBLIC HEALTH WORK

Part Four

THE CONTROL OF INFECTIOUS DISEASES

Part Five

VITAL STATISTICS AS A BASIS OF PUBLIC HEALTH WORK. SPECIAL STUDIES IN VITAL STATISTICS

Part Six

THE SAFEGUARDING OF DEVELOPMENT AND GROWTH

DIAGRAMS

ILLUSTRATIONS

PART I

MEDICAL AND SOCIAL TEACHERS AND TEACHING

CHAPTER I

PERSONAL AND FAMILIAL

Haworth and Brontë associations—The influence of Grimshaw and Wesley—Religious revivals

I WAS born in 1857, the year of the Indian Mutiny. My father was a wool-stapler, a merchant in wool, and my mother, his second wife, the daughter of a farmer. My father's office was in the Piece Hall, Halifax, then the headquarters of the Yorkshire textile industry. His father had been a textile manufacturer at Mytholmes, near Haworth, and not far from the village of Newsholme. This grandfather had been largely responsible for the introduction of Sunday schools into this moorland part of Yorkshire, and a local tablet commemorating his work for Sunday schools is still to be seen in the village of Oakworth, near Haworth.

Sunday schools in those earlier days were centres of general elementary as well as of religious instruction; and I may narrate an illustration in my own boyhood. I attended the Haworth Wesleyan Sunday School, the last quarter of an hour of each session being devoted to "spelling." I remember the word "quay" being given to be spelt, and only one boy spelt it correctly. But there was an official in that Sunday school whose duty was to pass from class to class and assist in maintaining order. Hearing this word correctly spelt he intervened, protesting the absurdity of the notion that it could spell "ke," and the dispute on this point between the teacher and the supervisor was the source of joy to at least one scholar in that class.

Haworth, my birthplace, is a village on the edge of the moors forming the Pennine range between Yorkshire and Lancashire. Its population, including outlying farms, probably never exceeded four or five thousand. Dotted along each mountain stream flowing to form the River Worth, an affluent of the River Aire, were mills run by water-power, which was gradually being superseded by steam. Haworth itself crept up a steep Main Street, from the Worth valley to near the hill-top and the village church, which was surrounded by a cluster of houses, including three or four public-houses, one of them the "Black Bull," too much frequented by Branwell, the talented brother of the Brontë sisters. As I lived for a considerable part of my youth not far from Haworth Church, it is about it that many recollections revolve.

My father died when I was under five years old, leaving my mother with her five children, the youngest a girl, and I the youngest of four boys. We owed everything to her devotion. Her strong and vigorous character, her self-abnegation, her lofty ideals of duty and life were influences which determined in large measure her children's future lives.

My father had been churchwarden to Rev. Patrick Brontë, the incumbent of Haworth. Brontë was a native of Ulster, who changed his name from Prunty, about the time when Lord Nelson and Brontë became a national hero. His wife was a Cornish woman. Many stories of the Brontë family were told in my hearing, although Charlotte, the last survivor of the family except the father, died in 1855, two years before I was born. The story of Branwell Brontë, the talented but dissolute son of the incumbent, is well known to all Brontë students, especially since the two Brontë plays which have been acted in 1933-34. They give a fair idea of the historic facts and their setting, but exaggerate the eccentricity of the father. Branwell was a not infrequent visitor at our house, and a heavy old-fashioned tumbler out of which he drunk his beer has passed into my possession. So also did a large oil-painting of my father by an artist, whose work Branwell—also a painter in oils—had attempted to improve, but still left it an inartistic and unpleasing picture. It remained in the family for many years, and then it was imposed on me as the youngest of four brothers. It subsequently disappeared.

I recall vividly one story relating to Branwell Brontë. Dr.

Ingham, the local doctor, attended the Brontë family, and occasionally I was under his care; but for minor ailments my mother, like the village generally, consulted Mrs. Betty Lambert, the woman druggist of the village, and I recall the brimstone and treacle and other "spring" remedies which came from her shop. She was a noted local character, and she was sent for not only in sickness but also to make the last toilet of the dead.

One day she called on my mother, and I remember the conversation between the two, the small boy sitting on a hassock at his mother's feet being overlooked. Betty was telling my mother the circumstances of Branwell Brontë's death some twenty years previously. Even now I can recall the details. Let me state in preface that this erratic, dissolute but talented brother was a source of almost continuous anxiety and distress to his immortal sisters, Emily and Charlotte, and especially to Emily, who did much to shield him. To his alcoholism he had added laudanum drinking, and he died September 24, 1848, at the age of thirty. The certified cause of his death was chronic bronchitis and marasmus; but probably he had phthisis, his end being hastened by his habits. Betty supplied him with his weekly quantum of opium, which he fetched during Church-time on Sundays; and it was on one of these occasions that he boasted to Betty, as she informed my mother, that a man could do anything by force of will: he could even die standing.

One dark night Betty was sent for, because Branwell was dying. As she walked through the churchyard to the parsonage she wondered, she told my mother, whether he would remember his boast. She entered the sick-room, and, on seeing her, Branwell got out of bed and stood on the floor, saying, "it is coming." He sank to the floor, was covered with a blanket, and died before he could be lifted into bed.

The story of the Brontë family is well known. It raises the old question as to whether tuberculosis increases talent or genius, the association being so common. But tuberculosis has been an extremely prevalent disease, and the association need not be causal. In the Brontë days bronchitis and consumption were the banes of life on the bleak Yorkshire hillsides, and diagnosis between these two lethal agents was less accurate than it is now. Emily Brontë's lines, written in a homesick spirit at Brussels, illustrate the local climatic conditions in which she was reared:

> There is a spot, mid barren hills,
> Where winter howls, and driving rain;
> But, if the dreary tempest chills,
> There is a light that warms again.

Rev. Patrick Brontë was incumbent of Haworth from 1820 until his death in 1861 at the age of eighty-four, apparently from bronchitis. His wife died in 1821 in her thirty-ninth year, leaving six young children. Her death is said to have been due to an "internal cancer." This may be so, but doubt may be entertained. Four years later two of her children died, aged eleven and twelve respectively, probably in "decline." Branwell, as we have seen, died in 1848 aged thirty years; his sister Emily three months later, aged twenty-nine, in a "decline," and another sister, Anne, in 1849, aged twenty-seven, also in a "decline." Charlotte survived to marry, in June 1854, and died on March 31, 1855, at the age of thirty-nine, apparently from exhaustion due to irrepressible nausea during pregnancy. One can speculate as to whether the present more advanced obstetric science might not have saved her life. But her death-certificate gave phthisis as a cause of death, and it is likely that impending motherhood had fanned the flame of latent tuberculosis with which she, like the other brothers and sisters, was heavily infected.

The Rev. Patrick Brontë lived to the age of eighty-four, dying in 1861, the certified cause of death being chronic bronchitis, from which he had long been a sufferer. The pathetic history of his family is not inconsistent with the hypothesis, I believe not previously advanced, that the unwitting father had suffered throughout his adult life from tuberculosis, and that at intervals he infected his whole family with the same disease. Such chronic fibroid forms of phthisis are well known, and are consistent with survival to advanced years. It is the role of modern preventive medicine to seek out these chronic patients especially when a case of more acute tuberculosis is recognised in a family. They are not very ill, and their intermittent infectivity can be reduced below the level of danger when hygienic personal habits as to coughing and spitting are scrupulously maintained.

A further note on "chronic" carriers of infection may be added here. Illustrations of the fact that some few exceptional children, after an attack by scarlet fever, may continue to infect others with scarlet fever are given on page 185; and in diphtheria the same exceptional semi-chronicity of infection is displayed (p. 185). The same phenomenon is seen in exceptional cases of typhoid fever; in this instance the carrier-capacity may continue for many years (p. 185). In this disease, and still more in tuberculosis, it can truly be said that the chronic carrier is a chief reservoir from which further cases of illness are derived.

Although milk from tuberculous cows produces tuberculosis (not of the lungs) in young children, human sputum is the chief source of tuberculosis (both pulmonary and non-pulmonary) in children and in adults.

In family life—especially in circumstances like those of the Brontë family, in which spittoons were in use, and only imperfect precautions would be taken in spitting or in coughing—each member of the family receives frequent doses of infective material. The result depends in part on the vital resistance of the children, much more on the frequency and the dosage of the infection by sprayed or expectorated phlegm. The prevention of tuberculosis consists to-day in removal of the patient to a sanatorium, giving the family a holiday from daily exposure to infection, and training the patient in hygienic methods of coughing and spitting before he returns home. The alternative to this is removal of the children, temporarily or permanently, from the source of infection, and especially the avoidance of fondling or other obvious means of infection.

For most people interest in Haworth centres round the Brontës; and I remember well the chuckling with which my mother recalled Charlotte Brontë's description of the curates in *Shirley*. They were unmistakable portraits, the originals of which she identified. So also the story of the heroine in *Shirley* burning with a red-hot iron her hand which had been bitten by a suspicious strange dog is an incident in Emily's life. Emily was devoted to her own dog, and to a stray dog passing the kitchen dcor she offered a basin of water. The dog bit her, and realising the risk she at once took the action which is attributed to the heroine in *Shirley*, in the chapter entitled "Phoebe," and thus described by her:

> I walked straight into the laundry, where they were ironing. . . . While the maid was busy crimping or starching, I took an Italian iron from the fire, and applied the light scarlet glowing tip to my arm; I bored it well in: it cauterised the little wound.

The Brontë girls were intensely shy and the villagers scarcely knew them socially. They can have had little sympathy with the local manufacturers, and except for Sunday-school teaching, other social contacts were scanty. The father's religious teaching was "sound," but did not influence local life so much as the teaching in the Wesleyan and other chapels of the district. Early in his charge at Haworth a devastating storm had occurred, which was sometimes mentioned in my boyhood. It formed the subject of a sermon by Mr. Brontë, published "by request," in which the catastrophe was claimed to be a direct Divine warning to the people. What happened was this. There had been steady rain for weeks, and the peaty soil of the moorland heights in the hills above Haworth had become supersaturated with moisture. One day a mountain-side of peat slid down into the valley below, destroying farm-houses and other buildings in its torrential course down the valley. This catastrophe has been utilised in one of Halliwell Sutcliffe's novels (himself a Haworth man), in which a "border" fight between Lancashire and Yorkshire was effectively stopped by a similar land-slide.

For the Haworth people themselves an earlier celebrity had

a much greater influence than the Brontës on life in the district —the Rev. William Grimshaw, who though he became incumbent of Haworth in 1742 and died in 1763, was still remembered and revered in my boyhood. Two years after his induction at Haworth he was the subject of a sudden "conversion," associated with great rapture, which entirely changed his outlook on life. It was similar to the change which occurred in a multitude of early Methodists, and we may recall the sudden conversions of Saul the persecutor and of Francis of Assisi. Grimshaw became an itinerant preacher somewhat like his friend John Wesley, but his travels were limited to Yorkshire and Lancashire. He retained his charge at Haworth. In summer, crowds came to Haworth to hear him preach, and on the occasion of visits by John Wesley many thousands collected in the churchyard to listen.

Many stories concerning Grimshaw were current in my boyhood. He was a stern disciplinarian, and on occasional Sunday mornings he would give out a long psalm, and during its singing visit the three or four beer-houses within a stone's throw of the church, horsewhip in hand, bringing into church all who had not escaped over back walls or hidden in outhouses.

A Sunday traveller through the village found that his horse had cast a shoe. The blacksmith refused to do the needed work without Mr. Grimshaw's consent. This a visit to the rectory secured when it was elicited that the traveller was on his way to fetch a midwife!

On the moors there was annual horse-racing and betting. Mr. Grimshaw prayed earnestly that there should be a heavy rain on the day fixed for the races, and a deluge of rain came which effectively prevented the racing that year. It was never resumed.

Grimshaw died of a "putrid fever" in his fifty-fifth year, having forbidden friends to visit him, as he knew his condition was infectious.

It may appear a far cry from this sketch of Grimshaw to

the influences of my boyhood between 1860 and 1872; but this is not so. John Wesley and Grimshaw were in fact colleagues, and Grimshaw did much to build up Methodism in Haworth. He was responsible for building its first chapel, and his old oak chair—in which I have sat at a semi-centennial celebration—is still preserved there. It was recently borrowed on behalf of the Bishop of Ripon for a local church celebration. For many years local Wesleyans continued to attend Sunday morning service in the church and to attend service in chapel in the evening; and this in earlier years was the practice of my parents. It was consistent with my father's position as a churchwarden. But my mother's leanings were Methodist; for among the Wesleyans her mother, Mrs. Mary Binns, was a shining light. And in time the separation between Anglicanism and Methodism became definite, as it was in my youth. But the combined influence of the teaching of Wesley (1703–91) and of Grimshaw (1708–63) left its deep impress on local life, as Wesley's teaching did throughout the world—for "the world was his parish."

Although it may appear foreign to the main aim of this volume, which is to trace health progress as seen through my eyes, I am impelled to comment on this Evangelical revival as a potent factor in determining the social and hygienic as well as the moral uplifting of the nineteenth century.

This spiritual awakening was in reality a reawakening. Similar awakenings having occurred throughout the history of historic Christianity. Such an awakening was seen in the Lutheran Reformation, though intermingled with the dross of national and international politics. The same may be said of the great spiritual awakening in the Commonwealth era (say 1640–60). Wesleyanism furnishes the next great example, in this instance free from political side-currents. Such spiritual upheavals may be compared to biological mutations, for they were unforeseen and their occurrence could not be predicted.

Each resuscitation of Christian belief has been characterised by intense personal faith. The main element in the Wesley evangel was the emphasis laid on a personal certitude of a direct relation with God through Jesus Christ. This was Martin Luther's (and this was St. Paul's) doctrine of Faith elevated into an emotional certainty of salvation from "a wrath to come" and into a certainty of communion with the Divine. The goal was not the ecstasy with which this "flight from the alone to the Alone" was commonly accompanied, but the communion itself. In my boyhood I saw many examples of the ecstatic, and of the more stable religious experience in which ideal Christian lives were lived.

I can illustrate by an experience narrated to me concerning my maternal grandmother, and belonging to the early years of the nineteenth century. Mrs. Mary Binns (or Bynnes, as it was spelt in the Haworth records of the fourteenth century) was a leading Methodist, great in persuasive power. A notorious drunkard was locked in the stocks at the church gates while the Sunday morning congregation passed to church. Mrs. Binns took the opportunity to supply him with a cushion to sit on, and a cup of tea for refreshment. Needless to say he was talked to sympathetically and "for his good." He joined the Methodists, and not many Sundays afterwards my grandmother rejoiced to hear his testimony of conversion to the assembled congregation.

There were dangers in religion in which emotion played a supremely important part, but there were greater dangers in its absence; and that it produced God-fearing people of faultless integrity, always ready to help the weakly, and profuse in good works, I can testify. The results of their faith and works were even more striking than have been seen in the more recent experiences of the Salvation Army.

It is agreed that the evangelical movement was of great national importance. It was under its influence that the liberation of the West Indian slaves—purchased by a great national expenditure—was secured. Not only the work of Wilberforce (1759–1833) but also that of Lord Shaftesbury (1801–85) and other social reformers owed the same driving-power; and the prison reform of John Howard (1726–90) sprang from the same source. Evangelicalism meant an enormously increased solicitude for one's fellow-men and not merely or chiefly that "other-worldliness" attributed to it by Matthew Arnold. The Puritan movement led to the introduction of democratic government in religious communities among believers, and slowly and haltingly State democracy followed. The Wesleyan evangelical movement carried this movement towards democracy even further, perhaps more in the State than in Wesleyanism itself.

It is true that Charles Wesley in one of his hymns expressed the sentiment that

> Nothing is worth a thought beneath
> But how I may escape the death
> That never dies.

But this was poetic exaggeration. Methodists were good citizens, and during the vast upheaval of the French Revolution Methodism was a potent factor in preventing excesses in this country. The honesty and frugality, the abstinence from alcohol, the cherishing of the best family life promoted by Methodist teaching did wonders in mitigating the terrible sanitary and social evils of the earlier decades of town industrial life.

The relative importance of individual change of character and of the work of social amelioration is even now disputed territory. We encounter ministers of religion who appear to spend their energy almost exclusively in advocacy of making clean the outside of the cup and platter. The enthusiasm of some of them for "birth-control," a mechanical device for reducing overcrowding and economic difficulties, which can act irrespective of self-control is well known. So also as regards housing: not long ago I heard a cleric, after giving particulars of slum life in a central district of a great town in which public-houses abounded, ask his audience how could one expect the men and women living under such housing conditions to keep sober. He evidently thought—to quote an old adage—that the shortest way out of (old) Manchester was to get drunk. But he had neglected the fact that on an average one-fourth of the earnings of the people living in that particular slum area were wasted in its many public-houses. Having spent my life in securing improved housing and in allied efforts at social amelioration I regret that ministers of religion of this exceptional type do not appear to realise that their infinitely more important share in social amelioration is to evangelise the people and thus to reduce slum-life much more rapidly than any medical officer of health can do. Removal of the slum-dweller from the slum is a valuable auxiliary to moral reform; but unsatisfactory lives are not confined to slum-dwellers—a converted person is unlikely to need to continue to dwell in a slum. There is no antagonism between destroying slums and evangelising their dwellers. Both are needed, but as an expert on one side of the problem I would beg spiritual experts to appreciate and act on their greater possibilities for good.

CHAPTER II

PREPARATION FOR A MEDICAL CAREER, 1870–80

Grammar School of the old type—Pre-medical training in medicine—St. Thomas's Hospital in my student days—The educational value of blunders

I HAVE already testified to the supreme importance of my mother's share in my earlier training. Happily she was helped by the presence within two miles of my home of a grammar school, now extinct, known as the "Free Grammar School." This was one of many similar schools throughout the land, founded by the piety of a former generation. This particular school was endowed in 1638 in the reign of Charles I. In 1827 it had some two hundred scholars, in 1865 when visited by H.M. Inspector (Mr. J. G. Fitch, M.A.) the number was much smaller, and during the years when I was a scholar (nine to fifteen years old) there were seldom more than a dozen pupils. The headmaster, Rev. W. Patchett, M.A., was the master and sole teacher, and the teaching embraced almost solely Mathematics, Latin, and Greek. But these—to a willing pupil—were taught thoroughly; and when I was transferred at the age of about fifteen to a Science school in Keighley I found myself at no disadvantage, except in natural sciences.

The teaching in the new school was directed chiefly to securing certificates from the Science and Art Department for the pupils, on which monetary grants were based. This led to some cramming of undigested facts, not adequately supplemented by personal experimental work. The system has been greatly improved; and even then the school held a high position as a centre of "practical" training.

At this stage an uncle, a school-master in London, and an executor under my father's will, intervened, and for nearly a year I lived with him in Vincent Square, Westminster, attending daily Matriculation classes at University College in Gower

Street. I was left to my own resources; and, ambitious beyond my knowledge and judgment, I remember attending a course of Anglo-Saxon, as well as Professor Henry Morley's fascinating lectures on English literature, neither of which came within the scope of the Matriculation examination. I attended the chemical lectures of Professor Graham, of colloid chemistry fame, and did practical chemical work under Professor Williamson, who introduced a modified nomenclature, under which, for instance, sulphuric acid was named hydrogen sulphate. In the Latin part of the Matriculation course the London University had set a book of Livy which is omitted from ordinary editions of that author, and I only succeeded in getting a second-hand copy, bound in old leather, which was purchased in what was known as Booksellers' Row or Hollywell Street. The setting of this book for Matriculation students must have been inadvertent, for I remember the embarrassment of the teacher in translating some portions of the descriptions of Bacchanalian games.

I matriculated when just over sixteen years old, and not long afterwards *res angusta domi* compelled my return home to Bradford, where my mother then lived. My hope had been to prepare for the Indian Civil Service, but evidently this was not now practicable. My mother, fortunately, consulted her family doctor, Dr. Burnie of Bradford, who proposed that I should become his dispenser and surgery assistant for a while. I remained with him for over a year, and thus happily was among the, even then, limited number who received an admirable training in practical pharmacy, in minor surgery, and in the methods of private medical practice before entering a medical school. My time was occupied in dispensing the prescriptions of two skilled practitioners of the older school, in taking the numerous messages of a busy practice, in keeping its "books," and in acting as clinical assistant in minor accidents and operations. Happily also the doctor's qualified assistant interested himself in me, and taught me some physiology, and much about the "bones." To both Dr. Burnie, a Scotchman, and his assistant, Dr. Samuel Johnstone, a North of Ireland

Irishman, I have reason to be grateful. I had spare time during the day to study the subjects of the Preliminary Scientific Examination of the University of London and in the evening to attend local science classes.

I regard this period as most helpful in giving me an early initiation into practical medical work, and regret that similar opportunities are now rare. In a visit to Russia in 1932 I was interested to find that medical students are required to undertake similar work in their early medical student's career, including the work of a nurse in cleaning up after operations, in undertaking minor dressings, and afterwards in actual nursing, while pursuing their theoretical medical training.

By some such method the risk that a medical student's training shall be concerned predominantly with major diseases and operations is reduced, and his knowledge of minor ailments and their treatment and his skill in utilising pharmacy to the full extent of its possibilities are greatly enhanced.

In 1875 monetary difficulties were adjusted. A small inheritance coming to me when of age was made immediately available, and though this did not suffice to carry me through for four years, the venture was undertaken, and I paid my entrance fees at St. Thomas's Hospital Medical School, London, in October 1875. Why St. Thomas's was chosen I cannot remember, but it was a happy choice. I sat for an entrance scholarship, and I remember that Charles A. (afterward Sir Charles) Ballance and I were placed next in order to the two successful candidates. At the end of each term during the next three years I secured monetary prizes, which with the help of some private coaching of a few medical students enabled me to complete my training and become qualified. Realising the importance of becoming quickly "qualified" I took the L.S.A. (Apothecaries Society) after three and a half years' training; and in 1880 obtained the M.B. Lond., and was awarded the gold medal in medicine with a University scholarship for two years. A year later I became M.D., being qualified for the gold medal in this examination.

In looking back on my work as a medical student I consider that I devoted too much time to theoretical studies, helpful in examinations, and too little to practical work in laboratories and among patients. The teaching in the medical school and for the University examinations was good, but it is now greatly improved. Then it was apt to turn out doctors insufficiently trained in minor ailments and in various special departments of medicine. Had it not been for my pre-medical experience in a doctor's surgery, and still more for my St. Thomas's Hospital appointments after qualification, as house physician, resident accoucheur and house surgeon, followed by a year's experience as house surgeon at the Tottenham hospital outside London, and afterwards as registrar in the Evelina Hospital for Children, I should have been ill fitted for the multifarious requirements of general medical practice in a suburb of London, which occupied me during some five succeeding years.

On the clinical side of medicine one learns perhaps most from one's blunders, and I narrate two such blunders here in the hope that the story may be seen by some medical student or junior practitioner.

While house physician at St. Thomas's, I was asked to see the out-patients of one of the physicians, Dr. X, who was notably *difficile* in his human relationships. Being very busy in the wards, I saw these out-patients hurriedly, and in one case prescribed for a patient with stomachic symptoms without overhauling him. This patient next week was found by Dr. X to have cancer of the stomach, and as house physician I had to receive the patient into my ward and prepare notes of his case supplementary to the notes already written by Dr. X, which included observations reflecting on me. I deserved this, although I think Dr. X was the only member of the then staff who would have acted as he did.

The lesson was effective, and it is a lesson still relevant for those who may be careless or pressed for time. Never treat a patient without making a diagnosis based on as complete an examination of him as is practicable in the circumstances.

One further story about this Dr. X. In his out-patient department a patient regularly attended who was utilised for demonstrating to junior students a "typical" præsystolic cardiac bruit. Some time after the previous episode Dr. X came to me asking me to try to obtain an autopsy on this patient who had died suddenly at home. After much conversation with the widow I was permitted to examine the chest. I found that an aneurism of the descending aorta had ruptured into the left pleura, and that two vertebrae had been partially excavated by the tumour. Dr. X did not give a clinical lecture on this case to his students.

With altruistic motive I may here narrate also my wrong attitude in a case under Dr. Charles Murchison's care. I was Murchison's clinical clerk in the months immediately before his premature death, and like all who came under his influence admired his supremely fine teaching and revered him as a man. I can now see him standing at the patient's bedside, leaning with one hand on the wooden handle with an overhanging cord on which the patient could raise himself in bed. Murchison's carotid arteries could be seen by his crowded class to be visibly pulsating. He died when only forty-nine years of age of aortic regurgitation.

In this particular case I was asked to conduct the examination in front of the class. I avoided the well-known pitfall of asking leading questions; and was careful not to resort to a physical examination until the information derivable from symptoms and from the history of the patient had been exhausted. Parenthetically, this to-day is a pitfall which is too often fallen into. Physical examination and, still more, laboratory tests are resorted to long before the possibilities of enlightenment by intelligent interrogation have been exhausted. A saying of a great clinical teacher of Murchison's time emphasises this lesson. Students often begin examining a patient by asking to see his tongue. This teacher always said, "Tongue last and least"; and if the tongue be taken as symbolising all physical and laboratory tests, the teaching of this aphorism is valuable.

I had, so far, avoided criticism, and passing from the bedside

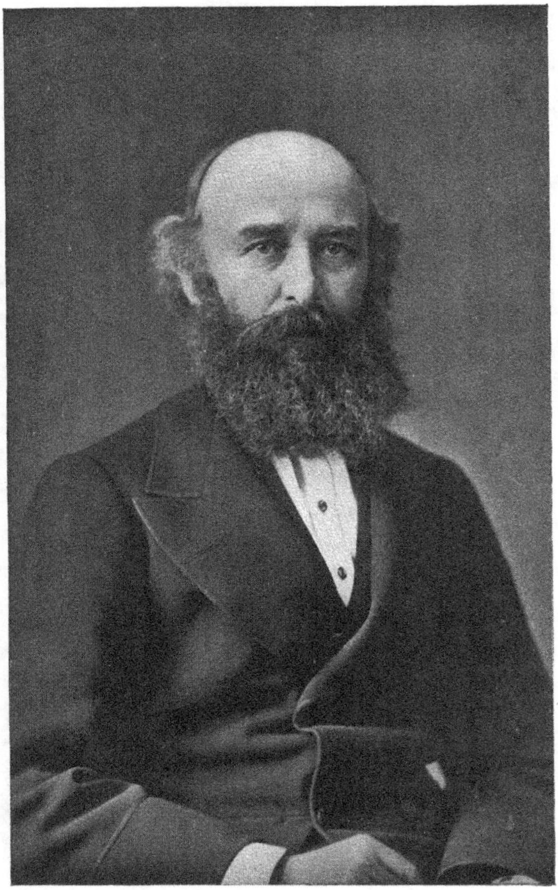

JOHN SAYER BRISTOWE

I gave the correct diagnosis of carcinoma ventriculi to the class. Murchison then asked my treatment. I unfortunately shrugged my shoulders, indicating my view as to the hopelessness of treatment. Murchison then gave a severe but kindly address to the assembled students, emphasising their duty to treat every patient to the hour of death, using every available means to maintain the patient's strength, to alleviate his sufferings, and to prolong life. And then followed his prescription, which is written indelibly on my mind.

R. Creosoti ♏ i. Extract. Opii, gr. i. Extract Nucis Vomicæ, gr. ¼ in Pilula, to be taken four times daily.

I must tell one more story illustrating the temerity of inexperience. A man was brought into the casualty department of the hospital with external dislocation of the knee joint. He was seen by me as casualty house surgeon, and I succeeded in replacing the dislocated parts without much difficulty. But the accident had produced a very rare form of dislocation, and the vivid language used by a senior surgeon who had missed the opportunity of taking a model of the displacement is still in my memory!

One's memory serves one best for exceptional or odd circumstances. In my second year as a medical student I one afternoon went round the hospital wards with Dr. Peacock's class, when I might have been better occupied at that stage of my medical training. Dr. Peacock was senior physician at St. Thomas's, a Quaker who was greatly respected and an authority on cardiac diseases. One student, senior to the others, who had recently come down from Oxford, was persistent in asking questions, until Dr. Peacock with some asperity remarked, "It appears to me that your questions are directed rather to air your own knowledge than to receive information."

A similar snub was administered by Dr. Bristowe—the kindliest of men—to a student who was notorious for his attempts to push his own opinion. "I have often noticed that a maximum of confidence goes with a minimum of knowledge."

A younger physician, an Irishman, was well known for his inability to resist the temptation to oppose the diagnosis of the examining student. Hence the following conversation:

Physician: "You say that is a case of mitral stenosis. Tell me now why I disagree with you."

Student (somewhat heated): "Of course you say No, because I say Yes."

Personal testimonials must have been a serious burden to teachers. I remember one given to a fellow-student who consulted me about a carefully inserted comma, the omission of which would have greatly enhanced the value of the testimony!

There were two brothers, great favourites in the school, who rejoiced in the initials F. W. and S. W. At school one of them told me they were known as "Fresh Water" and "Salt Water." A testimonial intended for Fresh Water was given to Salt Water, or vice versa, and disentanglement was called for.

I am tempted to mention Dr. Matthews Duncan, the famous obstetrician, who had migrated to London, as had also Joseph Lister—Duncan to St. Bartholomew's and Lister to King's College Hospital.

I was examined by Duncan at the M.B. examination of the University of London, and failed to receive distinction in his subject (as his co-examiner afterwards told me) owing to my inability to answer one question, the answer to which was contained in a volume of Duncan's essays not read by me. Duncan had a broad Scots accent and slow delivery which gave point to an incident in one of his lectures. He was, as a pupil of his recently informed me, deprecating hurried midwifery, and said, "Never hurry, except in one circumstance . . . (pause) . . ., when you are trying to catch a flea."

CHAPTER III

MY MEDICAL TEACHERS: BRISTOWE AND MURCHISON

JOHN SYER BRISTOWE (1829–1897)

To John Syer Bristowe and Charles Murchison I owe most that was of permanent value in my clinical training. They had widely separated characteristics; for Murchison taught dogmatically, while Bristowe was slow but very sure in diagnosis, perhaps in consequence of his very exceptional pathological experience. Murchison's general attitude in diagnosing illness was somewhat like that of a famous judge: "I may be wrong, but I have no doubts." Bristowe's diagnosis in doubtful cases was postponed, and an expectant attitude was maintained. Murchison was a master in teaching, especially for junior students; while Bristowe appealed especially to senior men. His Sunday morning round of the wards will always be remembered. At these, old students forgathered; and often Savage of Bethlem Hospital joined in the round, and the conversations between these two on nervous diseases were highly instructive.

But enthusiastic "youngsters" sometimes were concerned at the absence of active therapeutics; and I recall that a colleague, who afterwards became a distinguished surgeon (Sir Charles A. Ballance), and I were concerned about a syphilitic brain patient, who was then in fact moribund, and ventured jointly to ask Bristowe if the patient might have Iodide of Potassium. We had seen syphilitic gummata in less important tissues than the brain in other patients dissolve almost as by magic under the influence of this drug. Bristowe at once ordered the Iodide, but the patient died two days later! Of course the patient had come under treatment at a stage when this treatment must necessarily fail. I did not then know, but Bristowe was at this time the 7th President of the Society of Medical Officers of Health. (I became its 21st President in the year

1899–1900.) In his Presidential Address to that Society I have recently found the following remarks:

> I have to acknowledge, not for the first time, that I am one of those who look with a good deal of scepticism on most of what is generally inculcated with regard to the medicinal treatment of disease.

This incredulity as to the usefulness of a large part of the pharmaceutical armamentarium of that day was justified, but I doubt not he made some exceptions; for instance, as to the value of mercury and iodides in the treatment of syphilis, and as to the recently introduced treatment of acute rheumatism by sodium salicylate.

Through Bristowe came my first glimpse into public health work. Bristowe was medical officer of health of Camberwell, in the south-east of London; and occasionally he asked me to examine microscopically morbid animal tissues.

Bristowe in the year 1880, when I was his house physician, and afterwards was most widely known by his *Treatise on the Theory and Practice of Medicine.* The second edition, published in 1878, was familiar to me from cover to cover. It was most readable and eminently consecutive and scientific. It was, as his junior colleague, D. J. F. Payne, himself a profound pathologist, said, *the* pathological textbook on medicine, and in its literary quality it resembled Watson's earlier *Institutes of Medicine* and Osler's later *Textbook.*

Bristowe's handwriting, however, was not readable. I remember being asked to read to him notes on a case which he had written at a previous visit. I stumbled over some words and Bristowe himself could not decipher his own writing!

The literary quality of what Bristowe wrote had been evidenced in a volume of poems published in 1850, written by him in his pre-medical days, which I had read but could not buy a copy. He also wrote fugitive poems in later years, and I value much a copy of some of his later poetry printed for private circulation.

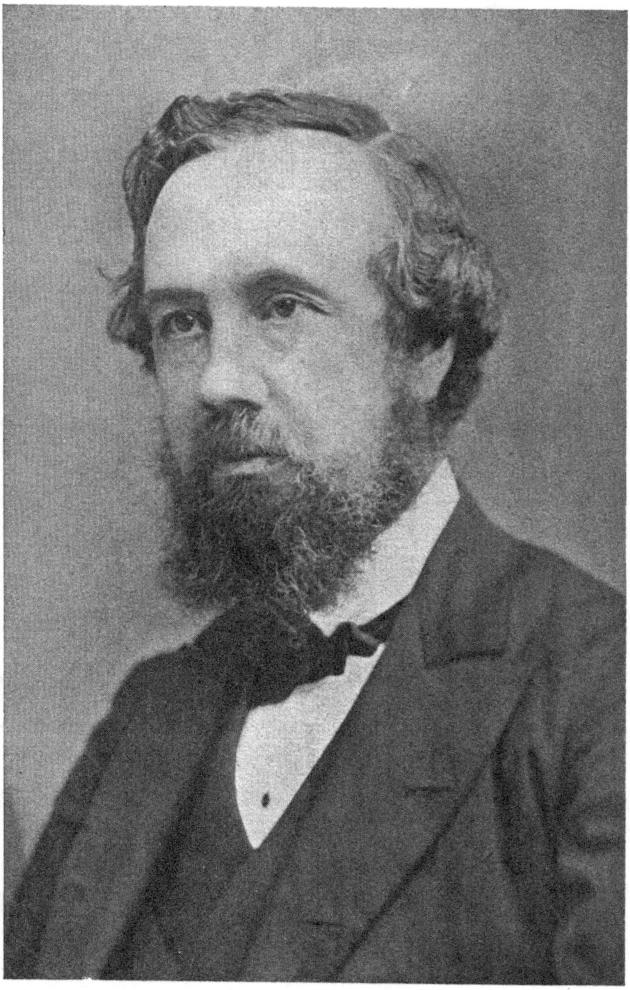

CHARLES MURCHISON

Bristowe was a member of the Royal Commission on Vaccination, 1889–96. In earlier years he undertook a number of scientific investigations for the Privy Council, of which his colleague at St. Thomas's, John Simon, was the Medical Adviser. In 1862 Bristowe reported on "Phosphorus Poisoning in Match Manufacture," and in 1865 on "Infection and Rags." With Burdon Sanderson he reported to the Privy Council on the Cattle Plague; and with Timothy Holmes he wrote a valuable report on "Hospitals in the United Kingdom" (p. 60).

I regretfully leave my reminiscences of Bristowe. He was universally respected and beloved. He was a highly scientific physician, a wise counsellor, a good friend, and, to quote the words of J. F. Payne, "unselfish, devoted, helpful, faithful, and candid." In 1887 his term as physician at St. Thomas's was extended for five years, and until his retirement he was its chief figure and the inspiration of all his colleagues and pupils.

CHARLES MURCHISON (1830–1879)

Undoubtedly the most potent influence during my student life was that of Charles Murchison, whose particular genius I have already contrasted with that of Bristowe (p. 35). Murchison's views on the pythogenic origin (i.e. the origin from putrefactive changes in the absence of a preceding case) of enteric fever are criticised on page 124 in the light, in part at least, of fuller knowledge than was available to Murchison.

Murchison was born in 1830 and was only 49 when he died. As a medical student in Edinburgh he had typhus fever and had a further attack when he became physician to the London Fever Hospital, where he obtained most of the material for his classical work on *The Continued Fevers of Great Britain*, of which the first edition was published in 1862 and the third in 1884 after his death. In this work and throughout his marvellously impressive teaching at St. Thomas's he utilised Louis's rule, whenever practicable, to reduce his "observations to a numerical expression." I have already mentioned (p. 35) his surpassingly great powers of teaching. In his formal lectures and in his clinical lectures alike the student who could take notes with fair rapidity had exact and vivid information more readily useful than could be obtained from textbooks.

His teaching, both at the bedside and in his systematic and clinical lectures on medicine, was, I believe, based on Professor Hughes Bennett's method of teaching in Edinburgh. In forming a diagnosis of each patient's illness he insisted that after a careful survey of the patient's history and present condition every possible diagnosis should be enumerated; and that then, by careful analysis, the symptoms favouring and antagonistic to each of these possible diagnoses should be considered. By this method Murchison succeeded in systematising the student's clinical knowledge and in widening his outlook on illness. In a relatively short time the whole range of medicine was thus brought under review. Of course, the method has the drawback that the enumeration of possibilities may have been incomplete; this might be so on any system of clinical diagnosis. But there emerged from his bedside teaching the great lesson that—apart from inadequate inquiry and examination—a chief source of error in diagnosis was the failure to consider all the possible diagnoses before reaching a reasoned conclusion. It was an inspiration to the crowd of students who surrounded him to see the courage and pertinacity with which he continued his exacting work, notwithstanding the aortic disease from which he suffered, and which ended in his sudden death on April 26, 1879. *Nec silet mors.*

Murchison treated typhus fever in the general wards of St. Thomas's Hospital. I suppose I was one of the last to see a few typhus cases sparsely distributed among non-infectious cases, and without any spread of infection. The reason for this safety became obvious in later years; but the current explanation was that the poison of the fever was diluted to a non-dangerous point by free circulation of fresh air. It is a remarkable fact that in British civilian life typhus fever became almost extinct before Nicolle and his co-workers in 1909 reported the transmission of typhus to monkeys and by them to other monkeys by body-lice which had fed on a human typhus patient. Evidence accumulated that the body-louse was the vehicle of typhus infection, but it did not follow that the stress laid by public health officers in their efforts to stamp out typhus, on clearance of slum areas, on reduction of overcrowding, and on measures of cleansing and disinfection was wasted; for all these activities meant discouragement to the life of the infecting louse, and otherwise tended to promote health. When the rôle of the louse in spreading typhus was discovered it served to re-emphasise the already realised importance of isolation in hospital of every known case of the disease; for this isolation ensured personal cleanliness and minimised the possibilities of dangerous parasitic activity. For other aspects of Murchison's life-work, see page 123.

CHAPTER IV

OTHER MEDICAL TEACHERS AND TEACHING

Cory and arm-to-arm vaccination—Greenhow, first lecturer on public health in a medical school—The salicylate treatment of rheumatic fever—W. M. Ord and myxœdema—Prevention by treatment

CORY AND SAFEGUARDS IN VACCINATION

ROBERT CORY (1845–1900) was Assistant Obstetric Physician when I was a student at St. Thomas's; and when I was resident accoucheur (R.A.) he was the consultant called in for very exceptional midwifery complications in the maternity districts of the hospital. He made a special study of still-births and of deaths occurring immediately after live-birth, a study in which Ballantyne of Edinburgh was a great pioneer. But Cory's chief relationship to us medical students was as Teacher of Vaccination. He held the post of public vaccinator for twenty-five years, and had a record of eighty thousand successful vaccinations with only two failures. I well remember his teaching. Arm to arm vaccination was then the universal practice, and he taught that this was free from risk of conveying extraneous disease, when due precautions were taken, the main one being that only healthy children should be used as vaccinifers. But in proving the absence of risk he went beyond this, experimenting on himself. On four occasions he vaccinated himself with lymph taken from syphilitic infants. In the first instance he took lymph from "an emaciated child, unquestionably syphilitic," but without active symptoms at the time. No result. He then vaccinated himself from a child with some active symptoms of syphilis. No result; and this was repeated in a third instance. Some two years later he selected for auto-vaccination an infant with open syphilitic sores and a skin eruption; and alas, three weeks later he developed a primary chancre at the point of vaccination.

Cory's subsequent history was that of a scientific martyr, for after a long illness, including hemiplegia, he died in 1900 at the age of fifty-five. A civil list pension was awarded to his widow.

The importance of his case was that it fitted in with allegations made by anti-vaccinators that syphilis could be spread by vaccination. These allegations were investigated on behalf of the Royal Commission on Vaccination appointed in 1889; and although it was found that the risk of producing syphilis was almost nil in actual practice, and that the occasional septic complications of vaccination occurred only when precautions had been neglected at the time of vaccination or afterwards, the final report of the Royal Commission published in 1896 recommended the substitution of calf lymph for human lymph in official vaccination; and this has since then been the universal practice. The Local Government Board accepted the duty of cultivating vaccine lymph in calves for use in vaccination by public vaccinators.

DR. E. HEADLAM GREENHOW

It will be noted that I write chiefly on teachers who, directly or indirectly, were concerned in the development of preventive medicine. Among these, mention must be made of two Lecturers on Public Health at St. Thomas's Hospital Medical School.

The first of these was appointed in 1855. Such an early acceptance of the importance of Public Health in the training of medical students is not surprising, for Simon, the leader in official public health work, was then surgeon at St. Thomas's.

Greenhow was born in 1814, and had practised medicine for eighteen years in North Shields and Tynemouth before he came to London at the age of thirty-nine. There he had also actively engaged in promoting public health reform while continuing in private medical work.

Greenhow was employed by Simon on behalf of the Privy Council (then the Central Authority for Public Health) very largely in making local inspections and in the preparation of comparative statistics of causes of death in various districts. The most important of these inquiries was into the local incidence of excess of lung diseases during the year 1860 and thereafter. These inquiries were ably summarised in Simon's reports; they not only threw a flood of light on local causes of excess of mortality, but also illustrated Simon's acute aliveness to the social and industrial conditions behind these excesses.

Thus in his 4th Report (1861) Simon said:

> It is true that the workpeople might rebel against needlessly unwholesome conditions of labour . . . but this theoretical power of the workman is in present practice a nullity,

a not obscure reference to the need for combination of workers or for adequate legal control by Government inspectors to rescue the workman from his helplessness.

Meanwhile, as Simon said:

> The canker of industrial diseases gnaws at the very root of our national strength.

In reports between 1859 and 1862, made to the English Board of Health and to the Privy Council, Greenhow, after analysis of local statistics of lung diseases in agricultural and manufacturing populations respectively, arrived at the important generalisation that:

> In proportion as the male and female populations are respectively attracted to indoor branches of industry, in such proportions *ceteris paribus*, their respective death-rates from phthisis are increased.

a conclusion which holds good to the present day, though the difference in the incidence of phthisis in industrial and in agricultural and other spheres of work has greatly diminished.

As bearing on the progress made in subsequent years, a paper by Dr. Greenhow "On a Standard of Public Health for England" may be mentioned. It was read before the Statistical Society of London in June, 1859. This paper has added interest to me because on the cover of my copy is John Simon's characteristic autograph signature.

In this paper Greenhow referred to the desirability he had found "as a teacher of Sanitary Science" of having "a Standard of Reference showing what may be termed the normal mortality produced by particular diseases in healthy places"; and he proceeded to analyse the vital statistics of three groups of rural populations, northern, southern, and south-western, which we need not further examine here, except to give one illustration showing the value of the method adopted by him. Pulmonary diseases of all kinds, including phthisis, on an average were responsible for 98,969 deaths in England and Wales in each of the nine years 1847–55; but had the deaths from these diseases, in each sex and at each period of life, been at the same rate as those in the northern group of rural districts in the same years, the average number of deaths in the whole country would have been only 54,098.

One conclusion from this state of things has already been given in the extract from Dr. Greenhow's report to the Privy Council. With characteristic insight, Simon generalised a further conclusion as follows:

> Anyone who will candidly consider what are *the possible meanings of those differences of death-rates*, can arrive, I think, at only one conclusion. The diseases which are known to prevail in different districts with such surprising degrees of inequality are eminently the diseases which can be prevented.

DR. ALFRED CARPENTER was lecturer on public health in my student period, and I attended the twelve lectures which under this appointment he gave each summer.

Of the lectures I remember only the pleasant oratory of the lecturer, but I recall that Dr. Carpenter invited us all to lunch at his house in Croydon, where he was medical officer of health as well as a busy private practitioner. We were shown the local sewage farm at Beddington, on the broad irrigation plan, which at that time was a "show place" in public sanitation. It is now realised that town sewage is so greatly diluted as almost to annul its value for fertilising land, and that for avoidance of nuisance and production of an effluent fit to discharge into a river, other plans are more successful.

I remember also that Dr. Carpenter ascribed local outbreaks of scarlet fever and of typhoid fever to sewer emanations from the street grids over sewers. In this respect he was like most of his contemporaries, and even of the next generation of sanitarians (see p. 155).

A personal incident illustrates the lack of interest then taken by the average medical student in public health. While serving as Dr. Bristowe's house physician and at the same time working for my M.B.(Lond.) examination, I acquired a "septic throat" and was sent for a week to the Isle of Wight. Hygiene formed part of one paper in this examination, and I had read no hygiene, except what is incidental to all medical studies. I therefore took with me Wilson's *Hygiene*, then the only really good small textbook available, and read it through in my train journey. I passed my examination, and obtained distinction in medicine; but I had only read "hygiene" for a couple of hours!

Two further events occurring during my student life may be cited as conducing to the progress of preventive medicine in its widest sense. One of these was a new and extraordinarily successful treatment of rheumatic fever, and the other the recognition and description of the disease which was christened myxœdema.

THE SUCCESSFUL TREATMENT OF RHEUMATIC FEVER

So long ago as 1865 Sir William Gull, writing in Guy's Hospital Reports, described a series of cases of this disease, which in order to ascertain its natural history he had treated simply with mint water. He compared his results with results from the current use of drugs supposed to be active, and concluded that the latter had no advantage, and that rheumatic fever "tends unaided to get well in nineteen days." But in my fourth student year I saw some of the earliest cases of this disease which were treated by sodium salicylate in 20-grain doses every two hours until the temperature fell, and was witness of the marvellous abortion of the ordinary course of the illness which was thus effected. My interest in this disease was aroused, and it was the subject of my Milroy Lectures in 1895. A chief difficulty encountered by me in this later study of the epidemiology of the disease for a series of years as measured by hospital statistics lay in the fact that cases formerly sent to hospital were now treated at home, and thus the ante-salicylate period was not strictly comparable with the post-salicylate period; and that, furthermore, the national death returns for the two periods were scarcely comparable. It is likely that a further factor has now come into play, and that irrespective of salicylates there has been a remarkable decrease in the total amount of rheumatic fever.

The story of the introduction of the salicylate treatment deserves to be recalled. There are, in fact, two stories. In Germany it appears that the new treatment was suggested by a hope to extend Listerism beyond surgery and in fact to disinfect the patient's blood while in circulation, an idea which probably arose from the fact that salicylic acid is easily resolved into carbonic acid and carbolic acid. The English story is told by Dr. T. J. Maclagan in his book *On Rheumatism*, 1881. His conclusions were based on the assumption that rheumatic fever, like ague, is "of miasmatic origin" and allied to, though distinct from, ague; and he was thus led to search for a remedy for rheumatic fever, as the Jesuits found one for ague in the bark of the cinchona, which grew on the marshy banks of the Amazon river, where malaria was prevalent to an exceptional extent. Inasmuch as rheumatic fever is "apt to occur in low-lying damp localities," salicin derived from the willow bark seemed likely to meet this end, as did the Peruvian bark for malaria; and Maclagan's trials showed that this anticipation was correct. Under treatment by salicin, the course of rheumatic fever was curtailed.

Now malaria does prevail excessively in marshy districts, but not exclusively so; and, contrary to the teaching in my student days and to the common opinion even to-day, I was able to show in the Milroy Lectures (p. 217) that rheumatic fever was most prevalent in dry years, and occurred excessively in some countries characterised by a small rainfall and great soil dryness.

So in both malaria and in rheumatic fever we possess successful empirical remedies, which were discovered by reasoning based on an erroneous hypothesis of the pathogenesis of each disease.

There are very few specific drugs in medicine. The two just named stand out, alongside of colchicum in the treatment of gout, and of mercury and potassium iodide in the treatment of syphilis; possibly also of iron in the treatment of chlorosis and arsenic in that of syphilis; but in recalling the triumphs of modern pharmacology, especially by the administration of glandular extracts, we cannot afford to forget the triumphs of empiricism, clinical trials on the hit or miss principle, which have enriched medicine and succoured mankind.

WILLIAM M. ORD AND MYXŒDEMA

W. M. Ord (1834–1900) was joint lecturer on Physiology and Assistant Physician when I joined St. Thomas's, and as such gave us up-to-date instruction, while his colleague in that course, Dr. John Harley, leaned to the "old ways."

Dr. Harley represented an earlier school of thought in other respects (p. 61). A patient under the care of Dr. Harley was found in the post-mortem room to have died of actinomycosis. The case had been fully investigated both macroscopically and microscopically by S. J. Sharkey, assisted by T. D. Acland; and there could be no doubt that it was a real instance of the parasitic disease, whose nature had been established by Bollinger in 1876. The new growths in the liver were, however, stoutly maintained by Harley to be tuberculous, in a discussion in the post-mortem room, at which I was present.

When Murchison died suddenly in 1879, Ord, who had become full physician two years earlier, undertook "clinical" teaching on an extended scale; but although Ord taught well, he did not approach Murchison as a great clinical teacher. He was a man of much talent, and a classical scholar. He did much to extend George Rainey's prior investigations on the influence of colloid media on crystalloid forms.

I was an onlooker on Ord's clinical research into a somewhat rare condition which he named myxœdema, in view of the excessive amount of mucin found in the subcutaneous tissues of patients suffering from it. These patients had a characteristic facies. The face was as if set in wax. All creases were erased and the hair of the scalp was very scanty. The mind was dull and speech slow and hesitating. Some years later one had the opportunity of seeing the almost miraculous change in mentality and physical condition produced by the administration of thyroid extract.

Ord's inquiries were made in 1877. In 1873 Sir William Gull had described the same condition in a paper on "A Cretinoid State Supervening in Adult Life in Women," which he pointed out was associated with atrophy of the thyroid gland; Ord worked out its pathology and symptomatology.

As in other instances, further advances were slow.

In 1883 Theodor Kocher (1841–1917) showed that after surgical extirpation of the thyroid for goitre there sometimes followed a condition like myxœdema or cretinism—"hypothyroidism"; and Victor Horsley in 1885 found that when the thyroid gland of monkeys was experimentally extirpated a similar condition resulted. Although Schiff in 1884 had proved that transplantation of a thyroid gland from another animal of the same species would safeguard against some of the consequences of thyroidectomy, and Horsley in 1890 made the same suggestion, it was not until 1891 that G. R. Murray introduced the successful treatment of myxœdema by the hypodermic administration of a glycerol extract of thyroid. Earlier attempts (1889 by Buchner and 1893 by Kocher) at grafting thyroid gland had been partially successful. In 1892 Hector Mackenzie found that administration of thyroid gland in small doses by the mouth was equally successful.

The history of this disease is a good illustration of the gradual growth of knowledge. It shows also how the art of medicine may advance the science of physiology, as well as the converse. This is also a good instance of therapeutics as a means of prevention of disease, in the sense of preventing its continuance. The treatment of diabetes by insulin, of syphilis by arseno-benzol preparations, the cessation of infection secured by the hygienic treatment of pulmonary tuberculosis and the treatment of pernicious anæmia by liver extract are well known further instances.

CHAPTER V

TWO EASTERN MEDICAL STUDENTS

Sir Ho Kai and Hong-Kong Medical School—Baron Takaki and beri-beri—Protracted incubation period before knowledge is applied

HERE and there in this volume are given illustrations of the slow growth of our knowledge of the causation of disease, and the more tardy adoption of measures of prevention or of preventive treatment thus made possible.

In the present chapter the work of Takaki, one of the two Mongolians who were my fellow-students at St. Thomas's, illustrates the fact that sometimes incomplete knowledge of causation may suffice for the prompt adoption of effective preventive measures. The illustration is as striking in its way as that of typhus.

HO KAI

Ho Kai, one of my two Eastern fellow-students, was a young Chinaman, the son of a Chinese missionary; the other, Kanehiro Takaki, a Japanese of more mature years, who had already become qualified medically in Japan. He had been sent for English medical training by the Japanese Government.

I knew both of them well. They visited my home. I gave my felicitations to Ho-Kai on his marriage to a charming English girl; and I had an offer from Takaki that if I would return with him to Tokio he would guarantee me a good practice.

While a medical student in London, Ho Kai was also "eating his dinners," and he was called to the bar. He took the degrees of M.B., C.M.(Aberd). Then he went with his young English wife to Hong-Kong, and for thirty years played an important part in the public life of the Colony. Until the death of his wife from enteric fever he practised both medicine and law. At her death—leaving one daughter—he founded a memorial hospital in her name, and subsequently, I believe, practised law only.

The management of this Alice Walkden Memorial Hospital he handed over to the London Missionary Society, of which his father was an active member. It had a European medical staff, among whom were Patrick Manson and later James Cantlie. Out of this hospital, which was founded in 1887, the College of Medicine of Hong-Kong grew; a five-year course of study was imposed, and the first diploma was given in 1902. The staff for some years taught without fees. This institution stimulated the foundation of the University of Hong-Kong, in which the College was incorporated.

For many years Ho Kai was a member of the Sanitary Board of Hong-Kong, and for twenty years he was a prominent member of the Hong-Kong Legislative Council. He lectured on Forensic Medicine in the College of Medicine. In 1902 he received his C.M.G. and in 1912 was knighted.

He died in 1914.

KANEHIRO TAKAKI

In 1872 Takaki entered the Japanese Navy as a surgeon, being promoted two years later to the rank of staff surgeon. In 1875 he was sent to England to study English medicine, and became L.R.C.P. in 1878 and F.R.C.S.(Eng.) in 1880. In that year he returned to Japan and was forthwith promoted to the rank of Deputy Inspector-General of the Imperial Japanese Navy. A few months later he became Director-General. At that time the Japanese Navy had much "kak'ke" or beri-beri. It accounted for three-fourths of the total cases of sickness. The seriousness of this disease among Japanese sailors recalls the devastating effect of another food-deficiency disease, scurvy, in the British Navy, until in 1795 lemon juice was made a compulsory ration.

Takaki investigated "Kak'ke" and came to the conclusion that it was due to the inadequate proportion of nitrogenous to carbonaceous food in the sailors' dietary. He succeeded after much opposition in securing an improved dietary. A test

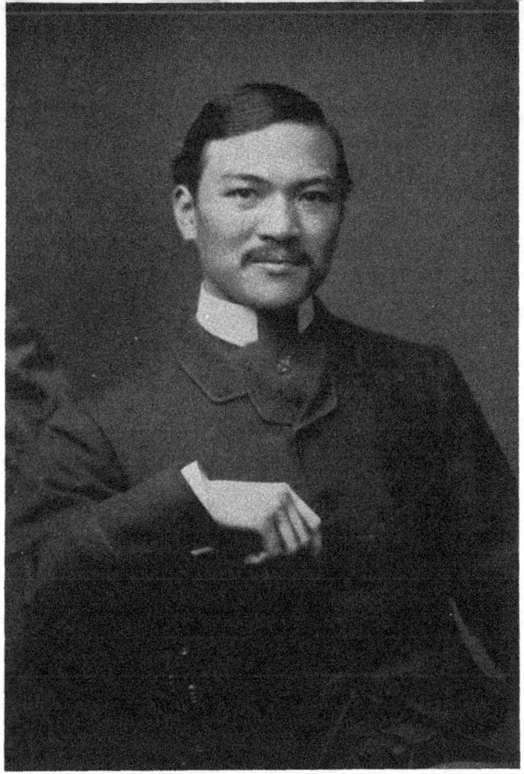

HO KAI

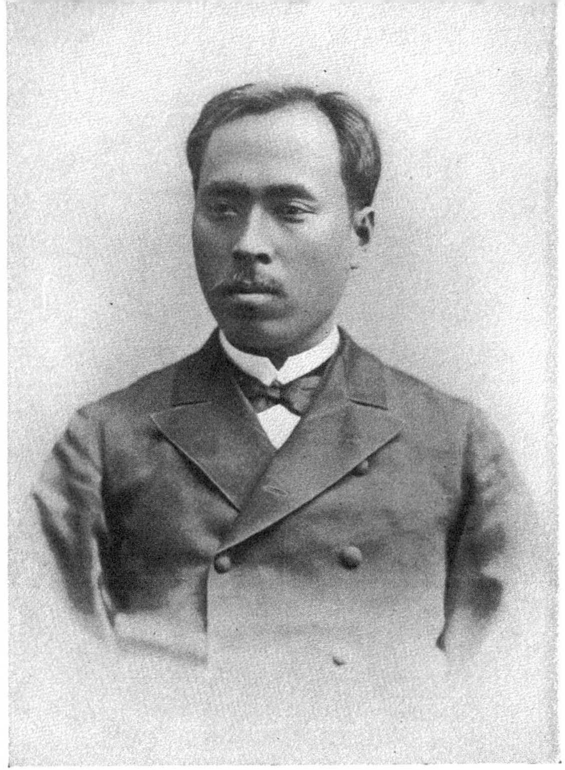

TAKAKI

experiment was made analogous to Captain Cook's circumnavigation of the world in the year 1772. It may be recalled that in that voyage, which lasted over three years, not a single case of scurvy occurred among the crew, which numbered 118, careful hygienic precautions, including an allowance of lemons and anti-scorbutic foods, being adopted.

Similarly, in 1883 the Japanese warship *Rynjo* was sent on Takaki's recommendation on a voyage of 271 days to New Zealand and South America, with 350 persons on board. The ship's crew had ordinary diet, and over a hundred cases of beri-beri occurred. Another ship, the *Tsukuba,* was then sent on exactly the same course, and under the same conditions, except that a new diet scale was arranged, which avoided an excess of rice, barley being used to a considerable extent as a substitute for the polished rice which had been the staple food.

On this trip no cases of beri-beri occurred. The general reforms introduced by Takaki included a more liberal supply of nitrogenous food, much less rice, and general hygienic improvements. In the light of further investigation we know that substitution of other foods for the devitalised polished rice was the essential reason for the success of Takaki's check experiment; but without this further scientific knowledge Takaki succeeded in eliminating beri-beri from the Japanese Navy. The results of an improved dietary were soon seen in the navy sickness figures. In 1879 beri-beri accounted for 38 cases of illness for every 100 sailors, in 1889 the proportion was only 0·03 per cent. Stated otherwise, the invaliding caused by beri-beri soon fell from $\frac{1}{2}$ to $\frac{1}{63}$ or even less of the total invalidity, and in a few years the disease had almost disappeared from the navy. In the subsequent war with Russia, Takaki's reforms were a large factor in the Japanese success. The Japanese Army's medical advisers were reluctant to adopt the naval reforms; and in the same war it is stated that nearly half the army sickness was caused by beri-beri.

Takaki came to England in 1906, by which time he had been

raised to the Japanese House of Lords as Baron Takaki. He lectured at St. Thomas's on the results obtained by his reforms. He visited me in Brighton with his son, a head taller than his father. The son was then a medical student at St. Thomas's. Takaki readily gave his view as to why his son was tall. It is interesting, even if one cannot completely accept the explanation. He had determined that his children should not be made to sit on their heels, or (as often happened) balanced in a similar attitude without support by the heels. He therefore had stools provided for them, and thus he had avoided partial stoppage of the circulation of blood to the femurs with resultant dwarfing of growth. Nor was he convinced when it was suggested that greatly improved dietary or the occurrence of a "throw back" to a taller ancestry or both might have been concerned.

Takaki died in 1920.

Takaki's special research had points of general interest, apart from its hygienic success with an incomplete analysis of the causal factors. He succeeded with marvellous promptitude in securing the practical dietetic reforms advocated by him. He was living in a more scientific age than when the means to cure and prevent scurvy were well known but failed to be adopted in the British Navy.

The contrast with the history of scurvy is striking. As early as 1564 the Dutch recognised the value of fresh fruit and vegetables in preventing and curing scurvy; and early in the seventeenth century Purchas and Woodall independently were advising lemon juice to this end. Dr. James Lind (1716–94) urged that vegetables and ripe fruit protected against scurvy; but it was not until forty-one years later that Lind's teaching was applied in practice, lemon juice being made a compulsory ration to the British Navy in 1795. Another half-century elapsed before a similar obligation was imposed on the Mercantile Marine.

This obligation on sailors was, I believe, the first instance of compulsion in the feeding of a large number of men. In recent years in the United States of America we have seen an example of attempted enforcement on a gigantic scale of prohibition of the manufacture and sale of alcoholic drinks, which has failed because the majority of the people who had voted for it were not prepared to apply their votes in their personal lives. In the one instance there was compulsory addition to the dietary of a large body of men under discipline, in the other, an attempt to deprive the entire population of beverages which often were detrimental to health.

The prevention of beri-beri on a large scale in Japan illustrates how prevention sometimes anticipates the complete knowledge of causation, the best starting-point for prevention. I have instanced typhus fever as a remarkable example of this (p. 38); but typhoid fever is quite as striking an illustration of the same point (see p. 89).

Takaki's investigation has a further claim to a special place in the history of preventive medicine, for beri-beri was the second disease—scurvy being the first—which was definitely shown to be due to a dietetic deficiency. Disease had repeatedly been associated with the action of positive enemies—parasites or toxins—invaders from without or self-generated—but the notion that deficiency of some element of nutrition might also cause disease was new, and for long found no favour. Even when Lind in his *Treatise on the Scurvy* (1st edition, 1754), testified to the preventibility of this disease by the eating of fresh vegetables and fruit, he also said "a most powerful and principal cause of scurvy is the moisture of the air, and consequently the dampness of the sailors' lodging." A similar line of thought was visible for beri-beri, until Takaki made his great experiment in 1882–86 and proved that given a more varied and improved dietary beri-beri disappeared. But the special vitamin in food which prevents scurvy, and cures it when disease has already occurred, has only been isolated a few years ago, and even more recently this vitamin has been synthetically produced by Haworth. The causal relation of vitamin B to beri-beri has an almost equally recent history.

Experiments on pigeons and fowls showed that multiple neuritis like that in beri-beri was produced when they were fed on boiled rice, and was cured when their diet was improved (Eijman and others, 1890). It may be that in this disease a toxic element is also involved, but the general fact demonstrated on a national scale by Takaki remains true.

CHAPTER VI

THE EARLY DAYS OF LISTERISM

FROM the standpoint of Preventive Medicine the most important event in my student life was the introduction of antiseptic surgery, and I had full opportunity of watching surgical work carried out by Listerian methods and corresponding work on old-fashioned lines. I can endorse the contrast between the two given recently (*British Medical Journal*, May 26, 1934) by an old fellow-student (now Sir Charles Ballance), that when he entered St. Thomas's very few operation wounds in the London hospitals healed by first intention, and that there was a general lack of surgical cleanliness in the operating theatre on the part of the surgeon and patient and their entire environment.

In my fourth year (1878–79) as a medical student I became a "surgical dresser" under Mr. Sydney Jones, the senior surgeon of St. Thomas's, a very able operator who had recently adopted Listerian methods, which were then attracting general attention. Prior to this I had done casualty surgical work, where antisepticism was the rule to the extent that all minor wounds were dressed with lint soaked in a chlorinated soda solution.

At first Listerism was often imperfectly practised by those who adopted it, and this occurred in some of the earlier operations in which I assisted. The knives and other instruments, it is true, lay in trays immersed in alcohol, but the person in charge handed them to the surgeon while taking snuff at frequent intervals! And I saw a surgeon pick up a forceps from the floor and use it again forthwith. The coats in which some surgeons operated were old frock coats, used repeatedly without adequate cleansing. Sponges were still used occasionally. I distinctly remember when visiting another large hospital with a student friend seeing sponges used in swabbing a patient and then thrown by a distinguished surgeon to a distant sink, where they were rinsed for further use. And one saw threaded needles with silken threads hanging down attached to the well-worn coat of the house surgeon, ready for the surgeon in the later stages of his operation.

The carbolic spray had been recently introduced at St. Thomas's, and like others I suffered from chapped and bleached hands, and occasionally from the slighter symptoms of carbolic poisoning.

Dr. J. D. Leeson, in his little book on *Lister as I Knew Him*, 1927, gives recollections of Lister from which I take the following story of events of which he was an eye-witness. It was in the early 'seventies, and Lister—a reserved and serious man, who seldom indulged in a joke—was about to begin a lecture to his Edinburgh students when one of them from the back of the theatre said loudly, "Let us s-pray." No one laughed. Lister looked steadily at the now-blushing student, and then without comment began his lecture.

I knew Dr. Leeson slightly in later life. He became a student at St. Thomas's in 1871, the year in which the hospital and school took possession of the new buildings close to Westminster Bridge. He recalls, as I can do, the septic block, to which surgical cases which developed erysipelas, gangrene, or pyœmia were transferred, and the occasional notice "ward closed for cleansing," which usually meant septic complications in the ward. Students might still possibly go direct from the dissecting and post-mortem rooms to midwifery cases, though there was a notice-board that they "must wash their hands in chlorinated soda solution before going to their cases." It is but fair to add that John Simon before operating had his instruments immersed in boiling water and that Le Gros Clark soaked the lint used by him in spirits of wine. But pus in wounds was still regarded as "laudable," so long as it was unassociated with fever and rigors; and healing of the incisions by "first intention," for instance, after amputations was exceptional.

There already existed definite knowledge which, had it been known and promptly appreciated, would have rendered incomprehensible the passive resistance to Listerism, still prevalent in my student days. Pasteur in 1860 had shown that spontaneous generation of yeast cells does not occur, and that there is no putrescence of meat so long as the dust from air is excluded. Even before this, in 1847, Semmelweis (1818–65), whose work was unknown to Lister, had shown that puerperal fever is conveyable either from a sick puerperal patient or from decomposed organic matter to healthy lying-in women; and Oliver Wendell Holmes (1809–94) in 1843 urged that puerperal fever was spread from patient to patient.

Spencer Wells in 1864 described Pasteur's work to the British Medical Association, but did not follow it up to its logical conclusions in practice, though he obtained great success in his ovariotomy and other operations by insisting on absolute cleanliness, as did also Lawson Tait in his further developments of abdominal surgery a few years later. Joseph Lister (1827–1902) had already been impressed by the fact that putrefaction did not occur in seriously injured parts when the skin remained unbroken, and was searching anxiously for means to reduce septic complications in the surgical work of the Glasgow General Hospital. In 1864 Lister's attention was drawn to Pasteur's memoir *sur les corpuscles organisés qui existent dans l'atmosphère*, published in 1862, showing how the air could be strained free from organisms able to produce fermentation; and this gave him the vital clue to his further investigations, and thus secured the greatest boon which medical science has given to mankind.

Burdon Sanderson showed that infective material was particulate and not gaseous, and Lister's methods were based on the dual principle of killing this particulate matter *in situ*, and of preventing the access of other germs during operation or afterwards. Watson Cheyne, summing up the work of the three men who placed antisepsis on a sound basis (in *Lister and his Achievements*, Watson Cheyne, 1925), said:

> To construct the building properly . . . Lister conceived and carried out its erection, Pasteur laid its foundation "well and truly,"

and Koch (1878) assisted very materially by his work on disinfection and also clarified the structural details by his work on infective diseases of wounds and on the cultivation of bacteria on solid media.

Listerism meant not merely immensely increased prospects of recovery after compound fractures and other injuries, and after operations rendered necessary by various diseases, but it made it possible safely to intervene surgically in many injuries and diseases of the trunk and brain which had hitherto been beyond surgical help. Extended surgery was made possible by Listerism, but not by it alone, for the discoveries of ether and chloroform as general anæsthetics emboldened surgeons to their extended triumphs. Even when I was a student rapidity in operating was still regarded as a triumph, and one counted the seconds elapsing between the first skin incision in a lateral lithotomy and the moment when the surgeon held up the extracted calculus for the admiring students to see. One can then enter into the spirit of relief with which Liston, a famous surgeon of University College, London, in December, 1846, performed his first operation on a patient anæsthetised by ether. It was an amputation of the thigh. The audience was excited with the success of the experiment and so was Liston. He had told the students before the operation: "We are going to try a Yankee dodge . . . for making people insensible." After it he exclaimed, "This Yankee dodge, gentlemen, beats mesmerism hollow" (*Lord Lister*, by C. J. S. Thompson, M.B.E., 1934).

As I have quoted a story of Lister in a serious mood, I will add another story, supplied by Thompson. He preferred chloroform to ether as a general anæsthetic, but used to quote:

> How happy could I be with "ether,"
> Were t'other sweet charmer away.

This reminds one of Oliver Wendell Holmes's quip, when asked the name of which of the rivals to the distinction of first using ether as an anæsthetic should be placed on the proposed statue on Boston Common, "Say, just 'Ether'."

CHAPTER VII

HOSPITALS AND LISTERISM

THE general adoption of Listerism revolutionised the professional and public estimation of the value of hospital treatment; and this change, which was occurring while I was a medical student, deserves more than a passing note. For long, hospitals had been regarded as death-traps, especially for surgical and obstetric patients, and experience oft-times confirmed this view. There were dangers in hospital practice exceeding those of private practice, and sometimes more than counterbalancing the advantage of the greater skill of the hospital surgeons. Early in the eighteenth century Pringle had said that the air of military hospitals killed more than the sword; and Sir James Paget, in an address to the British Medical Association in 1862, referred to the "tolerated barbarisms of practice," only justified by the belief that the risk of "a cutting operation is so great that there is nothing too bad to be substituted for it."

Erichsen, the author of the largest textbook on surgery when I was a student, quoted Cadge of Norwich, who said:

> I come to the conclusion in my own mind that pyæmia, if it does not find its birthplace, does find its natural home and resting-place in hospitals; and though a hospital may not be the mother of pyæmia, it is its nurse.

Florence Nightingale (1820–1910) added her powerful voice in agitation against hospitals as they then functioned. In the Crimean War she had witnessed the terrible mortality among soldiers treated in crowded insanitary military hospitals, and after her return to England she influenced public opinion on sanitary subjects and against hospitals more than any medical "expert." Writing in her volume *Notes on Hospitals* (3rd edition, 1863), she laid down as the first necessity for a hospital that "it should do the sick no harm," and she quoted the Registrar-General's figures giving the experience of the chief hospitals in England in the year 1861. These showed that in 24 metropolitan hospitals the bed-mortality was 90 per cent, in 12 large provincial hospitals it was 83·2 per cent, and in 25 county hospitals it was only 39·4 per cent; but a footnote shows her incipient realisation that in interpreting these figures various factors as to duration of treatment and character of cases would need also to be taken into account.

She had secured the powerful support of William Farr, first Superintendent of Statistics in the General Register Office, in her indictment of hospitals. In his 24th Annual Report to the Registrar-General (1861), Farr drew attention to figures compiled by him which appeared to prove that:

> The mortality of the sick who are treated in the large general hospitals of large towns is twice as great as the mortality of the sick who are treated in small hospitals in small towns,

and added that:

> it remained to be seen whether the mortality in small hospitals is not twice as great as the mortality of the same diseases in patients who are treated in cottages.

Mr. Simon, then Medical Officer to the Privy Council, arranged for an investigation by Dr. Bristowe and Mr. Timothy Holmes into Hospital Hygiene, and as to the relative merits of large and small hospitals and of home treatment of major cases of illness. This investigation was actuated in part at least by Farr's strictures on hospitals and by the even more drastic criticisms of Florence Nightingale, whose dicta secured general credence from the public. Farr had gone so far as to say that general hospitals had become "the ways of death to their inmates"; adding that they do "not benefit mankind directly" but only "as pathological observatories and medical schools."

Bristowe and Holmes had little difficulty in demonstrating the fallacies of the method of comparison used by Farr and by Miss Nightingale in giving hospital death-rates per 100 occupied beds, irrespective of the frequency or slowness with which patients were admitted and discharged, and without ascertaining the relative gravity of the cases admitted to different institutions. Thus a hospital having a bed death-rate of 50 per cent would be condemned as compared with a hospital with a bed death-rate of 2 per cent, when the difference might be and probably was accounted for by the amount of use of the beds for critical or for mild diseases or accidents! For once the statistical Jove had nodded.

But although the statistical bricks thrown at hospital practice were shown to be misdirected, many reforms in hospital practice were needed. This was accepted by Bristowe and Holmes, as also by John Simon in his exhaustive examination of the hospital problem as bearing on the public health, which is contained in his Sixth Report to the Privy Council. This can be read more conveniently in Volume II of the reprint of Simon's *Public Health Reports*, published by the Sanitary Institute in 1887. That there were dangers in hospital practice exceeding those of private practice, and sometimes more than counterbalancing the advantage of the greater skill of the hospital surgeons, was agreed.

How to reduce these dangers was the practical problem; and on this both Florence Nightingale, the authors of the above-mentioned official report, and Simon appeared to agree as to the supreme importance of free ventilation and of rigid cleanliness in hospitals. While Simon laid stress also on measures for the prevention of contagion, Florence Nightingale was a disbeliever in "germs," and she probably would have endorsed the statement of Dr. John Harley, physician to St. Thomas's Hospital, whose refusal to believe what he could not see was embodied in the following words, to be found in *St. Thomas's Hospital Reports* (N.S. Vol. III, 1872):

> The grovelling daughter of ignorance, the canker-worm of science, preys much on medicine. As men of science we should never forget . . . not to seek the explanation of a connected set of phenomena in

more causes than one, if that one be sufficient. . . . No doubt, if the specific poison exists it is a sufficient cause. . . . But I have never seen a specific poison . . .

Looking back, one is impressed by the insignificant reference to the cleanliness of surgeons' and nurses' hands, instruments, and dressings, or to the personal hygiene of the injured or diseased patient under treatment. Florence Nightingale in a footnote in her book quoted the following from an address given by Sir James Paget in 1862 to the British Medical Association:

Of all the remedies . . . I can find but one thing that I can call remedial for the whole disease, pyæmia; and that is a profuse supply of fresh air.

The new St. Thomas's Hospital built opposite the Houses of Parliament and first occupied in 1871 was an illustration in stone of the conviction that the safeguards needed to obviate sepsis in hospital treatment were cross-ventilated wards, built in pavilions separated by ample intervening space, allowing of adequate cross-lighting as well as ventilation, backed by scrupulous cleanliness of the wards and skilled nursing. And yet cases and sometimes epidemics of pyæmia and other septic affections continued to recur, notwithstanding these provisions; and in my time it was still sometimes possible to detect the smell of suppuration when entering a surgical ward. No wonder that in desperation some hygienists recommended that hospitals should at intervals be razed to the ground. And yet before the new St. Thomas's Hospital was opened, Lister was demonstrating in the badly arranged insanitary wards of the Glasgow Hospital that septic complications could be avoided by the adoption of means directed to two ends, to kill any germs *in situ* in the patient's injured tissues on admission, and to prevent access of germs during any operative intervention that might be needed.

Listerism and the use of anæsthetics have vastly extended the scope as well as the safety and freedom from pain of surgical work. The scope of cure of disease has been vastly expanded. Operations can now be performed at an earlier stage of disease, the number of inoperable conditions has been greatly reduced; and lastly, surgery has proved itself an important instrument of research in throwing light on obscure diseases. Hospitals, instead of being occasionally, as Farr put it, "ways of death to their inmates," are now institutions in which septic infection has been almost abolished, and in which nearly all major operations are successfully and almost exclusively performed. The pavilion system, regarded as an essential in hospital construction, has ceased to be so, though free access of light and air remains necessary in hospitals as in dwelling-houses for the healthy.

CHAPTER VIII

FLORENCE NIGHTINGALE

I HAD no personal contact with Florence Nightingale (1820–1910), but her name was universally revered in Britain in my youth, and when I became a medical student at St. Thomas's Hospital the Nightingale nurses were an important factor in life at the hospital. Our teachers taught also the nurses under training at the Nightingale Home, and Florence Nightingale's *Notes on Nursing and on Hospitals* were accepted as incorporating the highest teaching in hospital and general hygiene. A short sketch of her work must therefore be given here as a formative influence in my personal life and work in view of her influence on medical opinion, and still more because she was a pioneer in sick-nursing, and in advocating the work of female health missioners, who as "health visitors" have become in the last thirty years invaluable in hygienic work.

In previous pages I have criticised the statistical bricks which she threw at treatment in hospitals. There was ample justification for inveighing against hospitals as then conducted; but, as already shown, neither she nor the medical staffs of these hospitals understood the causes of excessive mortality in hospitals, nor the remedy that was needed. It was Lister who completely revolutionised hospital practice and vastly reduced preventible mortality and suffering in surgery.

Florence Nightingale early in her girlhood formed the ideal that "only in a life of nursing or other service to the afflicted could her being find its end and scope"; and in her fulfilment of this ideal she opened out a new sphere of usefulness for women of untold value to humanity.

Her work in the Crimean War showed that she had great force of will and powers of organisation. She had driving-power, even genius, in overcoming the difficulties often raised by army surgeons wedded to tradition. She had faith in the soldiers, and in the possibility of influencing their conduct. They were not essentially brutal and drunkards.

> Give them schools and lectures and they will come to them. Give them books and games and amusements and they will leave off drinking. Give them suffering and they will bear it. Give them work and they will do it.
>
> (*Life*, by Sir Edward Cook, 1913, p. 227.)

While she was a ministering angel to the Crimean troops, she had to contend against inertia, incompetence, and direct opposition, sometimes military, sometimes medical. She used her pen with irony on occasion. Referring to one dignitary who was a K.C.B., she supposed this meant Knight of the Crimean Burial-grounds!

But her Crimean work was "not so much a climax as an episode," and she proceeded to investigate Army statistics under peace conditions. Writing in March 1857 she said (p. 316, *Life*):

> The disgraceful state of our Chatham Hospitals, which I have visited lately, is only one more symptom of a system which, in the Crimea, put to death 16,000 men—the finest experiment modern history has seen upon a large scale, viz. as to what given number may be put to death at will by the sole agency of bad food and bad air.

There was much truth in this, though—as we have seen in the instance of hospital mortality—she may not have sufficiently recognised—as how could she?—the limited range of scientific hygiene at that time. One cannot but admire the clever way in which this "passionate statistician" handled statistics and threw stones into the glass-houses of both army and civilian administration. Her statistical diagrams were numerous and beautifully executed, and carried conviction even to unwilling politicians and statesmen. I have seen many of them, and can appreciate their effectiveness. Her diagrams of mortality in the British Army were named "Coxcombs" by her, because of the shape and colours of the diagrams; and she did not hesitate to describe them as "God's revenge upon murder."

She had a great share in securing the appointment of Edmund A. Parkes as Professor of Hygiene at the new Army Medical School, the inauguration of which was due to her. In doing this she initiated the teaching of hygiene for the British Army under the best auspices.

I have illustrated Florence Nightingale's caustic pen. Here is a further instance. Writing to Captain (afterwards Sir Douglas) Galton, her kinsman, she remarked:

> I understand that the Under-Secretary for War won't ventilate the Barracks in summer because the grates are not hot enough in winter. Why are the men to die of foul air in August because they are too cold at Christmas? I think the Under-Secretary must be an Army doctor!

Florence Nightingale's greatest gift to humanity was that she was the founder of modern nursing in Britain.

Her *Notes on Nursing* were published in 1859, and in June 1860 the Nightingale Nursing Home was initiated at St. Thomas's Hospital with funds given her by a grateful nation. Mrs. Wardroper, the first Superintendent of Nurses at the Nurses' Training School, I often saw in the wards of the hospital.

The former reputation of nurses may be gathered from the opinion of Mr. South, a distinguished surgeon, and twice President of the Royal College of Surgeons, that nurses were "much in the same position as housemaids, and require little teaching beyond that of poultice-making" (*Life*, by Sir Edward Cook, Vol. I, p. 445). As a man of the world he "found the world very well as it was."

Although Florence Nightingale would have repudiated this view of the qualifications of a nurse, she always emphasised the domestic side of a nurse's work. Thus in one of the annual letters which she sent for many years to the probationers and nurses of the Nightingale School at St. Thomas's Hospital (*Florence Nightingale to her Nurses*, 1914) she said:

> And don't despise what some of you call "housemaid's work." If you thought of its extreme importance, you would not mind doing

it. And you know, without thorough housemaid's work, everything in the Ward or Sickroom becomes permeated with organic matter.

The *Notes on Nursing*, as Paget well put it, formed an alphabet of household hygiene, as well as a treatise on nursing, and it must have had enormous influence in educating the general public in the value of cleanliness in all respects, including clean air by means of ventilation.

The nation subscribed £44,000 as a personal gift to her; and most of this was used in founding the Nightingale Home at St. Thomas's. A portion was also alloted to the training of midwives for the poor, the training for this purpose being centred at King's College Hospital; but this scheme was abandoned after six years, because of a calamitous epidemic of puerperal fever. No wonder that Florence regarded "hospitals as at best a necessary evil," and considered that "the secret of national health is to be found in the homes of the people." It could not then be anticipated that, after Listerism, parturition in hospitals would present fewer risks than in average domestic experience.

Florence was actively concerned in reform of workhouse nursing, and the appointment in 1866 by her of the Lady Superintendent for District Nursing in London was an important step in extension of skilled nursing in the homes of the poor.

Development of modern nursing.—Florence Nightingale's personal popularity gave speedy impetus to the replacement of unskilled by trained nurses. She co-operated in 1862 with Mr. Rathbone in Liverpool in initiating district nursing, and when Agnes Jones was appointed at her suggestion in the workhouse infirmary of that city, the nursing of infirmary patients by skilled nurses began in the provinces.

I cannot follow the stages of progress, except by mere enumeration. Skilled nurses for those who could afford them became available; and this provision was extended to a rapidly increasing portion of the poorer population by means of district and county nursing associations, supported chiefly by voluntary contributions. A description of the increasing scope of the work of these associations would fill a volume in itself. They have brought within the reach of the poor in nearly every district throughout the land the services of a skilled nurse, given either gratuitously or for a small fee. In recent years the work of these Associations in attending sickness, especially tuberculosis, has received financial support from Public Health Authorities; and this forms perhaps the most successful example in our midst of co-operation between private benevolence and official agencies for the well-being of the community.

On the fiftieth anniversary of Queen Victoria's reign in 1887, the women of Britain presented a large sum to her, which she devoted to the promotion of nursing by district visiting nurses. These nurses are divided into two classes, fully trained and "village nurses," the latter with not more than a year's training, but competent for most ordinary cases of illness.

An equally important development of nursing from the standpoint of public health was forecasted in Florence Nightingale's advocacy of "Rural Health Missioners." She supported the appointment of these under Dr. de'Ath, the M.O.H.[1] of a rural district in Buckinghamshire, and in advocating their extended use at the Women's Congress in Leeds in 1893 she said:

> The work that tells is the work of the skilful hand, directed by the cool head, and inspired by the loving heart.

The public health nurse or health visitor, unlike the sick nurse, has to seek out the dwellings in which she is needed, the information coming to her from varied sources. It may be given by a neighbour, or come from a hospital almoner when a patient is discharged from hospital—would that this source of information were oftener forthcoming. More often it comes from births or cases of tuberculosis that have been notified to the medical officer of health. As a rule the health visitor does not undertake actual nursing; but short of this, helpful advice, supplemented

[1] M.O.H. is used as an abbreviation for Medical Officer of Health throughout this volume.

when practicable by a demonstration of what is needed, is the best avenue for success in her mission. There is force in the principle behind the advice once given to a group of health visitors: "First do something, and then talk if you like." Not only medical and hygienic advice is needed, but the health visitor often opens up avenues of social help for the family, thus ensuring that her work shall prove completely successful.

The work following on notification of births is now carried on chiefly by health visitors, supplementing the skilled medical advice given at Infant Welfare Clinics. It would carry us too far afield to detail their work; but there can be no doubt that it is most fruitful in the prevention of illness, and in the improvement of child health, even though, as is illustrated on page 343, it may sometimes be impossible to measure this good by the imperfect statistical measures available.

EDMUND ALEXANDER PARKES

I append a note on the work of Dr. E. A. Parkes, who played a great part in building up modern hygiene, and in training (through his textbook) civilian medical officers of health, and as Professor of Hygiene in training army doctors in preventive medicine for home and for foreign service. His was the first great *Manual of Hygiene* written in this country, and must have done much in preparing others, like myself, for their public health work.

Parkes was born in 1819, and died of tuberculosis in 1876. Notwithstanding much illness he continued to work to the end, and his advice was sought not only by Florence Nightingale, but also by many of her contemporaries.

In 1849 he investigated epidemics of cholera in England, and in the same year became Physician to University College Hospital. In 1855 he did valuable work in organising hospitals in the Crimea; and in 1860, on Florence Nightingale's nomination, he was made Professor of Military Hygiene in the recently created Army Medical School. In undertaking this work, he had, as his successor (Professor de Chaumont), subsequently said, "almost to create the science he was to teach, or at least to reduce it from a chaotic condition to something like order." From the first he associated laboratory work and demonstrations with his teaching. In 1864 appeared the first edition of his celebrated *Manual of Practical Hygiene*, to which so many, like myself, have been indebted.

For many years Parkes was a total abstainer from alcohol and made experiments on soldiers to illustrate the influence of alcohol on the power to work. As Dr. Louis Parkes says in his memorial sketch of Parkes, he is rightly described as "possessing a character of singular beauty, sincerity, and gentleness."

In the words of two presidents of the Royal College of Physicians: "He made the world much richer by his life, much poorer by his death" (Sir Russell Reynolds); "He taught me as a student to desire knowledge for itself, and not for anything which might follow it" (Sir William Jenner).

PART II

PIONEERS IN STATE MEDICINE

INTRODUCTION TO PART II

THIS Part will be considered by some to be foreign to a volume of chiefly personal recollections. I am willing that it shall be so considered, and the reader may pass on to Part III if he holds this view. But I regard Part II as essential to the task I undertook in writing my recollections; for it gives the background of any work I have been able to do, and it elucidates the influences activating my own share in public health reform and that of my contemporaries. I hold strongly that a subject—in this instance *Fifty Years in Public Health*—is best understood when we know how public health during those years came to be what it became, and that this genesis can only be fully understood when one extends one's examination beyond the events of an individual life. This task is easier in regard to those whose work was finished in my youth than for those whose work has been contemporaneous with my own; and I remind my readers that the later chapters of this volume give chiefly personal recollections and do not profess to set out, except by way of occasional notes and references, the work done by many others also engaged in public health work.

In attempting to make this sketch of pioneers and leaders a living picture, I enumerate here some of the chief persons who need to be brought into it. It is an incomplete list, given in the order of date of birth. To it should be added some of the early workers mentioned in previous chapters.

Southwood Smith (1788–1861)
Edwin Chadwick (1800–1890)
William Farr (1807–1883)
William Budd (1811–1880)
John Snow (1813–1858)
John Simon (1816–1904)
Joseph von Pettenkofer (1818–1901)
Florence Nightingale (1820–1910)
Louis Pasteur (1822–1895)
Joseph Lister (1827–1913)
Benjamin Ward Richardson (1828–1896)
George Buchanan (1831–1895)
Richard Thorne Thorne (1841–1899)
Robert Koch (1843–1910)
William H. Power (1842–1916)

The three official heads of the Medical Department of the Local Government Board will be the subject of sketches in my second volume.

J. S. Bristowe and Charles Murchison have already been characterised. They influenced the progress of preventive medicine, the former especially by teaching the pathologist's attitude to disease, the latter by his classical work on continued fevers. It will be noted that I have included in my list the names of two great German and one French scientist, Pettenkofer, Koch, and Louis Pasteur, the two last named of whom founded the modern science of bacteriology, which has given increasing exactitude to the science of epidemiology and to the triumphs of Listerism. The list might be extended indefinitely; but as it now stands it includes the names of those whose work has been most fruitful in making public health an essential part of practical politics as well as of personal hygiene.

CHAPTER IX

JOHN SIMON

John Simon and St. Thomas's Hospital—Simon's early work for the City of London—His later career—Wide vision of preventive medicine—Relation of poor law to public health work

JOHN SIMON (1816–1904)

John Simon, the first governmental adviser for consecutive years of the British Government, may be first considered, for it was chiefly under his guidance that the earlier legislative and administrative reforms were initiated in England. I say this while remembering that Dr. Richard Mead, also on the medical staff of St. Thomas's Hospital, had received instructions in 1722 from H.M. Chief Secretary of State to advise on Pestilential Contagion "in view of the sickness now in France and fear of importation." In 1831, in the first outbreak of Asiatic Cholera in England, the Royal College of Physicians issued a memorandum of advice which, while endorsing Mead's earlier views as to the inutility of quarantine, advised separation of the sick and other measures. Their advice was criticised by Dr. Southwood Smith as laying undue stress on infection, and not enough on local conditions of filth, without which, in his view, cholera would not appear or spread. But it is gratifying to "an old St. Thomas's man" to find that during two hundred years members of the medical staff of its medical school have either held the chief advisory position or have been otherwise represented on the medical staff of the Government.

Two interesting recollections connected with Simon may be given in preface to a fuller outline of his life-work. He was partially of French—perhaps Huguenot—descent, and his name was (nearly) always pronounced with a strong accent on the last syllable (S'món). But at the Annual Prize Distribution

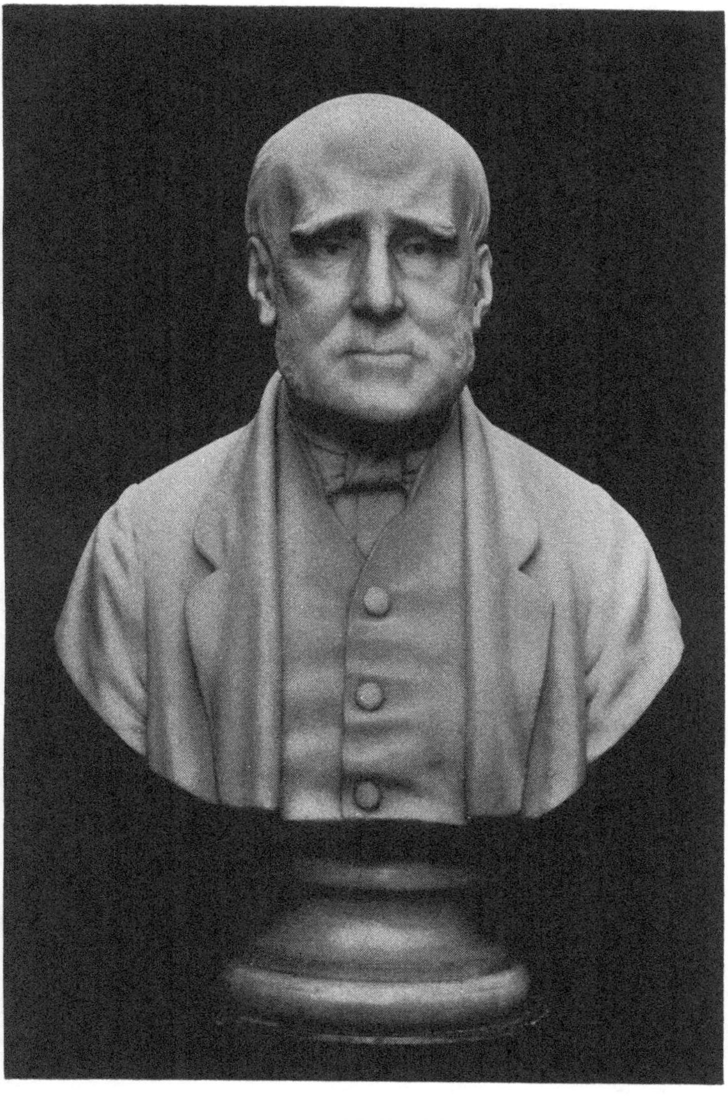

JOHN SIMON

in (I think) my first year, the task of distributing prizes and addressing the audience of students and staff of St. Thomas's fell to Arthur Stanley, the famous Dean of Westminster, and there was much tittering during his address at his frequent references to Mr. Símon.

Although only a second year's student I was fortunate enough to hear Simon's last clinical lecture, for he ceased to be surgeon to the hospital in 1876, the year of his retirement also from the public health service.

In the winter of that year the word went round that Simon was giving his last clinical lecture. Simon, when he was appointed the first medical officer to the Privy Council in 1855, was surgeon to St. Thomas's, and he made it a condition that he should be permitted to retain his surgical appointment. When in 1872 the appointment of medical officers of health and inspectors of nuisances was made obligatory on all local authorities by the Public Health Act of that year, Simon said:

> For the first time the medical profession throughout the country was to be brought into official use with a view to the better prevention of disease.

This remark applied with even more force to his own appointment in 1855 as Medical Officer to the Crown, for his was the first appointment of a central health adviser on a quasi-permanent basis.

But I digress from my recollections of Simon's last clinical lecture. The large operating theatre in the hospital was crowded to hear him. He entered from a side door: a lean man with a keen face and a bald head partially concealed by a black skull-cap. He sat down on a tall stool, unfolded a bundle of papers, and began a very deliberate talk on bone necrosis, illustrating his remarks from cases in his wards. Not a word was said as to his retirement, and the lecture to a novice was dull. He descended from his stool and walked towards the side door. But he was not to escape so easily. Someone shouted: "Three cheers for Johnny Simon!" Simon turned, lifted his hand, and said dramatically, "For God's sake, remember this is the hospital." And then he disappeared almost before the first cheer had ceased.

In later years I became familiar with his important public health work and writings, but had a further personal relation with him when the *Journal of Hygiene* was started in 1900, under the editorship of Dr. G. H. F. Nuttall, F.R.S., with whom were associated Dr. J. S. Haldane, F.R.S., and myself. He wrote an introductory note to the first number, dated October 22, 1900, in which he stated that he did this at the request of his friend, Sir John Burdon Sanderson, who in the partiality of his old friendship for Simon "had forgotten that I am eighty-four years old"; and he then referred to the past two centuries, and especially the last fifty years, which "have been beyond measure progressive" in hygiene, while "mare's-nests in science are tending to be a constantly diminishing quantity."

As early as 1848, when only thirty-two years old, Simon had been appointed medical officer of health of the City of London. This was the second of such posts created, the first being in 1847, when Dr. Duncan was appointed M.O.H. of Liverpool.

Simon led, and in large measure determined, the course of public health reform between the year 1855, when he left the service of the City for that of the State, and the year 1876, when he left the latter, although then only sixty years old.

Mention should be made of Simon's earlier work, before he left the City for Whitehall. His City reports were republished in volume form entitled *Reports on the Sanitary Condition of the City of London*. This was in 1854. The value of my copy is enhanced by its having formerly been in the possession of Dr. Edmund A. Parkes, whose signature it bears. The volume contains the following exquisite dedication to Simon's father:

To

LOUIS MICHAEL SIMON

of the Stock Exchange, London, and of Blackheath
I dedicate this Reprint of my Reports
Looking
Less to what intrinsic merit they may have,
Than to the years of anxious labour they represent:
Deeming it fit to associate
My father's name
With a record of endeavours to do my duty:
Because in this he has been my best example;
and
Because I count it the happiest influence in my lot,
That, bound to him by every tie of grateful affection,
I have likewise been able, from my earliest childhood
Till now—the evening of his life,
To regard him with unqualified and increasing respect.

To appreciate fully these early reports of Simon we must remember the sanitary circumstances of "the square mile" constituting the City of London, during the seven years when he was its medical officer of health. The City was then a city of homes as well as a centre of commercial life; and for the medical care of its poorer residents there were several poor law or district medical officers. Their services Simon succeeded in retaining as his medical assistants; and in doing so he adopted what, with a satisfactory system of administration, is an ideal arrangement. It will, I am confident, become the recognised practice in the medicine of the future. The medical attendants on the sick are the health guardians of rich and poor alike, and should be interested in preventing even more than in treating illness. Their training should be modified and extended to make them efficient for this purpose. They are already better equipped to this end than they were in the sixth decade of the nineteenth century; but even during Simon's City experience they were able to keep Simon advised as to "nests of disease," and thus sanitary effort could be directed where most needed. It may be added that this combination of public health work with medical attendance on the poor was continued throughout England when in 1872 all districts were required to appoint health officers. Poor law medical officers were made also medical officers of health. In many districts, without this combination health officers would not have been obtainable. Advised by Simon's successors, the practice of combination of public health and poor law functions was deprecated; the combination became rare and now has disappeared. During the subsequent decades, while the great struggle in public health was for domestic and municipal sanitation, for clean water supplies, and to secure isolation of the infectious sick, this change of practice was perhaps for good; but much was lost as well as something gained, and a prophet's mantle is not needed to forecast that when the general medical work of this country is satisfactorily organised there will be a return to Simon's City methods; and as I have elsewhere expressed it, "every medical practitioner will become a medical officer of health in the entire range of his medical work." This would, of course, not diminish the need for whole-time medical officials engaged in dealing with administrative health problems, with investigation of conditions adverse to health, and whole-time medical assistants engaged in certain special branches of clinical and hygienic work. The Local Government Act of 1928 has placed poor law medical work under public health authorities, and this opens up possibilities of realising the ideal which are only beginning to be appreciated.

The reprints of Simon's City reports embody the chief ideas subsequently expanded in his reports to the Privy Council and the Local Government Board. Even in these early reports he wrote in vivid and picturesque language and with an outspokenness which throughout his career enhanced the carrying-power of his recommendations. He laid "no claim to the merit of scientific discovery"; but in setting out "truths bordering on truism" he claimed it as no unworthy object "to make trite language bear fruit in common application." Writing in 1854, he animadverted on "our abortion of a sanitary system" and urged the appointment of a Parliamentary President whose department "should be, in the widest sense, to care for the physical necessities of human life. . . . For such a Minister, what a career!"

Although in the above quotation Simon may seem to have considered that public health was concerned only with the physical necessities of life, the quotation on p. 42 shows his wider vision; and the following extract illustrates this wider teaching, which is equally relevant to-day:

> Physical and moral conditions act and react on one another. . . . It has been my duty to make myself intimately acquainted with places respecting which it may with truth be said that vice and ignorance and brutality are among the chief causes of diseases . . . the people born in these slums must find it difficult not to be vicious and ignorant and brutal. . . . If social reformers of the two sorts addressed themselves jointly to these afflicting scenes, it would be no easy problem to determine whether, in their co-operation, the schoolmaster and moral teacher were doing more for the bodily health, or the sanitary improver doing more for the progress of education and the lessening of crime.

Simon's official health work prior to 1870 was done under the Privy Council, and he had a relatively free hand in advising and directing central public health administration. In 1870 the Local Government Board was formed, and the health duties of the Privy Council were transferred to the new Board, along with those of the Poor Law Board. Simon, who had a little of Chadwick's autocratic temperament, with the added capacity to express his views with a complete mastery of caustic as well as persuasive English, found himself hemmed in by secretarial conditions, which had become firmly established under the old Poor Law Board, and he resigned in 1876. He did this because he disagreed with the policy and procedures of the Local Government Board, which gave to its medical officer an inadequate part in the determination and guidance of public health work.

His principles in administration are well stated as follows in the obituary notice of Simon by his friend Burdon Sanderson. (*Proc. Roy. Soc.*, Vol. LXXV, 1905). These were as follows: he held that (1) the sanitary administration of the country should be under the direct supervision of the Central Medical Department; that (2) the relation of the department with local sanitary authorities should be such as to enable it to bring its influence promptly to bear on them in case of default of duty; and that (3) the saving of life by the prevention of disease should be regarded as the highest motive of official action.

The Local Government Board remained, as it had been in earlier years, preponderantly a Poor Law Board; and it was saturated with the deterrent procedures of the poor law of previous decades, which, however applicable to monetary relief, were contrary to first principles when applied to medical aid, or when children and the aged were concerned. It was not specially on this point that Simon resigned, but because in the central guidance of current public health administration Simon and his medical staff had little or no executive share.

I have mentioned Simon's annual reports. These, like his earlier reports to the City Council, were vivid pictures of sanitary and social evils, and embodied graphic and impressive accounts of the urgent sanitary reforms needed. They, along with Farr's statistical reports to the Registrar-General of Births and Deaths, were the chief motive forces of the steadily increasing stream of public health legislation and active sanitary administration.

In his earlier years Simon had himself been a pathological investigator, and in 1850 he published a *General Pathology*.

Throughout his entire official career Simon retained his earlier keenness to advance our knowledge of pathology, and most of the researches, for which he was able to arrange by means of an annual subsidy of £2,000 begun in 1870, were concerned with pathological problems, some of them apparently remote from immediate prospect of application in preventive medicine. In one of his earlier official reports is an especially important contribution on the "Preventibility of Certain Kinds of Premature Death," based on a statistical investigation by Dr. Headlam Greenhow (see Sanitary Institute reprint of Simon's Reports, pp. 427–488). Dr. (afterwards Sir George) Buchanan's investigation on the effect of works of sanitary improvement on the national death-rate illustrated an even wider outlook.

Simon's views and his work are further noted on pages 110 and 114. Young and old alike cannot fail to find inspiration in the record of his life and work, and in his noble expositions of the needs of public health. No health officer, general or special, can be regarded as having been adequately educated who has not read his *English Sanitary Institutions* (Cassell, 1890). The title of this work is somewhat misleading; for the volume is not only an historical study of slow approaches towards truth and knowledge concerning health, but also a philosophical exposition of the underlying principles of public health.

CHAPTER X

EDWIN CHADWICK

Beginnings of social reform—Belief in centralisation—Delay in reform with decentralisation—Personal recollections

EDWIN CHADWICK (1800–90) was concerned in the growth of public health earlier than John Simon, being actively engaged in what may be described as the ante-natal stages of its development. In its post-natal stages his phenomenal driving power led to his being pushed out of official life; but ere this happened he had set in action forces which, once started, became gradually irresistible in securing reform. Prior to his retirement he had more personal influence in launching the good vessel of public health on its long voyage than any other single person. Educated for the Bar, Chadwick as a young man wrote an article on Life Assurance, which attracted the attention of Jeremy Bentham (1748–1832). Intimacy with Bentham and his utilitarian philosophy largely influenced Chadwick's life. His first public work was as an Assistant Commissioner on the Poor Law. His exact methods and the skill and assiduity shown by him in ascertaining the evils of poor-law administration led to his appointment as a full Commissioner, and the Report of the Commission led to the adoption of Bentham's principle of strict centralised control over the relief functions of Boards of Guardians. Throughout his life Chadwick endeavoured to attack the causal factors of each evil and not merely to administer relief. Thus destitution must be treated in such a manner as to reduce its amount; disease must be diminished, because it caused destitution and so on. To other reformers of this period and in subsequent years, non-economic motives probably appealed more potently than economic. There was a growing sense of communal responsibility for injustice and oppression, and for bad housing and insanitary defects. The two currents of motivation, the economic and the humanitarian, ran concurrently, and combined they secured the social and sanitary reforms of the next few decades. The days of *laissez-faire* in respect of evils were gone, thanks to this dual attack.

In 1833 Chadwick with Dr. Southwood Smith and Mr. Tooke were appointed Royal Commissioners to consider the shocking conditions under which children were employed in factories. The Commission made what in its results was a revolutionary recommendation, namely, that professional paid inspectors should be appointed to ensure the execution of the needed reforms and regulations for protecting the children's welfare. Almost contemporaneously the Poor Law Commission, of which Chadwick was also a member, recommended an equally important departure in practice—the appointment of permanent paid officials as relieving officers, to undertake the giving of relief on a fairly uniform scale. Furthermore, largely and probably chiefly under Chadwick's coercive energy, the local administration of parochial relief was made subject to rigid regulation by the Poor Law Board in London.

A Poor Law Board consisting of three commissioners was created in 1834, with Chadwick as its secretary. This Board made drastic investigations, which hastened the initiation of the present public health organisation of England. To Chadwick and this Board it soon became clear that much of the illness producing destitution was caused by the wretched housing and insanitation of crowded populations; and these conclusions were driven home by Chadwick in his "Report on the Sanitary Condition of the Labouring Classes." This report was based on actual surveys of local conditions made by Drs. Arnott, Southwood Smith, and J. P. Kay; and here again Chadwick and his colleagues had made history by the novel appointment of medical inspectors or investigators for public health purposes. The fundamental principle implied in their investigations was that an investigation of causes should be made and that action for alleviation of distress, apart from investigation of its causes, should be at least partially abandoned (see my *The Ministry of Health*, Putnams, 1925, p. 10).

Other commissions and reports followed, in which Chadwick played an important part. In 1848 the first Public Health Act was passed. It created a General Board of Health of three members. This Board unhappily found its attempts to create local Boards of Health almost entirely futile, owing to opposition from many quarters, and the Central Board survived only until 1858. Chadwick—whose pertinacious and almost coercive activity had made him extremely unpopular—resigned from office in 1855, the year in which Simon left the City for State public health service. Chadwick's retirement at the age of fifty-five, when at the zenith of his power for good work, is regrettable but comprehensible.

He was a great believer in central governmental control by officials. Dr. Lyon (afterwards Lord) Playfair was a member of the Royal Commission appointed in 1843 to inquire into the sanitary conditions of towns. In his memoirs (p. 64) he states that one day he argued with Chadwick in favour of throwing greater responsibility on local authorities, and of regarding the function of central government as supervisory rather than administrative. Chadwick's stern rejoinder was:

> Sir, the Devil was expelled from heaven because he objected to centralisation, and all those who object to centralisation oppose it on devilish grounds!

Neither Parliament nor the people would tolerate the coercion which attempted to make them proceed at a pace for which they were unready.

Chadwick's views on centralisation developed early, and every event in his strenuous official life confirmed them. This is clearly seen in his brochure on *The Evils of Disunity in Central and Local Administration*, published in 1885, twenty years after his enforced retirement from official life.

I may mention as illustrations of his principles his objections to separate legislation for the different parts of the United Kingdom, especially his (I think wise) objection to separation of the offices for the collection of vital statistics for England and Scotland respectively.

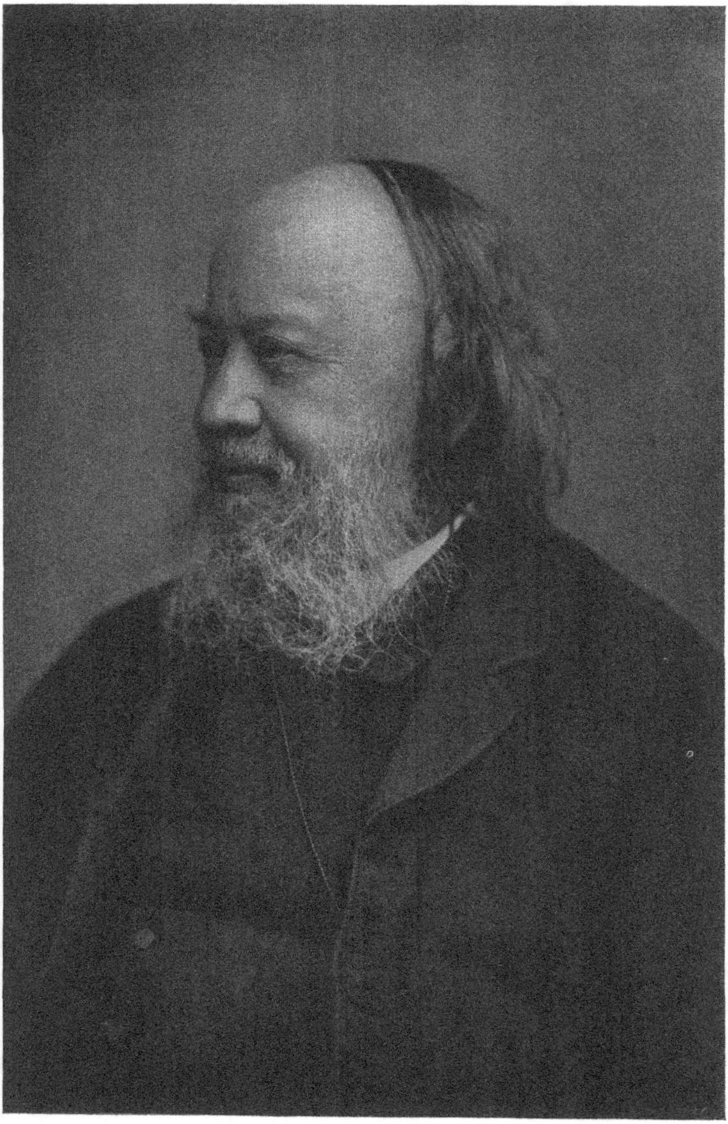

Edwin Chadwick.

(*By kind permission of Messrs. Longmans, Green & Co., Ltd.*

But when it came to questions of detailed poor law and public health administration in every area throughout England and Wales, he neglected the natural limitations of central enforcement of rapid local reform. Every one of these areas formed, or formed part of, the constituency of a Member of Parliament, and this meant that cumulative pressure could be exerted against the obnoxious centralised administration. It was exerted most effectively in respect of the newly centralised poor law and public health work. *The Times* regarded the new poor law as "worse than Egyptian bondage"; and Disraeli, the author many years later of the motto *sanitas sanitatum omnia sanitas*, described Chadwick as a "monster in human shape."

But before his retirement Chadwick had succeeded in bringing into existence or expediting the provision of new machinery of government both locally and centrally, in starting the work of paid inspectors and officers whose specific duty it was to discover and prevent dangers to health and social life, and in putting an end to *laissez-faire* policies. These were momentous accomplishments. If he fell foul of democratic government by his autocratic and peremptory methods, if he failed to appreciate adequately the personal element in the spread of disease and recognised almost exclusively environmental sanitary defects, this means that he had the limitations of knowledge of his contemporaries; but his special achievements remain as a permanent and essential part of the history of social progress.

B. K. Gray (*Philanthropy and the State*, pp. 309–10) has summarised admirably Chadwick's achievements:

> He was a prince of agitators. . . . While other agitators worked their will on individuals, he goaded corporations. His ideal of centralisation set him in opposition to the dearest faith of Englishmen, the belief in *laissez-faire*. He desired to strengthen the central control less for the sake of drainage or of health than for the sake of a strong administration. This was the height of his offending, and this drove him from office. But before he went he had shaken the old edifice of leave-it-alone to its foundations.

Chadwick's views on the technical side of sanitary reform were not always wise. He advocated the "separate system" of sewerage long after practical sanitarians had abandoned it. The system is theoretically sound; for obviously it would be well if rain-water were separately disposed of from sewage. But this has proved in large measure impracticable for large towns, and rain-water gathered from streets is very foul.

This leads me to mention in conclusion a pamphlet published by him in 1889 on *Circulation and Stagnation* in which he reprinted a paper read by his friend Mr. F. O. Ward at the Congress of Hygiene at Brussels in 1856, and prefaces it with commendatory remarks on the same subject. The paper advocated the use of steam power when required to ensure the carriage of town sewerage on to rural land, and to give a supply of water free from contamination from distant sources. The motto was to be "hygiene by steam power," and Mr. Ward described the circulation of pure and impure water as being an analogous and fruitful discovery in the social body, analogous to Harvey's discovery of arterial and venous blood in the individual.

My only contact with Chadwick was at a Conference of the Sanitary Inspectors Association, held in Brighton in the year 1888 or 1889, about a year after I had been appointed medical officer of health of that borough. Mr. Chadwick, as he then was (for he only received his K.C.B. from the King shortly before his death), gave a Presidential Address at this conference, which lies before me as I write. He first recalled his advanced years (he died in 1890 in his ninetieth year), and referred to this as an example of "exceptional hereditariness"; for his father had died at the age of eighty-four, his grandfather at ninety-five, and his two great-grandfathers as centenarians.

He then reiterated his reading of past experiences of the creation of partial sanitary Utopias, which he held could be almost indefinitely multiplied. He quoted the experience of various towns which, since he was the chief official of the First General Board of Health, had reduced their general death-rates, for instance, from 24 to 15 per 1,000 of population. He ascribed this reduction to the system, already mentioned, of "circulation versus stagnation," including a good water supply, efficient removal of fouled water and other waste products on to the land. And he claimed that

> by these factors alone, such certainty has been established, that a contractor might contract with safety for definable sanitary results.

This was no new thesis of his; to some extent he taught it during a great part of his life. The teaching embodied the great truths, that clean water, and prompt and effective removal of organic refuse from the vicinity of dwellings and its disposal without incurring risk to water-drinkers, were essentials for communal health; but we now know that the broad irrigation of sewage on land recommended by him is uneconomical and unnecessary; that complete separation of all rain-water from sewage in large towns is impracticable; and that the lowered death-rates quoted by Chadwick were in part due to sanitary improvements, which were not included in Chadwick's enumeration.

So earnest was Chadwick concerning his specific "for a complete sanitary cure" for Brighton that although then eighty-eight years old he wrote me the letter shown on page 88.

In this letter he expressed his desire to address the Mayor and Corporation of Brighton in advocacy of the separate system of sewerage (rain water being kept out of the sewers). Until a few years before the above-mentioned conference, Brighton's sewers had emptied into the sea near the centre of the town, and a medical journal had reported unfavourably on the town. The sewage was soon afterwards carried by an intercepting sewer to a part of the coast over four miles distant from the town.

My letter to Chadwick explained these points, while expressing appreciation of his offer to serve the cause of sanitation in Brighton. I have no doubt that I also expressed my profound appreciation of his great national work.

In the preceding pages I have attempted to indicate, however imperfectly, his position as one of the greatest builders of public health in Britain.

Park Cottage
East Sheen
Mortlake
S.W.

Sept 26. 88

"My dear Sir

I have requested the Messrs Longmans to send to you a copy of the Health of Nations, by Dr. Richardson in which you will find the best account yet given of my life.

I enclose a copy of the last photograph by Mayall: which is deemed the best. My hair has gone grey since I presided at the Brighton Congress.

I should be particularly glad, if the present Brighton town council forgetting the past, would ask Dr. Richardson to make a renewed sanitary enquiry. I deem Brighton an excellent case for a complete sanitary cure. I should like to pay a visit to the Mayor and the Council, and ~~tell~~ explain to them, the generalities of what may be done for it, especially as regards the schools; that would contribute largely to its prosperity.

Yours truly

Edwin Chadwick

Dr. Newsholme

Medical Officer of Health Brighton.

CHAPTER XI

OTHER BUILDERS OF PUBLIC HEALTH

Southwood Smith—John Snow—William Budd

IN the two last chapters I have attempted to indicate the great historical part borne by Edwin Chadwick and John Simon in designing and building the edifice of modern public health administration. Both of them—Chadwick much more than Simon—were imbued with the incomplete but fundamentally important generalisation that dirt produces disease. As Simon put it in 1874, "filth is the deadliest of our present removable causes of disease."

Simon accepted the specific pathogenesis of infectious diseases, though perhaps not exclusively; but he said very practically:

> Nowhere out of Laputa could there be serious thought of differentiating excremental performances into groups of diarrhœal and healthy. . . . It is excrement, indiscriminately that must be kept from fouling us with its decay.

On the other hand, Chadwick and the chief medical adviser associated with him (Dr. Southwood Smith) regarded favouring local circumstances as adequate alone to originate such diseases as cholera and typhus fever (typhoid was not then distinguished from typhus). If, then, we are to understand the position of preventive medicine in the 1880's, when my personal work began, we need to consider Southwood Smith's teaching and that of those of his contemporaries and successors who held the same views, and to compare their teaching with that of John Snow and William Budd, who lifted preventive medicine on to a higher level, placing it on a foundation of exact epidemiological research. Their great work is the more wonderful in that they did not possess modern laboratory aids to diagnosis and differentiation, nor had they that wide knowledge of the number and distribution of the cases in an epidemic which the compulsory notification of infectious diseases now supplies.

SOUTHWOOD SMITH

Southwood Smith (1788–1861) was Chadwick's chief medical adviser and expert on the technical side of public health reform. In his early manhood he was a minister of religion. At the age of twenty-four he entered Edinburgh University as a medical student, and after becoming qualified in medicine he continued as a Unitarian minister for some years. But in 1820 he removed to London, engaged in medical practice, and was soon appointed physician to the London Fever Hospital; and from this appointment we may date his career as a sanitary reformer. He practised very largely among the East End poor.

Strangely enough his sanitary career appears to have been determined by circumstances similar to those which brought Chadwick into the same field. In 1825 Southwood Smith contributed two articles on "Contagion and Sanitary Laws" to the first two numbers of the *Westminster Review*. Similarly Chadwick, while a law student, contributed articles to the early numbers of the *Westminster Review* which attracted Jeremy Bentham's attention, and there followed an intimate friendship between the two.

After Bentham's death, according to his instructions, his body was dissected, Southwood Smith undertaking this task. As is well known, Bentham's skeleton dressed in his ordinary clothes can be seen at University College, London.

It is scarcely open to doubt that Southwood Smith's articles were read by Chadwick; and Southwood Smith's treatise on fever, published a few years later, doubtless led to his being employed in official work.

The main contentions in Southwood Smith's articles and in his treatise on fever were that:

1. Epidemics prevail where there are sanitary defects;
2. The extension and spread of these epidemics is exactly proportional to the extent of bad sanitary conditions;

3. Epidemics are controllable by controlling these conditions;
4. Epidemics are not necessarily diseases of poverty; the want is one of pure air not of food;
5. Fever is pre-eminently a disease of adult age.

It followed that fever was the "great pauperiser of the country" and that it was preventible.

During the period 1833–54 Southwood Smith was employed intermittently in health inquiries for the official commissions which have already been mentioned. His report, published in 1837, "on the physical causes of sickness . . . to which the poor are particularly exposed, and which are capable of prevention by sanitary measures," had a powerful effect in expediting both poor law and public health reform. Southwood Smith had the background of six years' work, from 1824 onwards, as physician to the London Fever Hospital, which must have made him familiar with the spread of infection; but he held, as has already been indicated—and in doing so voiced contemporaneous medical opinion—that the spread of epidemics is determined by bad sanitary conditions, and that they could be controlled by remedying these local evils. As he said, "Our concern practically is with the known causes—the ascertained conditions," such as over-crowding, accumulation of filth, uncleanliness.

It was in the light of this teaching that the Augean stables of our great and rapidly growing towns began to be cleansed, with striking results in reduction of "fever." "Fever" then meant both typhus and typhoid; and typhus declined as the over-crowded nests of this disease were cleaned and cleared, and actual cases were hospitalised (that is segregated and treated in hospitals), and thus prevented from doing further mischief. Similarly, as scavenging improved and excremental removal became more satisfactory, and as water and food supplies became less prone to contamination, typhoid also decreased.

But this statement would not have satisfied either Chadwick or Southwood Smith, or most of their contemporaries and successors. It was held that effluvia from organic filth were capable of producing fever, and this was taught when I was a medical student, and continued to be the basis of action for some years later in practical public health work.

That this belief in the autogenous origin of contagion needed to be modified and corrected was realised by two British physicians, who—leaving Sydenham of an earlier century out of count—stand in my view supreme in the history of British epidemiology, John Snow and William Budd.

John Snow died when I was an infant, and my knowledge of his work is derived from his writings and from his intimate friend Benjamin Ward Richardson.

My personal knowledge of William Budd is derived in part from his sister, who gave me an almost complete set of Budd's reprints and pamphlets. She lived in her later years in Brighton. Budd lived until 1880. The two men working independently, each pursuing his epidemiological inquiries in his own way, came to the same conclusions as to the specific causation of infectious diseases.

JOHN SNOW (1813–58)

An admirable account of Snow's life and work was given by B. W. Richardson in *Asclepiad*, 1887. Snow was born in 1813, was a vegetarian in his youth, and an early advocate of total abstinence from alcohol. His first observations of cholera were in 1831–32, when he was a mere youth in Newcastle upon Tyne. Soon after 1846, the year in which ether was introduced from America as a general anæsthetic, he made a reputation in London as an anæsthetist. Throughout his professional life this was his chief source of income.

In 1848 he argued that not the inhalation of any effluvium, but the direct contact of the choleraic poison with the alimentary canal must be responsible for the disease. In 1849 he published his book on *The Mode of Communication of Cholera*, in which this view was urged, and in 1855 a second and enlarged edition of this book was published. Its publication,

Richardson says, cost Snow £200, and he did not realise as many shillings from its sale.

Snow temporarily laid aside much of his practice to pursue his study of the epidemic of cholera in 1847, and satisfied himself by carefully collected epidemiological facts that a portion of the metropolitan water supply was responsible for the disease.

In the 1854 outbreak of cholera he devoted himself to a more intensive investigation. In a special part of London near his home a sudden outbreak of cholera occurred, causing local panic. Snow obtained from the General Register Office special permission to take a list of the deaths from cholera in the special area, and found that there had been eighty-nine deaths within a single week, nearly all of them within a short distance of the pump in Broad Street. Charged with this knowledge, he inferred that the water from this pump was responsible for the outbreak; and although he was "merely" a private practitioner of medicine he acted on his conviction.

The local authority for this district was the Vestry of St. James's, and on the evening of September 7th, while the vestry-men were discussing this terrible visitation—it may be noted without any expert advice—a stranger, Dr. Snow, asked for a hearing from them. He urged that the Broad Street pump water was the source of the mischief and advised the removal of the pump handle. This was his great prescription. The vestry-men were incredulous, but sensibly they acted on his advice—it could do no harm! Further cases at once ceased.

Later investigations showed that between five hundred and six hundred cases of cholera had occurred among those who drank this well-water. Snow's bold induction was soon confirmed by the fact that a large number of people consuming water from other wells nearby escaped cholera. In one interesting case a woman living at Hampstead had water from the Broad Street pump brought to her home daily, because of her personal preference for it: she (alone in that district) suffered from cholera.

To Snow is due the immense credit of first discovering and announcing this great epidemiological induction, that cholera is conveyed by water.

In a Presidential Address to the Medical Society in 1852, "On Continuous Molecular Changes, more particularly in their Relation to Epidemic Diseases," he formulated his views as to the specificity of the poisons causing infectious diseases, their essential character being shown, as he pointed out, by the multiplication of the poison in the body, and by its conveyance from one person to another.

Snow's teaching controverted that of Southwood Smith, and the similar teaching which, for instance, was advanced in 1850 in a noteworthy report of the Massachusetts Sanitary Commission, based probably in part on Chadwick's teaching:

> Atmospheric contagion is usually harmless unless attracted by local causes; thus Asiatic Cholera derives its terrific power chiefly or entirely from the accessory or accompanying circumstances which attend it.

Both views embodied some truth; the codification of the two was necessary for complete conquest over "fever" and cholera.

Snow was attacked because he had stated that certain offensive trades "do not cause, or in any way promote, the prevalence and mortality of cholera, fever, and other diseases, which are communicated from person to person." He illustrated his view that dirt alone or gases given off by effluvia did not cause contagion, by the common contagious disease, scabies; though doubtless dirt favoured its spread. He vigorously protested that he was "no defender of nuisances"; but that these should be dealt with by law, "without using the word pestiferous, or otherwise dragging in and distorting the science of medicine."

WILLIAM BUDD (1811–80)

We may turn next to the second of the two great protagonists of specificity in infection. Budd was born in 1811, Snow in

1813, and Simon in 1816, so until Snow died in his forty-fifth year they were contemporaries, and all were doing immortal work in public health.

In 1841 Budd settled in Bristol, and practised and taught medicine there. His great life work was done in that city. According to Dr. E. W. Goodall, who has given a full account of Budd's life (*Proceedings of the Royal Society of Medicine*, November 1931), Budd appears to have arrived in 1843 at the independent conclusion that typhus and typhoid fevers were different diseases. Several independent observers reached this conclusion before it became common knowledge. In 1837 Gerhard and Pennock of Philadelphia established the points of difference between the two diseases. Dr. A. P. Stewart, of Edinburgh, shortly afterwards described these differences, and Sir William Jenner's researches, published between 1849 and 1857, removed all doubts as to their separate identity.

In 1849, Budd published his pamphlet on *Malignant Cholera: Its Mode of Propagation and its Prevention*, within a month of the publication of Snow's pamphlet on the same subject. Budd's conclusion in this publication was that "the cause of malignant cholera is a living organism of distinct species," these organisms being disseminated through society in impalpable particles in the air, or by food, but "principally, in the drinking water of infected places." He concluded that "the human intestine is the sole breeding-place of the poison." This, he said, was "the crowning truth of all, on account of the momentous practical consequences to which it directly leads." He emphasised the practical point that cholera need never have been epidemic in England "if the poison in the discharges of infected persons had been destroyed."

In a footnote in the same pamphlet, Budd states:

Dr. Snow, whose ingenious pamphlet fell into my hands while these materials were preparing for publication, has been led by the consideration of particular instances of some of the facts above alluded to, to the same conclusion as to the part which water plays in the diffusion of the disease. Of being the first to develop and to publish this very important conclusion he must, therefore, have the whole merit.

This extract and the rest of the long footnote from which it is taken show the generosity and fairness of Budd's mind. The last sentence of the footnote shows that he believed that a microscopic fungus found in the "rice-water" discharges of cholera patients was the causal agent of cholera, and he finishes the footnote from which quotation has already been made by the following remark:

> The detection of the actual causes of the disease, and the determination of its nature, were all that is wanting to convert his [Dr. Snow's] views into a real discovery.

In a later pamphlet reprinted from the *British Medical Journal* (April 1867), Budd agreed that a purer water supply had influence in bringing about the smaller mortality from cholera in Bristol in the recent epidemic.

He said:

> That the cholera germ is often transmitted through drinking water, the late Dr. Snow, by his admirable researches, long ago proved.

But Budd expressed the view that precautions as to water supply "single-handed" are insufficient to prevent a severe visitation. This "is entirely opposed by facts." He attached great importance to disinfection of the discharges from each patient and even more to "disinfection by anticipation," daily disinfecting the latrines and saturating the sewers of all threatened places with disinfectants. We now fully appreciate that the infections of typhoid and cholera may be conveyed by actual contact with contagious matter, whether this contact is direct or indirect by dust or flies.

Budd was a contagionist out and out, and maintained that contagion was due to a living organism, the contagium for each disease being special to it. His demonstration of this for typhoid fever is outlined in Chapter XVI, and to him

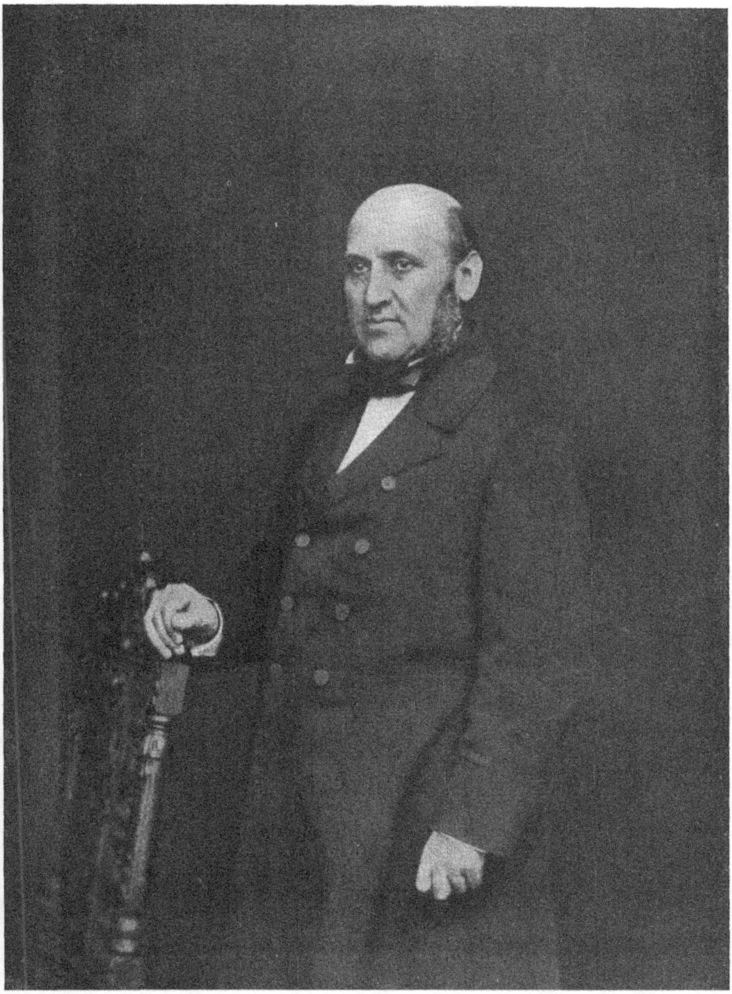

By kind permission of the] [*Council of the Royal Statistical Society*

WILLIAM FARR

must also be given the credit of first showing that the infection of typhoid can be conveyed by water. He taught that the infective material of typhoid (and of cholera) might be inhaled as well as swallowed, as shown by the following sentence from his *magnum opus* (*Typhoid Fever; its Nature, Mode of Spreading, and Prevention*, 1873, p. 93):

> To inhale, for an instant, the exhalations of a sewer; to walk down an infected alley, where there may even be no offensive smell to warn the visitor of his danger; to drink a draught of water which perhaps may only differ, to the senses, from any other drinking water, in being more sparkling . . . is often to be stricken with this fever unto death.

In a later paragraph he stated that the contagious particles must have been "resolved into the molecular state, and the infective molecules must have escaped from the liquid medium in which they were first eliminated, into the air we breathe."

The very limited extent to which typhoid germs or the germs of any other infectious disease can escape from the fluids of a drain or sewer in which they are imprisoned, was then imperfectly known: and "practical sanitation" of the next quarter of a century assumed that such an escape frequently occurs.

To Budd and to Snow, England is profoundly indebted. Eventually they swept away the older view that, without discrimination, sanitary defects, with resultant respiratory and excremental contamination of the air, determine respiratory and intestinal diseases. While not minimising the importance of these auxiliaries, they placed in its correct supreme position prevention of specific contagion as the direct aim of sanitary effort, the general removal of filth taking its place as an essential part of the effort to this end.

Their views were accepted officially only very slowly, and disease prevention was consequently delayed and decreased. The influence of Pettenkofer's views on the progress of modern pathology and preventive medicine is considered in Chapter XV.

CHAPTER XII

WILLIAM FARR

ALTHOUGH William Farr did not die before 1883, in his seventy-sixth year, I never spoke to him. I learnt much concerning him from the late Mr. W. J. H. Whittall, F.I.A., Actuary of the Clerical, Medical and General Insurance Society, a friend of many years, who was a relative of Farr. In 1923 Whittall gave money to the London School of Economics for a Farr Memorial Medal to be awarded to the best statistical student of each year. I was asked to give a public lecture at the school inaugurating the gift, and in preparation was given access to a trunk containing notebooks, letters, etc., left by Farr, which I utilised for the published lecture (*Economica*, November 1923).

Farr was one of the most potent influences in public health advancement, through his statistical reports, and the vivid and oft-times burning words in which his comments were made. These were momenta of great weight in securing national reform.

William Farr was born in 1807 of humble parentage. He was adopted by a friend, who in 1829 left him enough money to enable him to study in Paris for a year or two. While he was in Paris his love of statistics was probably inspired by Andral and Louis, who were the French leaders in the now blossoming subject of hygiene, and who taught the importance of securing accurate numerical statement of ascertained facts.

After his return he was for six months house surgeon at the Shrewsbury Infirmary, although at that time he had no diploma to practise; and I have seen a testimonial signed by the medical pupils at that hospital, expressing their appreciation of his teaching.

Farr took his L.S.A. in 1832, and this, the lowest of medical qualifications, was his only one, until later in life he received an honorary M.D. He proceeded, with the temerity of youth, associated happily with special knowledge, to give lectures on hygiene and medical statistics, and to write on the same subjects, thus laying the foundation of his subsequent supremacy in vital statistics.

The national system of Registration of Births and Deaths and the central General Register Office in London were initiated in 1837, and William Farr was appointed "Compiler of Statistics." This was an event of historic importance in preventive medicine. Not even Chadwick, who "discovered" Farr, and much less those responsible for the patronage of his appointment, could have known how momentous was the good thus initiated. For over forty years it was Farr who, in the words of my Farr Memorial Lecture (1923),

> devised the methods and supervised the actual compilation of our national mortality statistics, introduced methods of tabulation which have stood the test of time, and a classification of causes of death which has been the basis of all subsequent methods. And from these statistics, in reports year by year and in the classical Decennial Supplements written by him, he deduced practical lessons as to the causation and prevention of disease which have formed a most potent factor in determining the course of the sanitary history and the wonderful triumphs of public health in this country.

I must refer readers to Mr. Noel Humphreys' short life of Farr, which prefaces the collected edition of extracts from Farr's works (Sanitary Institute reprint, 1885), and to my lecture in *Economica*, November 1923, for particulars of Farr's life-work; but a few remarks on his statistical genius may be made before writing further on his wonderful influence as a missioner of health.

Farr was a mathematical genius, and his investigations in vital statistics went far beyond what was embodied in the Registrar-General's reports. He was an authority on life-tables, annuities, and life insurance, and achieved the solitary honour among doctors of being made an honorary fellow of the exclusive Institute of Actuaries.

Farr's great work in life, however, was to demonstrate how

statistics of life and death could be utilised to advance the public health. *The facts themselves*—more important than any deduction from them—he made significant as means of exposing the places and occupations which were lethal to man.

The *amount* and *localisation* of the mischief were thus revealed. He turned the searchlight of publicity on evils which could not then continue to be indefinitely neglected.

By means of differential statistics it was also often possible to trace *the sources of disease*. And this justified Farr's occasional assumption of the rôle of a prophet, *warning the public* of impending dangers. One example was his pointing to the Metropolitan water supply as a source of cholera in 1865. A parliamentary committee somewhat haltingly threw doubt on this reflection on the water supply of the East of London; and Farr defended his warning, even though the conclusion reached had not been completely demonstrated, as follows:

> The Registrar-General had to speak in the midst of a tempest, and on his words at the moment the fate of the ship to some extent depended;

adding words as to the need for accepting a judgment the elements of which

> existed in the accumulated experience of the previous epidemics, in the known laws of the disease, and in the facts of the case looked at comprehensively.

It may be noted that even in this instance, although the Registrar-General through Farr courageously gave a highly important forecast and warning, there was no statistical certainty, and the minds of both Farr and Simon, while leaning to the possibility of specific infection of the water supply, regarded it, at first, as supplementary to the evil influence of effluvia from organic filth.

Farr at an earlier date had prepared some elaborate statistics showing that cholera prevailed especially in the lower-lying parts of London; and considered that the influence of elevation above sea-level should be allowed for before measuring the effect of an impure water supply. This illustrates the limitation of utility of a statistical analysis, unaccompanied by field observations which give differential particulars of the individual cases. Farr's views on the relationship between density of population and general mortality form another instance (Chapter XXI).

Farr was primarily and always a hygienist, and in nearly all his reports there is, as stated in the above-mentioned address,

evidence of *eager desire for social service.* In his first annual letter to the Registrar-General he affirmed that "diseases are more easily prevented than cured," and that the first step in "their prevention is the discovery of their exciting causes." Farr's burning desire for social service was as marked as his statistical acumen; and he can worthily be placed in the company of Howard, who reformed our prisons, of the workers including Southwood Smith, Lord Shaftesbury, and others, who secured the mitigation of the evils of factory and mining life, and of Edwin Chadwick and John Simon, who were pioneers in Poor Law and sanitary reform. In the earlier reforms affecting prisons, factories, and mines, it was not the economic motive—although this was a powerful instrument in Chadwick's hands—so much as pity and religious motive which secured reform; and similarly, in the most severely scientific discussions in Farr's reports the humanitarian motive and driving power constantly emerged.

For remarks on Farr and hospital statistics, see p. 60, and on density of population, see p. 301.

Farr, as we have said, was a close friend of Richardson. He was also one of Florence Nightingale's "slaves," and we have seen how in this connection he went astray (p. 60).

CHAPTER XIII

BENJAMIN WARD RICHARDSON

PREVENTIVE medicine was fortunate in its early protagonists in the nineteenth century. Of the three who were most influential in establishing its fortunes, Chadwick, I admit, had a pedestrian style, and his writing lost much effect through its diffuseness; but he more than compensated for his halting words by his terrific driving power. Farr and Simon both wrote effectively, oft-times eloquently. In Farr's writings there emerged an occasional fervour which compels one to regard him as a missionary as well as an educator; while Simon's writings, though not lacking in earnestness, and never in dignity, appealed especially to the intellect.

Benjamin Ward Richardson does not occupy so high a position as these three in the hierarchy of public health; but he has a place among the mighty, and it may be said of him that for many years he was a chief agent in securing and retaining the attention of the public, and in educating them in the hygienic gospel.

My first personal experience with Richardson was in 1889. He was president of a local sanitary exhibition and conference organised by the Mayor of Hastings; and as a neighbouring M.O.H. I was asked to be one of the judges of the exhibition. At a public dinner I found myself seated next Richardson. He was then in his sixty-first year, and he was a delightful companion. But what captured the heart of one of a younger generation was his remark that he had just completed his review (*Asclepiad*, June 1889) of *The Elements of Vital Statistics*, a volume which had recently been written by me with infinite difficulty. No previous manual of this subject had appeared, and there was little to guide one beyond official Blue books. Richardson assured me that I might await the review with complacency; and this was correct, for when his three-paged review appeared it contained the following remarks, which I shall quote, although thereby I lay myself open to the charge of egotism.

> The author has spared no labour, has introduced no crotchet, has advanced no theory, has taken no extreme view, has become no partisan, and has claimed no originality; but, from the beginning to the end, has upheld the position and authority, firstly, of an honest and faithful compiler of facts; and secondly, of a judge of evidence derivable from the facts, without bias, prejudice, or other failing that might lead him from the truth. This is just what was wanted for all classes of readers, etc.

And yet on one page of my new book I had referred to Richardson's *Hygeiopolis*, deprecating the statement in it that its inhabitants would have a death-rate of only 5 per 1,000; and in another place I had illustrated the dangers of basing conclusions on total death-rates by asking the reader to compare the death-rate in a community of curates aged twenty-five to thirty with that in a workhouse for aged persons.

Richardson was least happy when using statistics; and Chadwick, whose erroneous methods of using statistics were also illustrated in my book, was a great statistical sinner, since figures he must use. William Farr, like Chadwick, was a friend of Richardson for twenty or thirty years, and all of them were possessed, one might say obsessed, with the spirit of missionary fervour.

Richardson presided at many sanitary congresses, and always chose attractive subjects for his addresses. In 1878 he gave an address on "The Election of a Minister of Health," and in 1883 on "Felicity as a Sanitary Research." He it was who coined the phrase "National Health is National Wealth," now become a universal proverb. At one congress he presided at a breakfast meeting at which ham was a dish. In his own slice he discovered trichinæ, and at once warned those present. Some of them had already finished their ham, and there was some alarm; but as it was well cooked no harm resulted.

In Germany before its rigid system of meat inspection was

enforced, trichinosis was a common and serious disease, owing to the practice of eating uncooked ham or pork.

Trichinæ were first discovered, I believe, by Paget (afterwards Sir James) in two bodies in the dissecting-room at St. Bartholomew's Hospital, and the name *trichina spiralis* was given by Cobbold. This was in 1835. Its life-history was then unknown. Its occurrence in epidemics was only recognised some years later. The symptoms produced by its invasion were sometimes confused with typhoid or rheumatic fever.

Richardson (1828–98) throughout his professional life engaged in very varied labours. He was a specialist in several directions. In physiological experimental research he early made his name. He discovered several new local and general anæsthetics, and in this subject he and his friend John Snow sometimes collaborated. He ascertained the physiological effect on the circulation of nitrite of amyl, and Dr. J. D. Rolleston tells an amusing story of the meeting of the British Association in 1863, at which Richardson described his investigation on amyl nitrite. He affirmed that the amount of amyl nitrite which he had poured on a piece of blotting-paper and left on the table would quicken the heart-beat of every person in the room. The chairman (Professor Rolleston of Oxford) smiled incredulously, and forthwith inhaled from the paper. His face almost immediately became blood-red and the results previously described by Richardson were obvious. The chairman at once stated to the audience that his experiment showed the folly of being incredulous!

Throughout his career, Richardson was in touch with Chadwick as well as with Farr, and must have shared much of their anticipations and hopes. He himself was an ardent writer on health subjects. In 1875 he gave a lecture at Brighton on "Hygeia: a Model City of Health," which although fantastic in some particulars attracted much attention to the possibilities of healthier life. Before this he had edited a sanitary journal of his own, and for many years edited and wrote a quarterly journal, called *The Asclepiad*, each number of which contained a charmingly written memoir of some medical worthy of the past. These memoirs are models of information and style. At an early date he advocated and took part in an attempt to collect weekly records of sickness, and was concerned in the early stages of the history of the Epidemiological Society. His views on zymotic diseases are stated on p. 122. Like Southwood Smith and Chadwick he held the undiluted doctrine that these diseases were the nemesis of unwholesome life and environment —in short, of sanitary shortcomings.

But his memory will live longest through his work on two problems of great public health interest. One of these was the Humane Slaughtering of Animals for food. In giving the second Benjamin Ward Richardson Memorial Lecture (October 13, 1923) I made the following remarks:

> I limit myself in the present lecture to one of the many subjects in which Richardson was a pathfinder, and which he illuminated by research and by advocacy, in writings which in eloquence and grace form a model for all medical authors. There ran through all Richardson's writings the unusual combination of suggestive research and of a powerful and vivid imagination, along with an always present desire to serve his fellow-men, and to improve the conditions of life, not only of mankind, but also of the animals over whom man exercises control. His research work and his writings alike showed his anxiety to prevent cruelty, both in man and in man's humbler associates, two problems which are intimately interrelated.

He made many experiments on methods of humane slaughtering, and in 1886 he established and became the first President of the Model Abattoir Society. The subject of sanitary and humane slaughtering was fully discussed in my lecture in 1923; but it is unfortunately true, notwithstanding considerable improvement, that private slaughter-houses continue in England and that over them the satisfactory supervision possible in public abattoirs cannot be exercised.

But Richardson's highest contribution to public health work consisted in his powerful advocacy of abstinence from alcohol. This was a chief outlet of his zeal as a hygienic reformer.

The social evil of alcoholism was greater then than now, though still lamentably great. He left others to advocate abstinence from a moral and social standpoint; it was attacked by him on its physiological side.

His investigations showed that alcohol did not raise the bodily temperature. Sir W. Collins states that when Richardson made this statement in 1866 at the meeting of the British Association it was received with incredulity. He also taught that alcohol was a drug not a food, a narcotic and not a stimulant; and by such teaching as this, which is now universally accepted, he gradually bent public opinion. It was slow work, and meanwhile Richardson suffered loss in medical practice and some partial medical ostracism. But he lived to see a revolution in medical and public opinion, and were he now alive he would see that—largely as the result of his work—the daily taking of alcoholic drinks has become the exception rather than the rule in some classes in the community.

Very few sanitarians have made anti-alcoholic educational work a large part of their life-work, though even now the remaining magnitude of the evil would justify this. All the more honour to one who, through evil and good report, was a chief advocate of the improvement in alcoholic habits which has already occurred.

CHAPTER XIV

MAX VON PETTENKOFER (1818–1901)

PETTENKOFER'S views on the relation of ground-water to disease had great weight in biassing the views of sanitarians on the relation of contaminated water supplies to cholera and typhoid fever, and they determined the trend of several years' work which I devoted to investigation of the causation of rheumatic fever and diphtheria. It is therefore desirable in these recollections to explain Pettenkofer's position in the history of Epidemiology and Public Health.

In an obituary notice by Dr. John S. Haldane, F.R.S. (*Journal of Hygiene*, Vol. I, July 1901), Pettenkofer is rightly described as "a great leader in our science, and as the pioneer who has been mainly instrumental in bringing about the recognition of hygiene, especially on its experimental side, as a separate subject of investigation and university instruction."

He held the first Chair of Hygiene (but see also p. 41), which was founded for him in Munich University in 1865, and he retained it until 1894. In his earlier life he made important investigations on problems of physiological chemistry and nutrition; and his work on the ventilation of dwelling-houses, on clothing, and on the soil entitles him to the title of founder of experimental hygiene.

He is best known, however, by his researches on conditions of the soil as affecting the occurrence of cholera and typhoid fever. These occupied him for over forty years, and his views on this subject were for many years regarded as authoritative by public health workers. Pettenkofer's investigations were pursued in Munich, which suffered severely from typhoid fever. When he began to investigate, Pettenkofer expected to find that contaminated water supplies were responsible for this state of things. Munich was built on gravel over impermeable clay, and its soil was permeated by cesspools, while private wells supplied its water. There were "some fifteen acres of ashpits out of the total area of Munich." The numerous supplies of water rendered inquiry into the water supply in cases of typhoid or cholera fairly easy; but Pettenkofer failed to discover any connection between the two.

He found that the infected localities had a porous soil polluted with organic matter, and these conditions, when they were associated with a certain state of the ground-water, were regarded by him as necessary for the causation of the two diseases. His observations on the level of ground-water began in 1856, and he showed that this prevalence of typhoid and of cholera varied in accordance with the statement that:

> Spread of cholera and typhoid fever depends upon the movements of the subsoil water, the prevalence of these diseases increasing after a fall in the level of that water.

In 1853 the cesspools were emptied and main sewerage was initiated, and after 1865 a safe public water supply replaced the local wells, and later experience when the use of well-water had ceased showed that the level of ground-water ceased to form an index of the diminishing prevalence of typhoid or cholera.

Pettenkofer did not exclude the importation of infection from a cholera patient as forming part of the causation of an epidemic of that disease. Indeed, in his own words he held fast to "the principle that the distribution of cholera from place to place is effected by human intercourse"; but he maintained that the spread of the disease is conditioned by the fact that "the soil has a certain condition of porosity affected by temperature and moisture or by the rise and fall of the ground-water."

His views did not go unchallenged, although for many years they were regarded as authoritative by most hygienists. Among the unconvinced was Dr. (afterwards Sir George) Buchanan (1831–95), who (*Medical Times and Gazette*, p. 283, 1870) in a paper read to the Association of Medical Officers of Health in February 1870 pointed out that the nature of the evidence upon which Pettenkofer had persuaded himself that it is not by pollution of wells that the subsidence of soil water comes to have its relation to cholera and fever

seemed to point in the opposite direction, inasmuch as lowered soil water meant greater contamination of the water pumped out of wells. Buchanan further urged that evidence of this relationship between typhoid and fall of soil water was lacking when the water supply of a community was derived from without the city, and he cogently demanded that strict proof should be advanced showing that

the distribution of fever and cholera has not in the cases examined coincided with the distribution of bad drinking water.

Pettenkofer, replying in the same medical journal, quoted instances of places

with the worst drinking water, but there is at the same time immunity from epidemic diseases.

This fails to carry weight in view of Budd's classical investigation (p. 124) showing that specific infection must be imported before an outbreak can occur, an experience which has been repeatedly confirmed.

It will be noted that both Buchanan and Pettenkofer appear to have regarded the choice of source of infection as lying between *soil and water*. Little knowledge was then possessed of other sources of infection, such as milk, and none of shellfish or carrier cases.

Pettenkofer's theory is now only a sign-post in the road of progress towards scientific certitude. The notion that there is some mysterious reaction between the typhoid excreta and the soil, constituting a *tertium quid* necessary to mature the contagium and give it striking power, has gone for ever. But in reviewing public health during the last fifty years it is incumbent on us to balance the teaching of Southwood Smith, of Snow and Budd, and of Pettenkofer, if we are to understand the slow process of enlightenment.

In 1856 Simon stated his views at that time as to specific infection as follows:

> Under the specific influence which determines an epidemic period, fecalised drinking water and fecalised air equally may breed and convey the poison [of cholera].

We have noted Buchanan's confutation of Pettenkofer's theory. But Pettenkofer's opinion that "cholera was neither wholly a contagion nor wholly a miasm, but a bastard of the two," persisted and continued to influence the policy of sanitary advisers in this country, and the interpretation which I placed on the epidemiology of rheumatic fever and diphtheria.

Simon was himself greatly influenced by Pettenkofer's views on typhoid, which are consistent with the view emphasised by C. Murchison that (as Budd put their case) "the poison of typhoid fever is not cast off from the body in a finished state," a process of subsequent maturation being required. Similarly, Simon contrasted smallpox in which direct infection occurs, and cholera in which "if truly the disease be contagious, foulness of medium seems indispensable."

Writing in 1866, Simon confirmed his appreciation of Pettenkofer's teaching, and emphasised the importance of study of soils and of exact observation of the heights of wells "as it seems established that these are two great governing influences in relation to the spread of disease."

In his report to the Privy Council, 1866, Simon regarded the distribution of cholera in London as illustrating and explained by Pettenkofer's ground-water theory. In summarising this subject elsewhere (*Evolution of Preventive Medicine*, 1927), I said:

> Pettenkofer's views . . . must, I think, be credited with responsibility for the inadequate emphasis which in the earlier years was placed on the special sanitary improvement, viz. a perfectly safe water supply, which would bring about the most rapid reduction of disease. On the other hand, it is arguable that the general campaign against filth urged by Simon, and forming the main item in the

sanitary work of Simon and Southwood Smith, was remarkably effective also in securing clean supplies of water for the public.

We may add a reference to a footnote in Simon's report for 1858, in which after summarising appreciatively Snow's teaching in 1849–55, as to the direct propagation of cholera, he adds:

> Whatever may be the worth of this theory, it has been of use in contributing to draw attention to the vast hygienic importance of a pure water supply.

This sketch of progress towards the light, as regards the causation and prevention of cholera and typhoid fever from 1849 to 1880, may, I think, be regarded as necessary if the sanitary events of the last fifty years are to be understood; but the subject will emerge in later chapters.

CHAPTER XV

"EPIDEMIC CONSTITUTION"

The x *of epidemicity—Ground-water observations—Further comments on Pettenkofer's views—Epidemicity of rheumatic fever and diphtheria—Disturbed epidemiology*

PRECEDING chapters have been concerned chiefly with those who taught me the elements of preventive medicine, and who formed the background of all subsequent progress. They need, I think, to be supplemented by a further statement of the epidemiological views held round about the year 1880, and their relation to two branches of personal investigation in later years. In doing this I must be allowed to include in my review investigations and facts which belong to more recent years.

Let me begin by mentioning the views held before the "germ theory of disease," which was being actively discussed when I was a medical student, partially superseded earlier views.

For long centuries, even from the time of Hippocrates (about 460–377 B.C.), health was regarded as largely influenced by air, climate, and season; and in the causation of epidemics the idea of contagion was largely ignored. Although Sydenham (A.D. 1624–89) regarded the remote causes of epidemics as "wholly inscrutable," he taught that in certain years there was an "epidemic constitution" which led to cyclical outbursts of epidemics.

This conception still survives, and I do not doubt that it embodies a truth of magnitude, although, in large measure, we must still describe it algebraically as x.

Without attempting to trace the history of this general notion, some reference is needed to that part of its history which belongs to the nineteenth century, as it influenced greatly the course of sanitary reforms and materially biassed the views of modern sanitarians, including my own for some years.

When in the years rapidly following 1875 the germ theory of disease became established, involving not only the general notion of contagia but also that of a probable specific contagium for each infectious disease, the early impulse was to reject altogether the conception of "epidemic constitution." But this did not happen; for the germ theory failed to explain why at long intervals diseases like smallpox or influenza swept round the world. True, they are infectious, but why vastly more so in these epidemic storms? The same question arose in respect of typhoid fever, and of the group of diseases comprising scarlet fever, diphtheria, erysipelas, rheumatic fever—in which, as Longstaff found, the annual death-rates in England varied to a large extent inversely with the annual rainfall of the year. Subsequently, in a series of international studies beginning in 1894, and continued for five years, I investigated intensively and exhaustively the annual incidence of rheumatic fever and diphtheria, and showed that the inverse relationship between rainfall and disease held good on an international scale.

But in order to realise the gradual process of enlightenment we must recall the intermediate stage between the blind acceptance of the unknown influences included in "epidemic constitution" and the—perhaps too unlimited—bending of the knee to the acceptance of specific infectivity, untempered by any consideration of environmental factors other than infection. The difference between epidemic and inter-epidemic years may, of course, be explicable by changes in the virulence or striking power of the germs of disease. But this still leaves us without explanation of this occasional change in the life-history of these germs.

The first sixty years of the nineteenth century were years of active efforts towards sanitary reform—attempts to prevent the accumulation of filth, especially excremental filth, in and around dwellings, and attempts to reduce the herding of persons in crowded rooms.

I need not repeat what has been written in earlier chapters concerning the great work accomplished by Southwood

Smith and Chadwick and their co-workers, which was extended and made more effective under the influence of John Simon's and William Farr's reports, and of sanitary administration based on the various Nuisance Removal and Public Health Acts. John Snow and William Budd stand out as pioneers of the more advanced sanitary science, which was based on specificity, at a period when the micro-organisms causing any of the acute infectious diseases were still unknown.

But before the specific micro-organisms of cholera and typhoid fever had been identified there was a period in which a doctrine without the driving power in the prevention of disease, embodied in the aphorism "dirt makes disease," became a partial impediment to the pursuit of activities conducing to the prevention of the spread of infection. With this doctrine the name of Pettenkofer is associated. His views as to the relation between ground-water and disease are outlined on p. 108. They delayed acceptance in England of the supreme influence of water-infection in the dissemination of cholera and typhoid fever. Direct infectivity in cholera and to some extent in typhoid fever, even in the case of attendants on the sick, was denied or doubted, while the possibility of "carriers" of infection by apparently healthy persons was not yet recognised.

I have already quoted (p. 110) from Simon's report in 1866 remarks which indicate his appreciation of Pettenkofer's views on the relation between soil and disease. In the same report Simon expressed his "deep sense of the value of Professor V. Pettenkofer's researches" and added, "it seems certain that henceforth no local health officer will be properly up to the standard of his scientific duties unless . . . he also maintains such systematic and exact observations of the height of wells as will enable him always to speak with precision as to the movements of water-level in the soil; for it seems established that these [i.e. water-levels and stratification of soils] are two great governing influences to the spread of disease."

It was under the partial influence of Pettenkofer's teaching that medical officers of health were educated during the quarter of a century under review in this volume, though gradually the importance attached to ground-water levels faded, as direct infection became more emphasised.

Among medical officers of health who kept ground-water records for a series of years were the late Dr. M. A. Adams (Maidstone) and myself (Brighton). Among non-medical observers the late Mr. Baldwin Latham kept long series of weekly observations of well-levels, copies of which lie before me as I write. In an address as President of the Meteorological Society (1890) Latham stressed the condition of ground-water as influencing the course of many epidemic diseases. Among these in his view was smallpox; and in the Jenner Centennial number of the *British Medical Journal* (1902) I partially confirmed this, so far as concerns smallpox in Britain during the last century. Sir Leonard Rogers has recently collected facts pointing to the same conclusion in the experience of India.

I give at this point a few sentences from my paper in 1902. After partially verifying Latham's observations I quoted his remark that

> smallpox is always preceded by a long period of dryness of the ground, measured by the absence of percolation;

and in concluding my review of the epidemiology of smallpox, I wrote:

> Although the chief governing factor is personal infection . . . there is, however, some further factor responsible for the causation of the greater epidemics and pandemics of smallpox, which, for lack of a better term, we must still designate by the old-fashioned name of "epidemic constitution." As the expression of a fact without being committed to a theory, we may admit with the older epidemiologists that there is a *constitutio epidemica variolosa*. What is meant by this is that at irregular intervals smallpox, as judged by its wider spread, is more infectious than it is in other years with equal opportunities for its dissemination.

When I gave the Milroy Lectures on Rheumatic Fever (1895) I collected a vast amount of information, which showed that deficient rainfall over two or more years favoured its epidemic prevalence; and in my brochure on *Pandemic Diphtheria* (1898) I showed that a similar relationship held good for this disease.

I still hold that both of these are "dry-year diseases," becoming epidemic by preference in years of deficient rainfall, though as this connection cannot be regarded as a *sine qua non* in their causation, deficient rainfall must be reckoned among the auxiliary, not the essential, factors in their prevalence.

When I published the results of my investigations on the two above diseases I attached greater importance to the occurrence of a low ground-water than I should now do, but I always regarded ground-water level as simply an index of some condition auxiliary (it may even be necessary) for the origination of a widespread epidemic of either disease. My views are those stated on p. 227.

Looking back on the toilsome months and years I spent in collecting rainfall and ground-water observations in many countries, I do not regard the expenditure of time and toil as altogether wasted. I still hold that in explaining epidemics of these two and some other diseases, the doctrine of specificity of infection "is not enough." There are unrecognised and neglected factors which will emerge as science advances. I therefore regret that the study of meteorology and of ground-water levels, as recommended by Simon, is not now much pursued. It may still throw some light on the dark corners of causation.

Disturbed Epidemiology.—My protracted study of rheumatic fever and diphtheria has left me with the conviction that the future course of these two diseases can no longer be followed with an approach to accuracy or historical comparability.

When I wrote on them in 1894 and 1898 their natural course was already being disturbed by therapeutic intervention by salicylates and antitoxins, although to a much less extent than now, and the peaks of their intermittent epidemics were consequently becoming truncated. These influences have since operated to an increasing extent, and to them has been added in more recent years the effect on prevalence which is being produced by the security against attack by diphtheria, produced by the use of toxoid antitoxin.

We can gratefully appreciate the increasing success in controlling these diseases—rheumatic fever by salicylates and by improved oral hygiene, diphtheria by antitoxin and toxoid-antitoxin—while nursing an undercurrent of regret that study of the natural history of these diseases has become more difficult, and we are left somewhat in doubt as to whether there has not been, irrespective of events as affected by the above activities, some natural diminution in the occurrence or the virulence of rheumatic fever comparable to that which has occurred in scarlet fever. Personally I hold that this change in "epidemic constitution" has occurred.

After completing this chapter I found two articles which I think have interest. These were contributed as editorials to medical journals.

(1) The first of these is an annotation on one of Q's (Quiller-Couch's) Cornish novels. The plot is laid in a Cornish village; and its interest here consists in its photographic sketch of the sanitary and meteorological conditions which heralded an epidemic of diphtheria. The local doctor is talking:

> And you say it is good weather, and you are a fool. For it is a dry February, and this is already the third case of French Croup that I am going to.

Later on he describes the progress of events:

> No rain fell in February; very little in March; next to nothing in April, and again none in May. A hot May makes a fat churchyard.

And the epidemic spread and became more virulent.

(2) My second article involves almost a personal confession. I wrote an editorial on a paper read at a meeting of the Epidemiological Society on February 18, 1898. The author of this paper had used his recent experience in a military station in India to show the relation of malaria in the soldiers at this

station to levels of ground-water in the local wells. Fever occurred when the well-water rose to 16 feet from the surface and increased with its further rise in a manner fully stated in the paper. This association was consistent in consecutive years. The explanation offered was that the rainfall drove the specifically polluted ground-air in piston-like fashion into the men's quarters, and when the level fell or failed to rise there was an absence of this expulsion of the specific miasm from the soil.

I made this experience the text for remarks as to the rarity of exact observations like those under review and as to the lack of organized co-operation by observers at different Indian stations and elsewhere. This particular experience was regarded by the reader of the above paper as justifying a causal hypothesis "more likely than the more elaborate mosquito theory," and my article endorsed the view that there was "a causal relationship between certain movements and levels of the ground-water and the incidence of malaria." And yet Manson's suggestion that the agent for distribution of malaria was a mosquito or "a similar suctorial insect" already was being worked out by Ronald Ross, and in 1896 he had proved this as regards the malarial parasite of the sparrow.

I quote this article because it throws light on the views held by some public health administrators near the end of the nineteenth century, and because it suggests the question whether in rheumatic fever an insect vector of infection—whose life history, like that of the mosquito, may be affected by climatic conditions—may not be concerned in its causation.

In diphtheria we know that no such intermediary is concerned; but we are still in primal darkness as to why, apart from certain auxiliary climatic conditions, diphtheria after intervals of years becomes widely epidemic or even pandemic.

PERSONAL CONTRIBUTION

"The Epidemiology of Smallpox in the Nineteenth Century" (in a special Jenner number of the *British Medical Journal*, July 5, 1902).

Also see references in Chapters XXIII and XXIV.

CHAPTER XVI

PREVENTIVE MEDICINE AND EPIDEMIOLOGY IN 1880

THE year 1880 corresponds nearly with my admission to the medical profession, as it was only in the preceding year that I had become M.R.C.S. and L.S.A.

I shall not attempt to mention the many possibilities of preventive medicine already existent in that year; but rather to indicate in particular the fact that the specific nature of infection was becoming realised. For in the earlier years of my practice of preventive medicine it was tacitly assumed that public health was concerned chiefly if not solely with the prevention of infection. It was only towards the end of the nineteenth century—with the notable exceptions of the prevention of scurvy in the British Navy and of beri-beri in the Japanese Navy—that other fields of preventive medicine emerged, with our increasing knowledge of physiology and especially of nutrition.

Even in regard to infection, knowledge grew very slowly. It was not until the nineteenth century that it increased by leaps and bounds. Much earlier, fear of infection had led to measures of isolation and quarantine against two great enemies of mankind, leprosy and plague.

The first great feat of preventive medicine consisted in the almost complete abolition of leprosy from Western Europe by the merciless enforcement of segregation of palpable cases of that disease.

The second great battle of preventive medicine was against plague. This disease prevailed for several centuries, no effective methods of control being discovered. Nevertheless, in the nineteenth century it had ceased to trouble the Western world on a large scale, although rat-infected fleas were not proved to be responsible for its spread until 1906–10. Long before this, intermittent pandemic extensions of plague had ceased to affect

Britain to a calamitous extent. The history of plague has points of resemblance to that of another great scourge—typhus fever—which was endemic in the British Isles and especially in Ireland; but which, during the period 1850–80, was being gradually reduced to insignificance, long before it was ascertained that typhus is spread from patients to their contacts by body lice. The conditions leading to the almost complete disappearance of plague and typhus from Britain are not far to seek, in the light of our more recent exact knowledge of the methods of spread of each disease. In 1894 Kitasato and Versin showed that the *Bacillus pestis* is the cause of plague; and the work of the Indian Plague Commission (1906–10) made it clear that infected rats and other rodents were the chief source of human plague, through transference of their infected fleas to man. We can then be certain that the prevention of access of rats to human dwellings and the destruction of black rats have been the chief means of preventing plague, when its infection is introduced from countries in which plague is endemic. Valuable aid was doubtless given by the internecine wars between the black or domestic rat and the brown or Norwegian rat, mainly a non-domestic rat, which came as a "Hanoverian invasion" and remains the chief rat of the British Isles.

The micro-organism conveying typhus is still unknown; but in 1909 Nicolle and his co-workers showed that typhus could be conveyed to monkeys by the bite of an infected body-louse. It is eloquent testimony to the value of isolation of all known cases of typhus and the long-continued warfare against overcrowding and personal uncleanliness that "fever" almost disappeared from this country before the essential importance of action directed specifically against the body-louse had been discovered.

The course of the national "fever" statistics illustrates similarly the progress made in reducing disease, before its channels of spread had been fully elucidated. Even before 1870 there had been a marked decline, as the result of removal of patients to "fever" hospitals, cleansing of tenements, clearing of slums, and efforts to improve general sanitation, and to supply uncontaminated drinking water. Typhoid fever figures can only be given separately from typhus for the years 1871 onwards. In three successive decades, 1871–80, 1881–90, and 1891–1900, the death-rates from enteric fever per million living in England and Wales were 322, 198, and 174 respectively.

The actual deaths from typhoid fever in the country numbered 12,709 in 1871 (population under 23 millions), and only 258 in 1932 (population over 45 millions).

I have given in particular the figures for "fever," as this was the enemy against which earlier sanitary measures were chiefly directed. The problem as to whether infection was specific or could originate *de novo* in circumstances of filth and crowding had scarcely arisen before 1870.

When I was a medical student the germ theory of disease was already gaining ground. A series of discoveries were already being made in the new science of bacteriology, though the belief in epidemic constitutions—an exaggeration of a true conception—prevailed, and minimised the hope that human intervention could be useful. The battle around the conception of a *contagium vivum* was still being waged when as a medical student I read a paper in January 1878 to the Students' Society at St. Thomas's Hospital, known as the Physical Society, on "The Origin *de novo* of Zymotic Diseases," which I utilise in this chapter as a convenient though imperfect summary of knowledge at that time.

The two theories of the genesis of epidemics then prevalent were the germ theory and the physico-chemical theory, and these were intermingled with the controversy then being pursued as to the possibility of "spontaneous generation" of living matter. Evidently the proof or disproof of Bastian's theory of abiogenesis had direct bearing on the medical problem; and Tyndall's investigations on dust and Pasteur's demolition of Bastian's views were reviewed in my paper with zest. In 1878 the opposing views were regarded as still debatable. In summarising Pasteur's recent researches I mentioned their recent application in surgery at King's College Hospital, London, as of universal interest. It is illustrative of our imperfect knowledge that I mentioned, though without endorsement, the then sometimes taught intercommunication between scarlet fever and diphtheria, and the view of Dr. John Harley (then physician of St. Thomas's) that the poisons of scarlet fever and enteric fever were identical.

Relapsing fever and anthrax were next taken as two diseases in which the germ theory had been established.

In my paper (1878) I quoted Dr. W. Roberts who, in mentioning the resemblance of *Bac.Anthracis* to the harmless *Bac.Subtilis*, and of a harmless spirochœte to the spirillum of relapsing fever, thought this might point to a natural explanation of the origin of contagia, by variation or "sporting." In supporting this view I mentioned the "occasional sporting of diphtheria from scarlet fever" which was then taught—really, of course, an instance of double infection; and the occasional origin of cholera without apparent importation (again a fallacious instance).

The objections to the germ theory were then enumerated, and the views of B. W. Richardson, of Lionel Beale, and of Charles Murchison were discussed. Richardson argued that if germs could multiply with the rapidity assigned to them, how could man escape destruction? Beale taught a modification of the germ theory, which eliminated the conception of specificity. In his view a disease germ was "the degraded offspring of some kind of normal bioplasm." I quoted Burdon Sanderson on this point: "It is not possible for any bit of protoplasm to be separated from the organism to which it belongs without losing its vitality."

Richardson enunciated the glandular hypothesis of contagion. This rested on the assumption that all the specific fevers are the outcome of vitiated glandular functions, a "septine" being secreted. He drew an analogy between the normal differences of function of normal glands and the characteristic differences of the various specific fevers. Snake poison was regarded by Richardson as the type of the poisons producing specific fevers; but in my paper, evidently summarising current knowledge, I regarded the analogy as feeble, for snake poison is dangerous only in proportion to dosage, and does not multiply in the victim's system.

The physico-chemical hypothesis was then popular. Bastian compared the multiplication of contagion to that multiplication of crystals of sulphate of soda which occurs when a crystal of this salt is added to a saturated solution of sulphate of soda, though he regarded this as an imperfect illustration. It fails entirely, as I indicated, because whereas in the process of infection the infecting agent multiplies indefinitely, the amount of sulphate of soda is exactly the same at the end as at the beginning of the above experiment.

Dr. Chas. Murchison's illustration, which he had recently advanced at a discussion at the Pathological Society, London, carried more weight with me. The substance oxamide is transformed into oxalate of ammonium when boiled with dilute acids or alkalies. Murchison remarked, if the acid selected be oxalic acid, "a small quantity of this will convert an infinite quantity of oxamide into oxalate of ammonium. In other words, the excitant of the change—oxalic acid—will be greatly multiplied without the intervention of any germs."

But in this change there is no real analogy with the multiplication of a contagium; for any other acid, e.g. HCl, would serve instead of oxalic to secure the change which, as shown in the following formula, consists simply in the addition of two equivalents of water:

$$\left.\begin{matrix} C_2O_2 \\ H_2 \\ H_2 \end{matrix}\right\} N_2 + 2H_2O = \left\{\begin{matrix} CO_2NH_4 \\ CO_2NH_4 \end{matrix}\right.$$

the process being one in which ammonia and oxalic acid are formed by action of the HCl, the HCl and NH_3 neutralise each other, and oxalic acid is left to continue the action. Thus at each stage a small amount of oxalic acid decomposes only a small amount of oxamide, as in any similar chemical action. There is, I contended, no analogy between the conversions in this chemical change and the process of infection, and there is no formation of new material.

Dr. Murchison made the further suggestion that if the chemical explanation was not satisfactory, the process might be one, not of multiplication of a contagium, but that "the contagium particles may, like a pus or tubercle corpuscle, excite *by contact* a fresh formation of similar particles in the human body." This hypothesis was likewise rejected in my paper in favour of the germ theory, which "was supported by numerous facts and analogies."

A large part of my paper was concerned with the specific communicability of enteric fever, a disease concerning which Murchison had said, "although communicable, it is not certain that it is contagious in the strict sense of the term." The apparent discrepancy between the experience that in rural districts it commonly spread from house to house, and only exceptionally so in cities and large towns, was claimed by me to have been explained by Dr. William Budd's investigations. Budd's experience may be summarised here in the following sentences written by me in 1878. Further references to the same subject are made in Chapter XI.

Budd found that in villages where there was practically no sewerage, where behind each farm-house there was the usual manure yard and the inevitable pig-sty, for years there was an entire absence of typhoid, but that after importation this disease rapidly spread. And it was found that labourers who were sent home ill, carried the disease to other hamlets, and thus it spread throughout the whole district.

Budd's explanation of the more sporadic incidence of typhoid in towns, apart apparently from any previous case, deserves quotation here, as in my paper in 1878.

In a rural district, in his words:

> Among the poor, when this fever breaks out in a family, the dejections are thrown either into a common privy, or upon a dung-heap, or even into the open gutter.

They thus remain near at hand, or are carried considerable distances, and "disease and death are carried into unsuspecting households." In towns, on the other hand, dejections are carried by water-closets into common sewers, and the immediate danger to the single family is thus limited. But in reality, as Budd put it:

> The sewer is the direct continuation of the diseased intestine,

and in the condition of sewerage systems of his time formed a centre from which the disease radiated.

Murchison's views that typhoid evacuations were only contagious after putrefactive change in them, and that "the poison of enteric fever is contained [also] in the emanations from certain forms of putrefying organic matter" were controverted by me with the audacity of youth; and the explanation I advanced of the relative non-contagiousness of fresh typhoid evacuations was that just as granite must be broken into dust before it can be inhaled, so the contagium of typhoid in dejecta needed liberating by drying, fermentation, or otherwise, from the entanglements in which it was embedded. This obviously was an imperfect explanation, as no account was taken of the safety occurring through cleanliness in nursing. Nor by any controversialist at that time was the supremely important part recognised which is played in spreading typhoid fever by specifically contaminated water, milk, or other foods such as shell-fish. Nor had the occurrence of healthy "carriers" yet been discovered.

PART III

MEDICAL PRACTICE AND PUBLIC HEALTH WORK

INTRODUCTION

Having described the public health history of the period which preceded what may be described as the bacteriological period of Public Health, I can now pursue a straight course in describing the further progress during the twenty-eight years in which I was engaged in private medical practice or in public health work in a large town. The advances made in knowledge and in its application to the prevention of disease during this more recent period have, we shall find, vastly surpassed those of preceding years.

I shall be unable to describe or even mention many events of interest in these twenty-eight years, in particular my highly appreciated contacts with public health colleagues at Congresses, at other meetings, and in correspondence with health officers, and perhaps best of all in reading their reports and their contributions to *Public Health*, the official journal of the Society of Medical Officers of Health, of which for over five years I was the honorary editor. In following chapters I attempt the simpler task of recalling those phases of public health work which in rapid succession engaged my interest and led me to undertake special investigations.

CHAPTER XVII

PRIVATE MEDICAL PRACTICE

Tetanus in the pre-bacteriological period—Friendly Society medical work—Defects in private practice

BEFORE illustrating the course of medicine and preventive medicine by recollections of the half-decade following 1881, when I was engaged in private practice, I give a further hospital experience. After holding the chief resident appointments at St. Thomas's I was for nine months house surgeon in the General Hospital, Tottenham, and an episode that occurred there is instructive. A workman was admitted for a comminuted compound fracture of the leg, which was amputated just below the knee. Tetanus followed, and at the autopsy I found a trunk nerve bound down over the amputated end of bone. The surgeon in charge regarded this, as I did myself, as an example of local nerve irritation producing tetanus, and a short account of the case was sent to a medical journal.

At that time tetanus was known to occur usually after injury, especially after compound fractures of limbs, but also after minor injuries. In some cases no injury could be detected, and the case was then dignified by the prefix "idiopathic," and "catching cold," or occasionally the rheumatic poison was invoked to furbish up imperfect knowledge of causation.

It was not until 1884 that Carle and Rattini produced tetanus in rabbits by inoculating them with pus from a human case of tetanus, thus showing that tetanus is an infectious disease. In the same year Nicolaier inoculated laboratory animals and found the tetanus bacillus at the seat of inoculation. In 1889 the Japanese bacteriologist Kitasato succeeded in growing the tetanus organism in pure culture, and showed that tetanus could be produced in animals inoculated with this culture. He also demonstrated that the tetanus bacilli remained at the seat of inoculation, the terrible symptoms of tetanus being caused by a toxin developed by the localised micro-organisms. This was followed in 1890 by the discovery by Behring and Kitasato of the toxins and antitoxins of both tetanus and diphtheria, which opened out an important extension of treatment and cure of specific infectious diseases. In the earlier part of the Great War tetanus was common, but after the institution of prophylactic inoculation it ceased to be serious.

At the International Congress on Tuberculosis at Washington in 1908 I sat next to Kitasato at the State Banquet, but as he spoke no English and I little German and no Japanese our conversation was limited.

After leaving Tottenham I "put up my plate" in the High Street, Clapham, and in the course of the next five years had gathered a good practice and a good insight into private practice in various grades of society.

In my second or third year in Clapham I was asked to be Medical Officer of a local sickness society (the Manchester Unity of Oddfellows). I was paid the usual rate of 4s. *per capita* for each member, and for this had to supply drugs as well as medical attendance to sick members. The experience may have been exceptional; but I do not recall that the club members were over-exacting in their demands, and the addition to my income was welcome. But for them there was also the open door of nearby hospitals, and it was fairly easy for me to obtain consultations with hospital staffs for this class of patient. My experience among my private patients, especially the small shop-keeper and clerk class, was less favourable in this respect. For them expert consultations when needed were less available, and there was lacking, as there is still to a large extent, that ready access to consultative aid which is indispensable if the standard of good medical work is to be maintained. For them, and also for well-to-do patients, private practice as usually conducted did not furnish the best conditions for optimum medical care.

My experience was that of a young practitioner. An older doctor might not have felt the same occasional deficiencies. True, I had been engaged in active clinical work in hospitals longer than comes to the lot of most young practitioners. Nevertheless, specialist difficulties arose in which a consultation was desirable, but in which sometimes this was impracticable for financial or other reasons. There were other cases where institutional treatment would have given greater benefit than could be obtained from a single-handed practitioner treating his patient at home, and often with inadequate nursing.

I may remark parenthetically that, in my opinion, excessive puerperal mortality, when it occurs in the midwifery practice of private doctors, is due in some instances to the fear that to call in aid from a neighbouring practitioner or to send the patient to a maternity hospital, whenever either procedure is desirable in the patient's interest, is apt to bring disrepute on the doctor in primary charge. He is regarded as fussy or incompetent, and so in the maintenance of professional prestige the two patients—the mother and the infant—sometimes suffer harm.

My experience in 1883–88 confirms the need for fuller access to consultants. I have discussed this problem more fully in my *Medicine and the State* (George Allen & Unwin, 1932) and have concluded that until these consultative facilities (personal and laboratory help) are made universally available for every practitioner, and a hospital bed is available for every patient whose condition demands it—whether for continuous skilled observation or for treatment—private medical practice for a minority of total patients must remain unsatisfactory.

Of course, the suggested arrangements, if made readily available, might tend to favour mental parasitism on the part of the private doctor, but this would be avoidable by regulations as to excessive use of necessary facilities, whether asked for by the practitioner or by his patient. It would be minimised, further, by the obligation of the doctor to furnish accurate records to the consultant or hospital; and the general standard of the work of a careless practitioner would be raised by the occasional inevitable discovery of avoidable blunders which consultation reveals.

I am not suggesting that the good private practitioner is incompetent to treat the majority of his patients satisfactorily alone. He is quite equal to this work. But there remains a minority, for whom further provision is needed, and the ordinary conditions of medical practice in Britain do not satisfactorily meet this great need.

I had not bought a practice, but I had no reason to complain. My patients steadily increased. My actual receipts from private patients in the second half of 1883 were only £126, in the next entire year they were £362, and in 1885 were £492, increasing to £758 in 1886, and to £897 in 1887. There was then no "panel" practice.

As a married man, occupying a large house at an annual rental of about £100, supplementation of earnings from patients was necessary, and fortunately article-writing for journals, the preparation of a textbook on hygiene, and considerable coaching of doctors for higher degrees filled up the gap in the earlier years. It will be convenient to defer comment on work undertaken in the teaching of hygiene to Chapter XIX.

But in 1884 I was appointed M.O.H. for Clapham, and my first sanitary report was concerned with the parish or subdistrict of Clapham for that year. My salary was £80 per annum, and I was a "part-time M.O.H.," as were then nearly all such officers in England and Wales, including London. At that time I possessed no special diploma in public health, and there was then no legal obligation on local authorities to appoint only officers with such a qualification. I obtained my public health diploma shortly afterwards at the University of London.

CHAPTER XVIII

PUBLIC HEALTH WORK ALONG WITH PRIVATE MEDICAL PRACTICE

Distal aerial convection of smallpox—Weakness of negative evidence—Early history of a metropolitan borough—Early evidences of a sanitary conscience—Corrected use of vital statistics—Dust destructors

BEFORE I give my experience in the dual capacity of private practitioner and M.O.H. I may refer to two earlier incidents bearing on public health work.

(1) In 1882 I attended several cases of typhoid fever in patients living on or near Clapham Common; and suspecting that the common milk supply was the source, wrote to the local M.P., who communicated with the Local Government Board. The investigations made by Dr. Parsons on behalf of the Board confirmed the ascription of the outbreak to infected milk; but, in accord with the views as to the origin of typhoid then prevalent, the M.O.H. of the division of Battersea in which that side of Clapham Common was situate, reported (in his annual report for 1882) that a drastic examination of the drains of the infected houses showed overflowing cesspools and blocked drains, and added, "here was a sufficient means of poisoning not only a family but a district with fever."

(2) In 1884 there was no compulsory notification of cases of smallpox or other infectious disease. A part of the area of my practice was separated without any bridge from another part by a railway cutting which extended between Brixton and Clapham suburban railway stations; and on one side of this railway cutting was the Stockwell Fever Hospital, then in use for smallpox cases brought from various parts of London. I noticed the freedom from smallpox of the part of this special district which abutted on Brixton, and was separated by the railway cutting from the hospital; and Dr. Vernon,

the M.O.H. of Lambeth, made a contribution on the subject to the *Proceedings of the Society of Medical Officers of Health* during the session 1884–85. He stated that in the part of the area cut off as regards both roads and sewers from the Stockwell Hospital, only three cases of smallpox had occurred within half a mile of the hospital, while within the corresponding distance from the hospital on the unprotected side sixty-one cases had occurred. Both districts were covered with houses.

The discussion at the Society of Medical Officers of Health here referred to arose from the important report by Mr. (later Sir William) Power on the recent experience of excessive smallpox around the Fulham Smallpox Hospital. The incidence of cases in the population living near this hospital was found to be graduated according to distance from the hospital, the quarter-mile circle being most affected; the half-mile circle less, and the one-mile circle least of all. The evidence appeared to point to the conclusion that this distribution was ascribable to distal aerial infection from the hospital and not to direct sources of personal infection.

The problem of distal aerial convection of smallpox divided medical officers of health into two camps, perhaps three, those who thought such convection had been almost completely demonstrated, those who regarded it as highly improbable, perhaps even fantastic, and those whose opinion was expressed in the following extract from a contribution I made to a full discussion of the subject in 1903 at the Epidemiological Society (*Transactions*, N.S., Vol. XXIV, 1904):

> My own position in the matter of distal aerial convection is that of an agnostic. I have no prejudice against it; I do not, however, regard it as proved. I wait for confirmatory evidence, and I incline to think that such evidence of a satisfactory character will not be forthcoming.

I believed in "hospital influence," that a smallpox hospital might easily be a serious risk to people living near it, if they were not adequately protected by fairly recent vaccination. But I knew that when exposed persons were thus protected, as in

Germany, cases of smallpox could be and were treated safely in separate rooms of hospitals containing many non-infectious patients in their general wards.

Dr. J. C. Thresh had described and Dr. (now Sir George S.) Buchanan more fully described (*Epidem. Soc. Trans.*, Vol. XXIV, 1904–5) a recent experience of the village of Purfleet on the Essex banks of the River Thames, which also supported the idea that smallpox infection had been aerially conveyed to the inhabitants of this village from hospital ships in use for smallpox moored near the opposite (Kent) banks of the river and at least half a mile distant by water from the village. Purfleet had some six hundred inhabitants, and they suffered from smallpox out of proportion to the incidence of this disease in other parts of Essex. And yet "hospital communication and traffic" across this half-mile of river "was non-existent. . . . The staff had nothing to gain by rowing across there, even if the ship's rules allowed it."

I may narrate at this point an incident throwing doubt on this statement as to no visits of the hospital staff ashore. Dr. Oliver Field, D.P.H. of Clapham, was in medical attendance on my mother, and not long after the above-named discussion I called on him to inquire concerning her. On seeing me he remarked, "I wish you had been here a few minutes ago. I was seeing an engineer employed on the hospital ships, who told me that he and others used to take a boat late at night and row to a public-house in Purfleet where they played cards!"

One swallow does not make a summer; but the story illustrates the risks of negative evidence.

It may be added here that the policy of treating smallpox in hospitals remote from inhabited centres has been justified whether we regard the risk as consisting in the movements of human carriers of infection, or believe that infective material has flown out of the hospital windows to people living a quarter-mile distant or even more remotely. The hypothesis of aerial convection has ceased to be a subject of public interest. Outside Britain it never received much acceptance.

In 1884 I became M.O.H. of Clapham, a sub-district of the then Metropolitan District of Wandsworth, the other sub-districts in the same administrative district being Balham, East and West Battersea, Putney, Streatham, and Wandsworth. Each of these sub-districts (or parishes) had its separate Board of Guardians for care of the destitute. The population of Clapham in 1881 was 36,380, of the whole district of Wandsworth 212,492.

Later on Battersea became a separate local governing unit, and in 1901 the rest of the district blossomed out as the Metropolitan Borough of Wandsworth, taking its place among the twenty-nine metropolitan boroughs then created.

Dr. Duncan of Liverpool was the first M.O.H. in England. He was appointed M.O.H. for the City of Liverpool in 1847 under the special powers given by a Local Act. The square mile included in the City of London was similarly endowed in 1848, when John Simon was appointed its M.O.H.

Other metropolitan districts followed. In 1855 Wandsworth already had six health officers, one for each of its sub-districts. They were all local private practitioners, and in 1884 when I joined their ranks, all except me were, I believe, also district medical officers, responsible for the medical care of the sick poor, as well as for the sanitary care of the entire community. An annual combined sanitary report was issued each year, comprising the report of each M.O.H. for his own sub-district, and in addition a prefatory statement written by one of their number. Earlier annual reports contain many items of interest.

As shown by his report for 1856, the significance of Dr. Snow's cholera investigations on the Soho epidemic (p. 93) was already known to Dr. G. E. Nicholas, the far-seeing M.O.H. of the sub-district of Wandsworth, with whom in 1884 I came into profitable personal contact.

The unpopularity of sanitary work, interfering as it did with "the rights of property," was realised by Dr. R. H. Whiteman, the M.O.H. of Putney, who in his section of the Wandsworth Annual Report for 1856 used words with the sentiment of which struggling health officers and sanitary inspectors have often had to comfort themselves.

> The calm approval of his conscience must for a long time stand him [the Health Officer] in the place of popularity.

I am tempted to quote from Dr. Whiteman's quotation from Thomas Carlyle in the same report, which shows how deeply the writings of Southwood Smith, of Chadwick, and of Simon had already (in 1856) become etched into the sensitive conscience-plate of contemporary thinkers.

> In all thoroughfares, and in all arenas and physical departments of existence, running water and Herculean scavengerism have become indispensable, unless the poor man is to choke in his own exuviæ, and die the sorrowfulest of deaths.

It is often erroneously assumed that child welfare work is entirely of recent origin. Its main accomplishments belong to the twentieth century; but, much earlier, exposure of the terrible facts and advocacy of remedial measures could be extracted from many annual reports of health from the date of Greenhow's and Simon's earlier writings onwards. There is an interesting reference in Dr. Whiteman's 1858 report for the Putney division of Wandsworth to the common occupation of married women in gardening and laundry work, and a mention of establishments known as "La Crèche" in Paris, "which would, if adopted in this country, save thousands of children from a premature grave." Dr. Whiteman evidently thought this work outside the scope of sanitary administration, and commended it to the attention of philanthropists.

The enlightened views on the relation of poverty to sickness, shown in the writings of both Chadwick and Simon, are seen in the following extract from Dr. Whiteman's report for 1860:

> My own experiences, in common with those of my colleagues, have long produced the conviction that to obtain the full benefits to be derived from sanitary legislation, "Pauperism" (to use the words of a much-admired living writer) is the corner where we must *begin*

—the levels all pointing thitherwards—the probabilities all clearly lying *there*.

There was in each of these reports a table of the cases of sickness among the parochial poor under the care of the Union medical officers. These sources of weekly information were already being utilised to some extent as "pointers," indicating where preventive work was specially needed; and it is a pity that when notification of cases of the chief infectious disease by private practitioners became available, the information as to parochial sickness became almost completely neglected. From 1884 to 1888 I weekly made my own extracts from the case-books of the poor law medical officer for Clapham.

That Dr. Whiteman was a student of the Registrar-General's Reports is shown by his reference in his local 1861 report to "the invasion of the faulty dwellings of the poor by disease." He characterises disease—surely in Farr's language—as

> a health inspector that speaks a language which nobody can misunderstand.

He adds:

> The oversights, the errors of persons who in responsible offices have charge of the health and lives of men, are proclaimed aloud by this inexorable voice.

In 1884 the birth-rate of the Wandsworth district was 35·7 and its death-rate 17·2 per 1,000 of population, ranging from 19·9 in Battersea to 12·1 in Streatham. The infant mortality in the same year was stated to be 28·6 per 100 total deaths at all ages. Up to this year infant mortality continued to be stated as a percentage of total mortality; but thereafter as proportional to the lives (infants) at risk, which in most years can be assumed to be the number of births.

My first annual report was for the year 1884. Clapham's infant mortality was then 160 per 1,000 births as compared with 155 for the whole of London and 174 for England and Wales as a whole. In commenting on this infant mortality I laid stress in this first report on malnutrition, and on improper feeding, especially the premature giving of farinaceous foods as important factors in the excessive death-rate. The following remark was added:

> The increased study of the laws of physiology and health in our public schools will probably lead to a great diminution of this premature mortality.

This educational side of hygiene, as will be seen later, already occupied a large share in my thinking and in my work.

In the same report I evidently held the prevalent beliefs as to the causation of infectious diseases, for, referring to cases of diphtheria, I remarked: "The close connection of diphtheria with bad drainage cannot be doubted"; and I appear to have shared the sanitary inspector's idea that a bell-trap having been found in the kitchen of an invaded house, which led to the sewer without an intervening intercepting trap, the causation of this particular case of diphtheria had been satisfactorily elucidated. (I am not even now certain that the offensive gases coming from an imperfect drain may not have contributed something in aid of personal infection.)

In this first report my mind was already exercised over problems of local and national vital statistics, density of population as a factor in excessive death-rates, and the need for local intensive comparisons of death-rates. Referring to large block dwellings (Peabody Buildings) in London, I commented on their low death-rate, notwithstanding the "crowding on area"; and I gave the results of a painstaking investigation of three special groups of houses in Clapham, in which the death-rates were respectively 20·9, 17·9, and 17·7 per 1,000 of population as compared with 13·7 for Clapham as a whole. I emphasised that the differences of experience were largely explicable by high mortality at ages under five. It was not until the following year, however, that I was responsible for a more nearly scientific comparison of death-rates for the entire Wandsworth district. I should explain that on my appointment my colleagues, to whose kindness and co-operation I owe much, insisted on my preparing the joint sanitary report for the whole district. It was in this capacity that the following table was prepared.

Death-rates per 1,000 living at each of the following age-periods, 1885

At ages 0–5,	lowest was	Streatham,	36·4,	highest	Battersea,	63·0
,, 5–10,	,,	Streatham,	3·04,	,,	Clapham,	7·1
,, 20–40,	,,	Clapham,	4·07,	,,	Wandsworth,	7·07
,, 40–60,	,,	Putney,	7·7,	,,	Wandsworth,	23·0
,, 60–80,	,,	Putney,	41·6,	,,	Battersea	72·4

The lowest infant mortality per 1,000 births was 110 in Streatham, the highest, 175, in West Battersea.

Here was an early local attempt to escape from the practice (outside Farr's reports) of resting contented with a statement of total death-rates at all ages, with their many openings for erroneous interpretation.

In the same report a reference was made to the good work of the Metropolitan Asylums Board in sending each M.O.H. a weekly list of cases of infectious diseases admitted to its hospitals for treatment. This Board (M.A.B.) had been constituted because of the impracticability of each local Board of Guardians in London providing satisfactorily institutional beds for various forms of illness, and especially for epidemic diseases. At first, admission to a M.A.B.'s hospital technically made the patient or his parent a "pauper"; but as years passed this restriction was limited and then removed, and the M.A.B. became the public health hospital authority for the whole of London. In this reform, and in other sanitary reforms in London, Dr. Orme Dudfield, M.O.H. of Kensington, took a leading part. The work of the M.A.B. has now been taken over by the London County Council.

The educational side of hygiene was again emphasised in my report for 1886 in the following words:

> The educative value of the visits made by the sanitary inspectors on the householders of Clapham should not be forgotten in any estimate of the sanitary work executed during the year.

This remark followed a tabular statement of sanitary work carried out during the year. The point is one which in later years I have repeatedly emphasised. Vast sanitary improvement has been secured as the result of notices of work required which have been served on owners and on occupiers of property; but still more extensive and important are the improvements in cleanliness, ventilation, etc., suggested and recommended by sanitary inspectors in friendly conversation with tenants and owners, and never needing to be supplemented by statutory demands.

This has been a very important factor in improved domestic hygiene during the last half-century. The more recent work of health visitors has exerted a still more marvellous influence in correcting and improving the personal habits of mothers and their children.

During my tenure of office as M.O.H. in Clapham I was responsible for three Special Reports, in two of which I was acting in co-operation with my five colleagues.

Each summer we were faced with the terrible mortality from summer diarrhœa, and in 1885 we produced a joint report in which we emphasised high temperature as a chief factor in its causation, showing by comparative figures that a high temperature of the River Thames and a deficient rainfall went with excessive diarrhœa. We stressed the importance of a constant supply of water (unstored in domestic cisterns) and of better flushing of sewers; and in a final sentence we stated:

> The fact that epidemic diarrhœa is almost confined to hand-fed children illustrates the lack of cleanliness in feeding children, and the importance of boiling all drinking water and milk.

In 1887 we wrote a joint report beginning with the remark that the extreme desirability of notification of all cases of the more serious infectious diseases was now generally recognised. In this report we set out the benefits derivable from such notification, and appended a table of the information collected by us from forty-four towns in England and Wales in which compulsory notification was already in force. Some years had, however, still to pass before this beneficent legislation was applied to London (see also p. 280).

The third special report alluded to above discussed a proposed destructor of house refuse in Clapham. It was prepared by me on behalf of the Clapham Committee. In this report the evils of the present position were emphasised. Mountains of house refuse accumulated in local depots until its removal into the country or on barges down the River Thames could be managed. As an alternative, the Committee recommended a local destructor, and I gave reasons in support of the proposal. But the local inhabitants thought otherwise. They were not satisfied that the destructor with the proposed addition of a Jones' Fume Cremator would, in fact, entirely obviate nuisance from smell, smoke, and dust. It became an election cry, and at the next local election in the following November I found that a third of the members of the Committee were new members. These had replaced the unhappy members who had faced the electorate! They did not dismiss me; but in the light of the investigations of more recent decades, had these then been available, I think they might have done so without blame; for "peppering" with fine dust has hitherto often been the lot of houses surrounding dust destructors, and I doubt if even now it is entirely eliminated.

I may now sum up my experience as a M.O.H. who was engaged also in the private practice of medicine. Theoretically, I have always thought the combination of the two functions in some respects desirable. My remarks concerning Simon's City experience make this clear (p. 77). The combination was inevitable, then, as for many years there were no doctors specially trained for public health work. The first body to institute diplomas in public health was the University of Dublin in 1870, and the possession of such a certificate of competency for public health work was only rendered a statutory obligation in 1892, and then only in respect of units of local government in which at least 50,000 persons dwelt.

Now that large units of administration are becoming the rule, the chief M.O.H. must be an official only; but he is the better official if he has had several years' experience of private medical work. Indeed, I remember committing myself to the too extreme statement that if I were an autocrat no doctor would be allowed to become M.O.H. unless this condition were fulfilled.

So long as smaller units of administration remain, the part-time M.O.H. must encounter the difficulties experienced by me as a practitioner M.O.H. in attempts to inquire into sources of infection. The almost unanimous opinion of practitioners themselves is in favour of whole-time medical officers of health, though there are large differences of opinion concerning minor sanitary posts in the department of the M.O.H., especially now that clinical practice is so large a part of child welfare work and of medical work for school children.

At this point is interpolated a chapter dealing with Sanitary Education, after which follows an account of personal experience of whole-time public health work in Brighton.

CHAPTER XIX

EDUCATIONAL WORK IN HYGIENE

From the early years of the nineteenth century the sanitary movement received increased momentum from active educational work. By this I do not mean mere propaganda which lacks a reasoned statement—as, for instance, scrappy circulars or great posters. Such propaganda has much, but a limited, value in inciting readers to do something when there already exists a body of knowledge to which public attention is desired. But infinitely more important than such propaganda is steady communication to the general population of the results of sanitary and social surveys, and of the results of scientific research, whether in the field or the laboratory. The dissemination of such knowledge, backed as it was by the growing sentiment of mercy and pity, was the activating force of the early sanitary movement in England. The reports by Southwood Smith and his co-workers on the terrible conditions of filth and crowding in towns and in country places alike, Chadwick's great reports to the poor law and sanitary commissions, and Simon's early reports as Medical Officer of Health to the City and afterwards to the Privy Council, impelled the creation of the machinery of reform, which, however much it creaked and groaned in its earlier action, has never stopped and has steadily become increasingly efficient.

And as has been illustrated by the extracts from early reports of the medical officers of health of the Wandsworth district (p. 136), the educational impetus was being communicated to every member of every local sanitary authority and to a large section of the outside public. The Local Government Board and Parliament builded better than they knew when it was made part of the duty of every M.O.H. to write an annual report, reviewing local vital statistics, and setting out sanitary defects and the action taken thereon. An annual stocktaking, if honestly carried out, is an excellent way to secure and maintain good work, and many of these annual reports have proved this. They are read by some members of the public—that is good; they are read also by the medical officers of health of other districts—that is still better; the points of excellence are imitated and so the educational work widens and deepens. On the statistical side many of them, unfortunately, were useless receptacles for crude and undigested figures, a valley of dry bones; and until they were breathed on by the spirit of fervour and zeal for reform, manifested for instance in Farr's reports, they remained so. Intellect and zeal are both needed, now as then, if statistics are to have living interest and influence; and a multitude of reports, happily, have been a measure of yearly progress and a shining light guiding to further reforms.

A second great line of educational work affected the general population through its younger members.

The Science and Art Department, South Kensington, initiated science teaching under its direction, technical and other schools throughout the country being encouraged to carry on science teaching, and a financial grant being given for each student who successfully passed a written examination after a six months' course of instruction. These grants for a series of years formed a chief source of income of technical and science schools. Among the subjects introduced was that of Hygiene, in the preparation of the syllabus of which Professor W. H. Huxley had a large part.

In a paper read at the International Congress of Hygiene and Demography, London, 1891 (Sec. IX), I summarised the arguments for the "Teaching of the Laws of Health in Schools," discussed the various means for teaching the public, and concluded that the main hope lay with the children in elementary schools, who formed one-fifth of the total population. In this paper the improper feeding of infants and the origin of rickets as a chiefly dietetic disease were emphasised, and the argument that infant mortality was in any sense selective in action was traversed. In particular it was urged that preventible sickness attacked healthy as well as sickly children, and that the survivals of damaged lives were almost immeasurably more serious than any theoretically possible benefit derivable from the weeding out of weaklings by preventible diseases.

In 1890 I had addressed a conference of medical officers of health on the same subject, advocating that the teaching of hygiene then given to some older students in secondary schools should be given in a modified form to the scholars in elementary schools. I remarked:

> By the teaching of hygiene is not meant instruction which will vainly attempt to make "every man his own doctor." Such attempts are irrational, and apt to be pernicious in their tendency and effect; but what is needed is instruction like that embodied in the syllabus of the Science and Art Department in Hygiene, adapted to meet the requirements of junior scholars. This teaching, in order to be successful and sound, must be based on an elementary knowledge of chemistry and physiology. But it would be a profound mistake to debar scholars from the study of hygiene until they have previously passed a somewhat severe examination in physiology. The amount of chemistry and physiology necessary to understand a really useful and practical course of lessons in hygiene can be incorporated in the lessons themselves. That this is so is now sufficiently acknowledged by the Science and Art Department, who have removed the restriction previously in force that no student shall be admitted to the hygiene examination unless he previously or at the same time passes the elementary examination in physiology of the Science Department. We all remember how in our student days anatomical facts which could receive applications in surgery or medicine were easily recollected, while facts which could not have such applications dovetailed with them escaped recollection; and similarly the teacher who is master of his subject will be able to teach physiology in its hygienic aspects, and to make every point clear by chemical and other experiments, thus introducing his scholars to a useful and practical knowledge, having immediate and most potent bearings on the public health.

Although much more is now being done in the directions thus indicated, it cannot be said that even in 1934 as much is being done as the national welfare requires.

The teaching of hygiene under the Science and Art Department must have had a valuable educational influence on a large section of the total population. I can speak of this as teacher, author, and assistant examiner for the Department for several years.

From 1882 onwards for several years I gave a six months' course of weekly lectures at the headquarters of the Y.M.C.A. in the Strand, the first hour each evening being devoted to physiology and the second to hygiene. Most of my students, usually numbering a hundred to one hundred and fifty, were keen teachers in elementary day schools, knowing how to teach, and how to take full advantage of teaching. My share of fees and grants thus obtained was considerable, and the mental impetus to my personal freshness of work was valuable.

This teaching led to the publication in 1884 of my *Hygiene: a Manual of Personal and Public Health*, which ran through many editions in subsequent years. Altogether some twelve thousand copies were sold; and a more elementary guide to domestic hygiene, which I wrote later, had a wider circulation, over forty thousand copies being sold.

The results of the teaching then carried out in various technical schools and classes throughout the country were tested by a written examination. I was one of seven or eight assistant examiners of the Science Department, and each May had from a thousand to one thousand two hundred papers to examine and mark. The answers showed a varying quality of teaching, and there was evidence of much memory work, and of teaching which had not been illustrated by experiments. But a majority of the papers gave evidence of good work, and by means of the instruction and examination thus given, tens of thousands of families must have been led to more healthy ways of living.

Occasionally amusing and absurd answers were given, and for some years I kept and collected the best instances of these. It must not be inferred from the following examples that they are other than exceptional. It will be remembered that some physiology was required; also, I should note, one question always dealt with ambulance aid.

One question was: What is the spinal column and where is it situated? And a candidate who drew on his imagination to cover his ignorance answered: "The spinal column is not confined to any one part of the body, but is uniformly diffused throughout."

Another answer was that "the vertebral column runs down the back of the head, branches off down the arms and back, and on reaching the lower part of the back it branches off down the legs."

One more: "The thorax lies behind the heart and near the chest."

A further answer illustrates the still persistent notion that muscular exercise does not also imply cerebral activity.

The brain should be exercised at the same time as muscle. Some people when they go for a walk take a book with them so that the muscle and brain may be exercised together.

Spelling, or the misuse of unaccustomed words, gave rise to odd blunders. Thus:

The object of clothing is to preserve an equitable temperature.

Let meat simper until it is finished.

Nitrogenous food and the waist of the body.

Burn out the wound with a cosmetic.

The air is drawn out—"asphyxiated"—by means of a revolving ventilator.

There are two kinds of hardness of water—permeable and impermeable.

When a vein is cut it collapses, when an artery is cut it forms an artifice.

First-aid questions occasionally supplied amusing answers. Thus:

In a case of carbolic poisoning, send for a doctor; and meanwhile give a teaspoonful of baking-powder, and keep up the patient's spirits as much as possible.

Perhaps the gem was the following answer to the question as to the right course of action if a child were bitten on the wrist by a suspected mad dog. The answer was:

Heat the poker red-hot, place it in the wound, talking pleasantly to the child, meanwhile, to divert his attention.

Another candidate, discussing the same contingency, said:

If a person can be found handy and foolish enough to suck the bite, let this be done.

Here is an answer which amusingly represented when it was written a fairly general view as to pulmonary tuberculosis:

If a young lady shows a persistent delicate flush on her cheeks, it is likely to be the hectic flush of consumption. Then her fiancé must be firm and brave the risks of a breach of promise suit!

Perhaps I should add an allusion to my studies in vital statistics. At an early stage I realised the importance of systematic examination of the Registrar-General's Reports, which Dr. Farr was making invaluable in measuring the vital conditions of the country, and an irresistible lever in pressing for sanitary reforms. These studies led up to the publication of my *Elements of Vital Statistics*, 1889 (see also page 274).

Reference should also be made to the International Health Exhibition held in 1884. For several months crowds attended this exhibition, and although military bands and amusements were attracting them, they could not fail incidentally to receive much valuable instruction in foods, domestic sanitation, recreative exercises, and many other branches of personal hygiene. Many Health Conferences were held and popular lectures on health given. My interest was especially aroused by the sickness statistics quoted by Sir James Paget, in the course of an eloquent address at the inauguration of the Exhibition. The figures were prepared by Mr. Sutton, Actuary to the Registry of Friendly Societies, who was a neighbour of mine in Clapham and a member of the local Vestry, under which I worked as M.O.H. I do not quote these figures in full; but, based on the average experience of over 300,000 members of the Manchester Unity of Oddfellows—the average sickness per annum in weeks was as follows: 0·67 for male workers aged 15–20; 0·74 for workers aged 20–25; one week for workers aged 25–45; and 2·7 weeks for workers aged 45–65. Sir James vividly showed the total loss of working-time from sickness for all industrial workers in a year, and the suffering, diminished national efficiency, and economic loss implied in this mass of sickness, much of it avoidable.

Many years later I found that the average certified loss of working time for sickness among insured persons had still further increased, while the death-rate among the same workers had declined. I deprecated, however, the conclusion that this necessarily meant an increased proportion of sickness in each age-group among workers in the more recent years. The problem is more complex than this, for it necessitates allowing for the altered standards of certification of sickness, which almost certainly have occurred.

CONTRIBUTIONS

Hygiene: A Manual of Personal and Public Health (George Gill & Sons, pp. 408, 1884).

School Hygiene: The Laws of Health in Relation to School Life (Swan, Sonnenschein & Co., 1887). Fifteen editions, 1887–1918.

See also references in Chapter XXXIII.

CHAPTER XX

WHOLE-TIME PUBLIC HEALTH WORK

Humours of elections—The health officer and his masters—Difficulties in sanitary and domestic reform—Meat inspection—Ejecting a Sanitary Committee—Value of sanitary inspectors' work—Water supplies

IN 1888, I left Clapham to take up the post of Medical Officer of Health of Brighton. This largest of British health resorts, often called London-by-the-Sea, then had a population of some 110,000, and I was the second M.O.H. of the town. My predecessor, Dr. Taaffe, had combined his official duties with private practice; but I was appointed as a whole-time officer. My salary was £500, but there was a prospect that ere long I should become medical officer to the fever hospital with an additional emolument of £150. This happened; and the Corporation of Brighton were so public-spirited and so appreciative of public health work that when in 1908 I left Brighton to become medical officer of the Local Government Board, my total salary had become £1,000, as compared with £1,200, the initial salary in the Government post. The latter, however, carried with it pension rights—which, in fact, meant merely deferred payment; whereas at that time Brighton had no such provision for pensioning its officers. Happily, pension arrangements are becoming more general in the local government service of England.

The initial salary of £500 meant a serious restriction of the family exchequer, as compared with my increasing income from private medical practice; and the determination to leave relative prosperity for straitened domestic conditions meant some anxious moments. But public health work was attractive in itself, and it opened up many fascinating problems on which exceptionally useful work was possible. Furthermore, it relieved one from the harass of night work and of being on duty continuously, and it removed the fret—which I confess weighed heavily with me—associated with sending in bills periodically for professional services. The relationship with my patients of payment by fee or by aggregate fees was hateful to me. Possibly I am exceptionally sensitive on this point. It should be added, *per contra*, that in public health work I missed greatly the confidence and even affection which the relationship of doctor to patient permits and evokes; and it was only when I resumed clinical work in the fever hospital, and later, on a large scale, in the institutional treatment of consumptives, that this side of one's nature was satisfied.

But the plunge was made, and I was successful against some fifty fellow-candidates. I remember the details of the candidature well. Canvassing was permitted and expected. Two incidents may amuse some readers. My canvass, so far as I could judge, had been rather favourable, though at each interview I made it clear that I had come not to ask for a vote but to state my case and to submit myself to personal questioning. I had, however, several times failed to see a certain alderman, a lawyer who, I was told, was most influential. At last I found him in his office. He accosted me by saying: "Well, young man, I have heard about you. Of course you are a Mason, or you could not have done so well in your canvass as you have done." And he remained incredulous when I assured him I was not a Freemason!

The local newspaper contained a full report of the discussion on the relative qualifications of the two candidates who were finally submitted to the Town Council by the Sanitary Committee, and I must recall a gem from this report. Mr. Alderman X (a wholesale grocer): "Yes, I agree, Dr. Newsholme is not a bad fellow, but he does not possess the brain power of Dr. T." (my remaining competitor). To which the next speaker, Mr. Councillor Z, retorted: "I am aware that Alderman X is a good judge of sugar, but I have not equal confidence in his estimate of intellectual gifts."

I secured a majority of votes, and then began my official

work for Brighton, which lasted over nineteen years. During it, owing to the almost uniform support I received from the Corporation, I was able to initiate new departures in public health administration to an extent not practicable in other towns in which reputation as a health resort was not involved. As I do not further mention my colleagues in the municipal service, especially Mr. Tillstone and Mr. Talbot, two successive Town Clerks, and Mr. Lockwood, Borough Surveyor, let me say here that they were models of public servants, in intelligence and devotion, from whom I learnt many valuable lessons.

The relation of a M.O.H. to the local authority served by him was then more intimate than now. New medical services on the clinical side have developed, and in towns like Brighton, with a population still well under 200,000, the medical staff of the Town Council is now many times the number during my time. Public health work was and is supervised by a Sanitary Committee of some fifteen members, whose resolutions became operative when confirmed by the Town Council, consisting of some fifty to sixty members.

The M.O.H., therefore, was more directly responsible to the Sanitary Committee, before whom his routine work and that of the sanitary inspectors came fortnightly for approval. This was not all; for the M.O.H. was expected also to make proposals for new or improved measures or methods of work when he thought such improvements desirable. The M.O.H. is the expert adviser, as well as the executive officer of the Committee charged with the public health work of the Town Council; and much of his success as an administrator depends on his persuasiveness and reasonableness and on his capacity to indoctrinate the members of his Committee with his ideals and ambitions for reform. In securing maximum success he has to deal not only with the Town Council, but even more with the Councillors as individuals, and to take every opportunity to secure their friendly interest in the work and to help them to master its principles. This educational side of the M.O.H.'s work (which is most effective when not recognised by its recipients as such) is of the highest importance; and the difference between the successful and the relatively unsuccessful M.O.H. lies in the measure of his capacity for it.

But however tactful and efficient the M.O.H. may be, his path is not always one of roses. In the early part of my work in Brighton, the sanitary inspectors were engaged zealously in testing drains, in requiring movable dust-bins in substitution for fixed receptacles, in compelling flushing cisterns to be provided for W.C.S, and such-like work, all of which involved expenditure of money by the owners of houses, especially of the dwellings of the poor. My earliest shock after entering on my duties was to find that a multitude of such "notices" had been served and not complied with, and that summonses against those in default applied for by the M.O.H., for various reasons had not been taken out by the legal department. I arranged with the Town Clerk that, as I could not be personally responsible for these arrears, they should be cancelled; and received a promise that, in future, summonses would be taken out against all recalcitrant owners. A few weeks' summonses in the Police Court convinced these owners that they must comply with reasonable instructions, and little further trouble arose. But even then the cost to small property owners was very heavy. An influential alderman, the owner of many small houses, called on me one day and showed me his builder's bills and his rent receipts for the last quarter. The balance was on the wrong side, and it was difficult for him to appreciate expressions of sympathy which did not include an undertaking to check the sanitary inspectors' activities.

A few months later I met him on the Brighton railway platform.

"Hullo, Doctor! Where are you going?"

"On holiday."

"How long are you going for?"

"A month."

"I say, Doctor, couldn't you make it six months?"

I can claim that I enjoyed the good-humoured joke as much as did the alderman.

Looking back on this period of "sanitary notices," in which the work of the inspectors bulked very largely, I sometimes ask myself, Did we overdo it? I think we did in some minor details; but the provision of watertight drains, of flushing cisterns, and of movable dustbins was necessary, and these and other similar improvements rendered life more comfortable, freer from nuisances, and healthier than it would otherwise have been.

As it was impracticable with the available staff to inspect every house each year, any house in which a case of the chief notifiable diseases (scarlet fever, typhoid fever, or diphtheria), or in which a death occurred, for instance from measles, whooping cough, or summer diarrhœa, was specially visited and its domestic sanitation overhauled. This might be regarded as implying a causal relationship between domestic insanitation and cases of the notified cases of infectious disease, and as being a survival of the views on the strength of which Southwood Smith and Chadwick initiated sanitary reform in England. The generalisation of these pioneers was true for intestinal diseases (typhoid, diarrhœa); and the clearing up of grosser filth conditions undoubtedly was a main agent in reducing the incidence of these, and probably also of other, diseases. But it took long to eradicate the notion that one could extend this generalisation to diphtheria, to puerperal fever, and even to scarlet fever.

Whatever the basis of the sanitary inspectors' work in securing improved domestic sanitation, I have no doubt that their detailed work not only increased the comfort, but also favoured enhanced health of the people.

A difficult part of one's work was deciding as to the fitness of meat for human food. Brighton had a number of registered private slaughter-houses, and cattle and sheep were brought to these by both road and rail. For the poor there was a trade in inferior beef of more than dubious salubrity, which was sold by street auction on Saturday nights. A few butchers were notorious for their purchases from farms in surrounding districts of cows oft-times emaciated and diseased, which were slaughtered in one or other of these small slaughter-houses; and it was almost a chance if the meat inspector succeeded in visiting the slaughter-house before the flesh of these animals was exposed for sale on a Saturday night.

Before long, however, a number of butchers were detected in the process of preparing for sale carcases unfit for food; and these butchers, on being prosecuted by the Town Council, were convicted and fined. A general notice was then given that a butcher who sent for the inspector when he found a given carcase was of doubtful quality would, if it were subsequently condemned, be exempt from prosecution. But the illicit purchase and preparation for sale of unsound meat continued, and further prosecutions were necessary. One butcher thus prosecuted was a town councillor and a member of the Sanitary Committee, and he succeeded in creating a feeling among many of his fellow-councillors that the M.O.H. and meat inspector were in fact persecuting as well as prosecuting him! At the next election he was made Chairman of the Sanitary Committee! Soon afterwards the fearless inspector came to inform me that he had discovered at the Chairman's private slaughter-house the carcase of a cow unfit for food, but prepared as for food. On visiting the premises I found an emaciated carcase, obviously unfit for food, and ordered it to be brought before a magistrate for condemnation, in accordance with the statutory procedure under the Public Health Act, 1875. The magistrate had no hesitation in condemning it; but knowing the storm which impended, I asked three members of the Sanitary Committee (including a medical man) to see the carcase before it was sent to the cremator in accordance with legal procedure.

At the next Sanitary Committee I reported the seizure and condemnation. The Chairman judiciously was absent, but he had been very active in canvassing his friends. The Sanitary Committee voted six for and six against the prosecution of the owner of this meat, which normally should follow the condemnation: and in accordance with usual procedure this deadlock was reported to the Town Council.

The facts had become widely known owing to the canvassing by the Chairman butcher's friends, and by a majority vote the Council decided to take no further action. This was almost tantamount to a vote of censure on the officials concerned. But the end was not yet: the six members of the Committee who had supported legal action resigned from the Sanitary Committee, and they were forthwith interviewed by local newspaper reporters. Reports of what had happened appeared in the London Press, and it became evident that the reputation of Brighton might suffer. The "rump" of the Sanitary Committee met and asked the Town Council to fill up the vacancies that had occurred. The Town Council then met and solemnly passed a resolution that they would not fill the vacancies until the rest of the Committee also resigned. This (with one exception) they did; and forthwith a new Committee with a new chairman was elected. I never subsequently had the slightest difficulty in condemning unsound meat, and I incline to think that Brighton may claim the distinction of being the only Sanitary Authority whose sanitary officials have been instrumental in ejecting one and securing the election of a new Public Health or Sanitary Committee!

In this chapter I have indicated two difficult sections of a medical officer's health work. In both of these he has the invaluable co-operation of the staff of sanitary inspectors, and if sanitary inspectors are not mentioned more fully in the following pages let me state here that if the M.O.H. be regarded as the commissioned officer of the Sanitary Authority, sanitary inspectors are the non-commissioned officers and rank and file of the Army of Sanitation, and to them the M.O.H. is indebted to an enormous extent for such success in his work as he may achieve. In the earlier Public Health Acts they were described as inspectors of nuisances, and their appointment, like that of the M.O.H., was imposed on Sanitary Authorities as a compulsory duty. The change in their statutory name to "sanitary inspector" is symbolic of a new ideal in public health administration; their chief duty, instead of being the detection of nuisances and their removal, has become—in part at least—action directed to securing such domestic and non-domestic arrangements as will prevent the occurrence of nuisances or of any other physical environmental conditions which are inimical to health.

WATER SUPPLY

Brighton has an almost unlimited supply of water from deep wells in the chalk, the upper part of the well being protected against surface soakage. From each well lateral adits are run to catch more of the subterranean streams of water travelling slowly to the sea. Following on the two episodes mentioned below, Brighton's area of supply of pure water from remote hills some miles from habitations has been vastly extended.

In a year of protracted drought another town on the south coast, supplied like Brighton from deep wells, found that its water was becoming very saline. Soon afterwards the chemist attached to a local brewery drew my attention to the fact that in Brighton also the water contained two or three grains of salt per gallon more than usual. I made confirmatory analyses, and the amount of salt very slowly increased, though it never became perceptible to taste. I reported on this to the Waterworks Committee of the Brighton Corporation, and remember the indignation of two worthy aldermen that I should dare to reflect on the water supply of which the civic fathers were rightly proud. What had happened was that the water in the chalk flowing seaward had become exhausted, and we were pumping into the water-pipes a small amount of sea-water.

Incidentally this led to my making for some years systematic monthly analyses, chemical and bacteriological, of water from each of the four or five wells then supplying Brighton; and this led later to an unexpected discovery concerning a well which was then a large source of water. I found on analysis that the "free ammonia" in the water of this well had increased, while there was no increase of "albuminoid ammonia" and no other evidence of contamination.

This puzzling result was cleared up on studying the geography of the well. It was not far from a small coal-gas producing factory of the railway company; and on wending my way through the adits of the town well I was able to prove that the ammonia had soaked from the gasworks. It was harmless; but the use of the well was discontinued, and we went further afield for an increased supply. Neither of these two "accidents" could now happen.

CHAPTER XXI

HOUSING OF THE PEOPLE

Stages in housing reform—Clearance of insanitary areas in Brighton—Economic rents?—Octavia Hill—State and municipal aid in housing—On what principle?—Can insurance be utilised?—Can undesirable family expenditure be controlled?

MEDICAL officers of health for a long series of years have made copious contributions to the vast literature on housing, for on them the legislature has imposed the statutory responsibility of condemning houses and groups of houses which are unfit for human habitation. Social reformers regard housing reform as a, if not the, most important element in social and sanitary improvement. From the standpoint of morals improved housing is even more important if we consider the difficulty of securing the decencies of family life when there is inadequate bedroom provision for normal families.

The history of the housing problem gives a cross-section of the social history of England during my lifetime. The problem—although it exists also in rural districts—is in large measure the product of the rapid and unregulated growth of industrialisation in towns. The ideal is that each family shall have a separate dwelling, with adequate room space for its occupants, and with a water supply and sanitary conveniences special to this dwelling. A wide departure from this ideal still characterises a large proportion of total "homes."

The struggle for better homes may be said to have begun in 1838 with the issue of Edwin Chadwick's first report on the sanitary conditions of the labouring classes in London; and then followed the campaign for the removal of organic filth, already mentioned in several chapters of this volume.

As usually happens in reform, voluntary preceded official activities. This was so in elementary education; and similarly, voluntary societies were attempting to provide better housing before official action began. Three Royal Commissions on Housing have reported, but the problem of housing is not yet solved. Its solution is now progressing with increased rapidity; but the problem is never-ending, somewhat like a recurring decimal. Improving standards of living will ensure its continuance.

The first Housing Act was passed in 1851 on the initiative of Lord Ashley, the future Earl of Shaftesbury. It gave powers to local authorities to build dwellings for the working-classes. In 1868 the Torrens Act was passed. It aimed at the reconditioning of single houses, and provided for compulsory purchase of houses by the local authority after compensation.

In 1875 the great Public Health Act was passed and in the same year Cross's Act became law; and by this Act, as Major Barnes has put it in his excellent *The Slum, its Story and Solution*, 1934:

> Slum dentistry had advanced a stage. It was useless to stop the tooth, the whole set must go.

Insanitary areas were to be dealt with.

There have followed provisions for the planning of houses, of areas, of towns, and of regions, which cannot be detailed here; but action, largely owing to the enormous expenditure involved, has been hesitant and slow.

In Brighton during my nineteen years as M.O.H. of the borough, improved housing engaged a large share of my time. Brighton, like other towns a large part of whose houses was built in the latter half of the eighteenth and the first half of the nineteenth century, had streets and alleys which were too closely crowded together, and which from the first moment of their existence must have been unsatisfactory and often unfit for habitation when judged by present-day standards. In those earlier days street and town planning and building by-laws did not exist, and modern sanitation had not yet been evolved. A former vicar of Brighton described the town as a ragged garment with a golden fringe—its magnificent esplanade! This was a picturesque exaggeration of the very real housing evils of the early Georgian period.

In 1879 my predecessor as M.O.H. represented two insanitary areas as requiring to be made the subject of improvement schemes under the Artisans' Dwellings Act, 1875, and estimates of the expenditure required to deal with them (estimated at £53,000 or alternatively £70,000) had been prepared by the Borough Surveyor, but the schemes of clearing and re-housing had not been carried out.

In 1888 I made an official representation respecting a small area, which contained 91 houses with 318 inhabitants, and in 1890 one relating to a second larger area, under the Artisans' Dwellings Act, 1875. The cost of the first scheme was estimated at £13,800, that of the second scheme about £40,000. A third area was condemned at a later date.

These three areas were cleared at great cost, and on them and on land further afield a population equal to the persons displaced was re-housed. The total inhabitants of these three areas was 2,158. This number may appear small, but it constituted nearly 2 per cent (1 in 58) of the total population of the borough.

This action was accompanied by steady condemnation of individual houses, which repairs and alterations under the powers of the Public Health Act could not render fit for habitation. The number of persons thus de-housed was about 1,044. In the aggregate, by clearance of areas and of single houses the number of persons de-housed and satisfactorily re-housed up to the year 1904 numbered about 1 in 40 of the total population of the town and probably 1 in 20 of its total working-class population.

Proceedings by the condemnation of whole areas under the limited powers then possessed by Sanitary Authorities were terribly costly per person displaced and re-housed. But under modern regulations and by-laws relating to dwellings the chief reasons for condemnation should disappear, leaving only sanitary repairs, which can be enforced, and decrepitude of individual dwellings the condemnation of which does not carry with it compensation to the owner.

In a special report to the Town Council written in 1904, I emphasised a fact now widely realised, that re-housing accommodation should, so far as practicable, be provided for persons of the same social stratum as the persons dis-housed; and for this reason urged the building of double cottages (one on each of two floors with entirely separate accommodation and conveniences) rather than single cottages, which are more costly and are often sub-let in part to lodgers. Sub-letting I characterised as striking at the root of family life. The contention still holds good that a local authority is doing invaluable work "in providing that form of housing accommodation which is urgently required by the poor, and which private enterprise fails to provide."

ECONOMIC RENTS

Apart from the residuum of very poor people who cannot pay an economic rent, whether the landlord be private or municipal, the present great housing problem is whether monetary aid in the form of a house at a rental below its economic value should be given to less needy wage-earners who are not far from the border-line of poverty. When a local authority builds a house either an economic rent must be charged, or a part of the rent must be paid for out of local rates or grants from national taxation, or from both. While it is true that the tenant of a municipal house pays in a camouflaged form (in direct taxation and in indirect taxation on his tea, beer, tobacco, etc.) a part of the rent which is out of sight, the fact remains that he receives a differential benefit to the extent to which this burden is borne by the rate-payers and tax-payers who do not live in subsidised houses.

That is the economic problem which is involved in housing. A large part of the wage-earning classes are now living in subsidised houses for whom *special* treatment cannot be completely justified. These houses do not suffice for all wage-earners, and so at present some wage-earners are being indirectly taxed to secure the low rentals of their more fortunate fellow-workers.

Ought this to continue; and if so, ought not municipal provision of housing at non-economic rates to be extended to avoid inequitable incidence of taxation?

The trend of events undoubtedly is towards further housing at public expense, a trend which cannot be regarded altogether complacently.

Another aspect of housing inevitably obtrudes itself on the M.O.H., a large part of whose time is occupied by housing difficulties. He becomes convinced that with good will on the part of both owner and occupier, and with fair dealing on the part of both of these, a considerable part of the problem would vanish. It is in part because neither tenant nor landlord always "plays cricket" in the fullest sense of the word that it has become necessary for the legislature to confer drastic powers on local authorities, powers which for the landlords of unfit houses include confiscation without compensation and in other instances, especially when the letting of single rooms to the poorest of the poor is concerned, should but does not yet involve compulsory drastic limitation of usurious rentals. A step in the last-named direction has been taken in the Rent Reduction Act, 1933.

What can be done by voluntary personal work is illustrated by the admirable work of Miss Octavia Hill (1842–1912). I only talked with her once, after I had given evidence in 1908 before the Royal Commission on the poor laws. Her economics were rigidly mid-Victorian, and she would have been horrified by the developments of housing policy at the expense of the public purse which have occurred since the Great War, and which have been endorsed by all political parties. Her work began with the management, including the weekly collection of rents, of a few houses which John Ruskin had placed in her charge for social experimentation. She started by telling each tenant how much she could afford weekly for house-repairs and improvements, and that if anything was over rents would be reduced. Week by week she gave sympathy and friendship, acting on the conviction that "he who gladly receives to-day will to-morrow give more gladly." She was certain that the poor would not be corrupted by beneficence if "the man be called out of himself by letting him know the joy of receiving and giving." And her policy and personal influence succeeded in converting an increasing number of houses into dwellings that she could be proud of.

It is pleasing to recall that Octavia Hill's mother was a daughter of Dr. Southwood Smith (p. 90) and that she copied his methods of work, and did much to advance the cause in which he had been a pioneer.

Octavia Hill's admirable work opened up new methods in the management of property. There is now an Association of Women House Property Managers; and some municipal housing estates happily are being conducted to some extent on the general principles, whose value Octavia Hila demonstrated.

She always held that dwellings should be self-supporting, and she maintained that "to subsidise rents was a rate-in-aid of wages, and open to all the objections of such a rate" (Barnes, *op. cit.*, p. 190). In thus remaining true to her principles she may have partially overlooked the fact that she could choose her tenants, while the class of tenants with whom municipalities often have to deal would never be chosen as reliable rent-payers.

The unwillingness to depart from economic maxims has been shared by many of us, and we may yet retain these partially in housing matters. I have mentioned similar personal misgivings in regard to children's meals at school (p. 385). In some branches of public utility work we have cheerfully abandoned individual and family payments, except through taxation. This is so for universal elementary education and for much of the technical education of all classes. Public health, services of sanitation, of prevention of infection, of vaccination, of hospital treatment, of treatment in child welfare work and in school clinics are provided gratuitously, or nearly so. Police protection is a State service, and the list might be greatly extended. So that one need not assume an attitude of "economic correctitude" in considering housing, if the reasons for housing at the expense of communal funds be satisfactorily established. One must determine one's aim. If it be agreed that housing for the entire population cannot, or is very unlikely to, become a public charge, then evidently the portion of the population for whom we agree to supply it should be defined and thereby limited.

In this year (1934) there have been pronouncements of the Government to the effect that the provision of houses for the lower paid workers has now become a national social service. The lower paid workers for whom this can properly be said may, I think, be defined as those who cannot afford to pay an economic rent without unduly encroaching on that part of the family income which is needed for supplying such food as will give satisfactory nutrition to every member of the family.

If destitution or partial destitution is the reason for inability to pay an economic rent, there can be no hesitation in providing housing from public funds. But in these and in other cases coming within the scope of the above definition, the providing authority cannot with social safety deprive itself of the right to determine each case on its merits. I do not see how this can be avoided, in justice to tax-payers and rate-payers.

And this condition being accepted, one can justify the investigation of family earnings and expenditure, carried through in a spirit following closely the general lines of Octavia Hill's work. But although the community makes various provisions in aid of family expenses (as for instance in education, school meals, and rent), and is therefore justified in regulating (which means in a few instances prosecution and punishment) wasteful expenditure on, say, gambling or drinking, the difficulties of such an undertaking can scarcely be exaggerated.

Can the number needing free housing or subsidised housing be reduced by any practical action on the part of public authorities?

In provision for sickness or for unemployment due to causes other than sickness, a partial escape from public assistance has been devised by sickness and unemployment insurance. By this means the insured person, his employer, and the State have all contributed a share towards a fund providing for future emergencies. A similar provision for housing has, I believe, never been contemplated, and the weekly payments would probably be so large as to render it impracticable for a large proportion of total workers. This being so, the only alternatives are self-help or housing at the public expense for many poorer workers.

One interesting departure from economic practices has recently been proposed by a large local authority, which has introduced the principle of charging rent for its municipally owned houses on a scale varying with the total weekly income of the tenants. This applies the practice followed in imposition of general taxation, a practice which the medical profession have always adopted in their professional charges. In both these instances charges are made to accord with means; and there is nothing alarming in the extension of this practice to rents. The practice may be extended to the provision of milk or other necessaries, if the community desires it in the interest of the communal health; and it is now (1934) in process of being adopted for supplying milk to poorer school children. The possibility of increasing ability to pay rent by diminishing wasteful family expenditure also emerges, though the difficulties of official control of wastefulness are too obvious to need emphasising, whether it takes the form of gambling, of excessive resort to cinemas, or of alcoholic indulgence, or other forms of unnecessary expenditure.

In the late Dr. James Niven's *History of Public Health Effort in Manchester* (1923) I find the following observations:

There seems no other way of securing light and air in central districts for the requisite number of people than to house them in tenements. *This cannot be done economically*, and the community would have to pay part of the price of erecting the tenements required. One question needs to be asked. . . . *Can there be any doubt that the liquor trade paralyses the hands of the social reformer and keeps the people poor?*[1]

Niven's remarks are strictly relevant to our problem, and the reader is referred to Chapter XL in which the same problem is approached from a different angle.

[1] Italics not in original.

PART IV

THE CONTROL OF INFECTIOUS DISEASES

CHAPTER XXII

THE PREVENTION OF MILK EPIDEMICS

Early history of discovery of infection from milk—Does scarlet fever occur in the cow?—Illustrations of detective work

Cows' milk in the experience of medical officers of health of my time has played an important part in disseminating scarlet fever, diphtheria, and enteric fever, as well as septic sore throats. Its part in the production of non-pulmonary tuberculosis in children is described in Chapter XXVIII.

In this chapter I give a short account of some outbreaks of epidemics due to infected milk, which illustrate an important phase of public health history and emphasise the importance of pasteurising milk.

During my experience in Brighton there occurred several outbreaks of scarlet fever and diphtheria which were traced to an infected milk supply.

In Chapter XXV it is shown how epidemics of typhoid fever gradually ceased to be ascribed to sewer and drain emanations as the importance of specific infection of water supplies began to be realised. The change of view was expedited when epidemics of typhoid fever and of scarlet fever and diphtheria were found sometimes to be caused by a specifically contaminated milk supply: and the final disappearance of the belief that typhoid fever could be traced to effluvia may be said to date from the later years when shell-fish was discovered to be responsible for much typhoid fever (p. 206), and when a little later apparently healthy carriers of infection were detected (p. 214).

Dr. Michael W. Taylor of Penrith appears to have been the first (in 1858) to trace any outbreak of infectious disease to infected milk. He described a small epidemic of typhoid fever caused by a milk supply derived from a house in which there was typhoid fever, the mother of the family who attended the patient having milked the cows. In 1870 Dr. Taylor showed that scarlet fever could be spread in the same way. In 1877 Dr. Jacob made a similar observation for diphtheria at Sutton in Surrey. In 1880 Dr. Ballard traced an outbreak of typhoid fever in Islington to a particular milk service, seventy attacks occurring in 140 families supplied from the dairy in question. In 1873 Drs. N. Radcliffe and W. H. Power proved that a large outbreak of typhoid fever had a similar source; and since then many outbreaks of that disease have been traced to milk, including outbreaks caused by infected cream and ice-cream.

The association of scarlet fever with infected milk has been commoner than that of typhoid fever.

In 1882 W. H. Power, reporting on an outbreak of scarlet fever in certain districts of London, suggested for the first time that many of the circumstances of the outbreak "accorded rather with some cow-condition than with the theory of milk-infection through any human agency"; and Klein, experimenting with human scarlatinal material, produced a disorder in cows which was transmissible to other animals, thus apparently confirming "field" observations. In 1885 W. H. Power investigated a further outbreak of scarlet fever occurring in a milk service supplied from Hendon. No pre-existing cases of scarlet fever could be discovered on the farm or among the milk distributors, and as stated by Thorne, "it was clear that it was the milk of certain cows—and of those cows only—that had to do with the diffusion of the disease." These cows were suffering from an udder disease which was found by Klein to be characterised by the presence of definite micro-organisms in the affected tissues, these appearing to be identical morphologically and in pathological properties with the organisms found in human scarlet fever. The findings in this outbreak have been supported in a few outbreaks, but not often: and they have been disputed by veterinarians and many sanitarians. It cannot be said that they have been adequately confirmed, and it is clear that if there is a disease in cows which can cause scarlet fever in human beings its communication is very exceptional. This disease when milk-borne can commonly be traced to human infection. The difficulty of tracing human sources is, however, considerable, and is increased by the fact that scarlet fever may occur without rash. In milk epidemics traced to a human source of infection, the cases without a rash may be in a majority. Milk is an excellent medium for the multiplication of the germs of scarlet fever and of diphtheria. It is also certain that purulent disease in a cow's udder has sometimes produced human epidemics of streptococcal sore throat with high fever unaccompanied by a rash. Recent investigations on the relation of scarlatinal to other streptococci may call for revision of judgment on this problem.

The following illustrations bearing on the preceding remarks are taken from my Brighton experience. The notification to the M.O.H. of each case of scarlet fever occurring in the practice of a family practitioner has been required under a general enactment since 1892. Each notification was at once entered in a register with ruled vertical spaces for a statement of name, age, address, name of disease, occupation, school attended, milk supply, observations.

Thus one could see at a glance whether more than one case of scarlet fever or diphtheria or typhoid fever had recently occurred in the same milk service. But difficulty had not ceased when one found several cases of fever notified whose milk supply was from a single dairyman. Often he received milk from several farms. For this reason I requested dairymen to keep records of these different supplies, and to arrange their books to show the particular farm supply of each milk-round. This was done to a large extent, and in several instances I was thus enabled to prevent the continuance of infection much more promptly than would otherwise have been possible.

Not infrequently extremely prompt action became possible by the co-operation of the family doctor. Thus one morning, while considering two notified cases of scarlet fever, Dr. Morgan called on me to state that at a certain boarding school he had three cases very suspicious of scarlet fever. The source of the milk supply of these cases I found was the same as that of two other cases already partially investigated. I at once drove to the local farm and succeeded in persuading the farmer to sell me the afternoon's supply of milk which was about to be sent on his town-round. This was poured down the drain. The farmer had no provision for pasteurisation and the action taken was inevitable. In another outbreak I was able to purchase 18½ gallons of milk on its way to Brighton, and continued to pay the farmer for his milk and to destroy it until the source of infection was discovered in the family of one of the milkers.

The following summary of an outbreak of scarlet fever, which occurred in 1905 during my absence on holiday, illustrates the complexity of the inquiries needed in tracing a milk outbreak to its source. It was investigated by Dr. Heggs, my lieutenant, afterwards M.O.H. of Baghdad. Altogether some 720 houses were supplied by the infected milk, and the total number of cases was seventeen. The milk vendor received milk from thirteen farms, and had thirty men engaged in the local retail distribution of milk; he also served five shops with milk. Fortunately X had kept his books in accordance with the recommendation named above; otherwise the tracing of infection to a single farm would have been retarded or even impracticable. Dr. Heggs promptly traced the outbreak as far as X's shop, when only six cases connected with his milk service had been notified, though much mischief beyond what was shown by these six notifications had already occurred without having been notified.

Then began the further detective work. In the following schematic statement is given (1st column) the date of onset of the disease in each of the six patients first notified, all of whom had drunk X's milk. There were three daily rounds of milk. In the second column is given the distinctive number of the six milk-carriers concerned, and the letters A B C D E F in the next four columns indicate the six farms which supplied the milk on each of the sixty-four rounds of these six men

ANALYSIS OF THE SOURCE OF THE DAIRY MILK SUPPLIED TO THE FIRST SIX CASES OF SCARLET FEVER

Case	Number of Milk Carrier	Initials of Farm whose Milk was delivered on July 8th,	July 9th,	July 10th,	July 11th	
1 (Onset 12th)	No. 21	**A**	C	**A**	D	1st round
		B	B	B	B	2nd round
			C		D	3rd round
2 (Onset 12th)	No. 16	D	B	E	F	1st round
		B and **A**	B and **A**	B and **A**	B and **A**	2nd round
		A	**A**	**A**	**A**	3rd round
3 (Onset 13th)	No. 3	E	B	F	**A**	1st round
		B	B	B	B	2nd round
		D or C	D or C	D or C	D or C	3rd round
4 (Onset 11th or 12th)	No. 12	E	**A**	E	D	1st round
		B	B	B	B	2nd round
		D or C	D or C	D or C	D or C	3rd round
5 (Onset 13th)	No. 19	D	G	E	**A**	1st round
		D or C	D or C	D or C	D or C	2nd round
6 (Onset 12th)	No. 24	**A**	**A**	**A**	**A**	1st round
		D or C	D or C	D or C	D or C	2nd round

during the four days July 8th–11th preceding the onset of the six cases on July 12th–13th. It will be seen that these six scarlatinal patients were supplied with milk from one, two, three, or more farms during the critical period; but a glance at the scheme shows that source A was the only one common to all the cases. Milk supply A was, therefore, probably the milk which conveyed the infection. This supply was derived from two farms in West Sussex, which were inspected on July 15th. Nothing wrong was found on the first farm; but on the second farm several previously unrecognised cases of scarlet fever were discovered. It has been noted that only six cases were known when the above steps were taken, not reckoning two cases in connection with the shop supplies of milk. Eleven further cases occurred, but the outbreak then suddenly stopped when the milk supply was stopped.

This outbreak illustrates the complexity of the detective work often required in tracing sources of infection of milk-borne disease even in dealing with a relatively small dairy. In more recent years the difficulty in tracing the source of milk supplies has been greatly increased, owing to the formation of large milk "combines" and the collection of milk from a large number of farms into a single depôt, from which it is sent by train to London or other large towns. Happily this increased complexity has meant that unless the milk is pasteurised at the depot it is apt to decompose before reaching the customer; and at the present time probably more than three-fourths of the total milk consumed in large towns has been commercially pasteurised. It is for this reason that milk outbreaks of acute infectious diseases are much rarer now than in the past. But they still occur. Not all the milk is pasteurised; sometimes the process adopted is unsatisfactory: at other times it may fail through carelessness or negligence of the workers concerned; and in smaller towns and rural districts small farmers continue to retail milk themselves or to sell it to small dairymen without pasteurisation. The time is ripe for compulsory supervised and standardised pasteurisation of all milk supplies. This would reduce to a minimum the distribution of disease germs by milk, including especially the distribution of milk containing tubercle bacilli of bovine origin.

The most extensive outbreak of scarlet fever due to milk infection in my experience occurred in 1906, and a full account of it was published in *Public Health* for that year. I need not enter into details of this outbreak except to state that the case incidentally illustrates the value of bacteriological examination of "swabs" taken from suspected sore throats. It illustrates still more clearly the immense value of co-operation by the family doctor when he places himself in touch with the M.O.H., not waiting for the formal notification required of him when he has duly recognised a definite case of notifiable infectious disease.

On October 15th two cases of scarlet fever were notified, and later in the day after visiting the two houses concerned the inspector reported that in both instances milk was supplied from A's dairy. On the previous day "swabs" from cases suspected of diphtheria had arrived, and after cultivation on blood serum had proved negative for diphtheria. Might not these have come from scarlatinal throats? Suspecting this, I at once telephoned to A, and found that his milk was supplied to each of the houses from which the "swabs" had come. Next morning a doctor informed me he had several cases of sore throat in his practice. The milk supply in these cases also was from A. Meanwhile the infected milk had been traced to one farm, and the farmer interviewed, and I had arranged—without waiting for the slower machinery of Sec. 4 of the Infectious Disease (Prevention) Act—for the farmer to destroy his milk for a week. He received altogether £93 for doing this. Thirty-eight cases of scarlet fever and 215 cases of sore throat without rash occurred before the stopping of the milk supply became effective. I need not particularise certain special complications in this investigation, owing to absence of co-operation of the M.O.H. in whose district the infected farm was situate. One fact is illuminating. A supplied a children's hospital having accommodation for fifty patients. All the milk thus supplied was boiled at the hospital and no cases of either sore throat or scarlet fever occurred. The exact source of infection could not be definitely traced.

CONTRIBUTIONS

On an Outbreak of Sore Throats and of Scarlet Fever caused by Infected Milk (*Journal of Hygiene*, Vol. II, No. 2, 1902).

On an Outbreak of Scarlet Fever and of Scarlatinal Sore Throat due to Infected Milk (Annual Report, Brighton, 1906, and *Public Health* (same year)).

CHAPTER XXIII

THE CONTROL OF SCARLET FEVER

Cycles of scarlatinal severity—Reasons for lack of success in isolation—Overlooked cases—"Return" cases

DURING a half-century of public health work medical officers of health have been actively engaged in a double campaign: the study of and attempts to control communicable diseases, whether acute or chronic in their course, and work directed towards maintaining and improving physiological conditions. The supremely important work for maintenance and improvement of the health of infants and young children exemplifies both types of public health work; for it remains essential that improved hygiene and nutrition should be associated with active measures to prevent infection from syphilis, diarrhœa, pneumonia, and tuberculosis, and other communicable diseases, if the young are to be adequately protected. The future like the past work of medical officers of health must always comprise and consist very largely of measures directed to the prevention of personal infection.

Of the infectious diseases some run a chronic course, especially tuberculosis and the venereal diseases; and we possess adequate knowledge to ensure their extinction, if everybody everywhere would utilise existing knowledge of the means available to this end. This is true also for typhoid fever which is rapidly diminishing in prevalence, and for smallpox. On the other hand there are also several serious infectious diseases, most of them transmitted by discharges from the throat and respiratory tract, whose control, hitherto, has remained difficult and imperfect.

The most extreme instance under this heading is *Influenza*, which I do not propose to discuss in this volume. At long intervals this disease spreads over the world more rapidly than a prairie fire, causing a terrible amount of illness and mortality. The pandemic in 1918–19 caused more deaths than all the fighting of the Great War, and that of 1889–93 was almost equally severe. Of the causes of these visitations we are profoundly ignorant.

Two other diseases, measles and whooping-cough, become epidemic regularly every two or three years. Happily there is now hope of their control (p. 193).

There remain (in temperate climes) scarlet fever and diphtheria, which are considered in this and the next chapter, and rheumatic fever in Chapter XXVI. Of the effective control of scarlet fever there is, as yet, a poor prospect. The clinical treatment of patients suffering from scarlet fever and the study of the problems of its prevalence have occupied a large share of my total years of work, and I propose to give here a short summary of my own and some collateral investigations on this subject.

Scarlet fever when I was first a M.O.H. was still a very serious, though declining, cause of death; but now it has reverted to the type which prevailed in Sydenham's days (1642–89) when it "scarcely deserved the name of a disease."

Why this great change? It cannot be ascribed to sanitary improvements, though these may have helped to reduce septic complications. We must conclude that either the type of disease has changed or the number of cases has greatly decreased. Most writers claim that there is no evidence of decrease of prevalence of the disease. I am not certain as to this, and in a contribution to the Epidemiological Society (February 1901) I gave reasons for my doubt. But even though there may have been some reduction in the number of cases, the disease is still widely prevalent, and the reduced death-rate from it cannot be chiefly explained on this basis. Scarlet fever undoubtedly has become a much milder disease. Such terrible cases as I saw in the period 1881–90 now seldom occur, and the milder type now prevailing repeats experience in the seventeenth and eighteenth centuries. Similar changes have also been observed at shorter intervals. In Dublin early in the nineteenth century the change from the virulent to the mild form of disease was attributed to cooling remedies and the use of the lancet for bleeding; but three decades later the virulent type returned, and was uninfluenced by the same type of treatment.

One must regard scarlet fever, then, as a disease liable to great changes in character, irrespective of methods of treatment. The milder type of scarlet fever which has prevailed from 1890 to the present day shows little or no tendency to "revert," but one cannot be confident that change of type will not occur. Even now the type of scarlet fever prevalent in different countries varies greatly in severity.

Dr. C. V. Chapin, the distinguished American epidemiologist, has expressed the view that treatment of scarlatinal patients in isolation hospitals may have helped to reduce the virulence of scarlet fever. The tendency is for the more severe cases to be hospitalised (treated in hospital), thus lowering their opportunities to propagate cases of like severity. This I accept, while holding that the main factor in reduced fatality of attack is a more general change in type of the causal organism.

The isolation of many of the recognised cases of scarlet fever in hospitals has been much less successful in diminishing the prevalence of this disease than was anticipated in the earlier years 1880–1900. There are many reasons for this.

(1) Not every known case of scarlet fever has thus been isolated. That there has been no recognisable relation between the amount of isolation in hospitals and the total amount of scarlet fever was shown in Dr. Killick Millard's paper in 1901 (*Public Health*, April 1901). We should not, however, expect an accurate relationship, for a few cases not isolated may, for instance, by school attendance or by infecting a milk supply disseminate much infection.

(2) The stage at which the disease is recognised and the patient isolated varies greatly. Not infrequently no doctor is called in until some complication arises. In a paper read before the Epidemiological Society in 1901 I gave figures

indicating that the number of secondary cases in a household varied with the expedition of notification and isolation.

(3) More serious is the failure to detect recognisable cases, and, still more important, the failure to recognise anomalous cases of scarlet fever, including those in which no rash occurs. The importance of this factor was dealt with in detail in two papers enumerated at the end of this chapter; and a few particulars may now be given on—

MISSED OR OVERLOOKED CASES

In two papers (p. 186) I have given abundant evidence of the importance of missed cases in reducing the value of official preventive measures. In an address at Victoria University (March 9, 1904) I drew a distinction between the latent period and the incubation period of an infectious disease. Persons may harbour diphtheria bacilli in their fauces for a prolonged period before developing, as they may subsequently, an attack of diphtheria. It is conceivable, of course, that this attack was caused by new extraneous infection two or three days before illness began; but sometimes it is more likely that intercurrent illness, e.g. a catarrh, has enabled the "resident" diphtheria bacilli to "take root" and produce the clinical disease. I have recorded cases of scarlet fever in which also—although in this disease one has no confirmatory laboratory test—it appears probable that such delayed development of disease has occurred. This evidently suggests one of the many ways in which scarlatinal infection is overlooked and propagated.

Another is the absence of symptoms in patients actually infected. The rash may not appear, and the sore throat which occurs may not be recognisable as scarlatinal. There may not even be any evidence of sore throat. An infectious disease is the resultant of an attack made by specific micro-organisms on the patient, to which is opposed his natural resistance to them; and this resistance varies with the natural resistance of the invaded person and with the virulence *and number* of the attacking organisms. We know that, both in scarlet fever and in diphtheria, immunity becomes more and more general with increasing age; and this may be regarded as resulting from invasions by the specific micro-organism in numbers not adequate to cause illness, but adequate to secure immunity against attack. We do not know whether these sub-clinical cases of scarlet fever may sometimes have communicated the disease to persons with relatively low resistance. When it is clearly practicable with a minimum dose of dead scarlatinal organisms to anticipate a clinical attack, hospital treatment of scarlet fever will cease to be a problem; and we shall then have advanced from effort at a secondary method of preventing further infection to successful initial prevention. Meanwhile it is clear that while hospital isolation of scarlatinal patients has not been successful in bringing this disease under control, it has, owing to superior treatment, saved the lives of many patients.

Its partial lack of success as a preventive measure does not imply that treatment in these hospitals should be abandoned. Many more cases might be treated at home; and hospital treatment may without risk be shortened in the majority of cases. But it is indubitable that, although reduced prevalence on a national scale cannot be demonstrated, spread of the disease in a family is often prevented, the family by means of hospital isolation can resume their occupations, and danger is avoided of spread through milk or shops in which food is sold.

"RETURN" CASES

After scarlatinal patients have returned home from hospital, in from 1 to 4 per cent of the cases another member of the family develops scarlet fever within a few days or weeks of the return of the first patient, and this phenomenon has been the subject of many investigations. The late Professor (Sir James) Simpson and afterwards Dr. Cameron investigated it on behalf of the Metropolitan Asylums Board, and among others the late Dr. James Niven, M.O.H. of Manchester, and I arrived at opposite conclusions after careful investigation of many cases.

These return cases occur usually in association with persistent or recurrent ear or nose discharges, but may occur in their absence. Desquamation, it is now agreed, has no etiological significance in these cases.

In several reports I have shown that these secondary cases occur also after the release from isolation of a patient who has been treated at home. And I have recorded cases in which this happened without any possible fallacy as to failure of disinfection or an overlooked case. Others have done the same. It is difficult to determine whether "return cases" are as frequent when the patient has been treated at home as in cases where the patient has returned from hospital, owing to other circumstances of variation, but the usual impression that recrudescence of infection is exclusively a hospital phenomenon is erroneous. I do not propose to give the evidence for this statement here, as it can be studied in the papers cited on page 186. Two views are maintained as to the causation of these "return" cases. One of these is explained in a letter from Dr. Niven to me (1904) and in his Manchester reports:

> By stating that return cases are a hospital phenomenon I go beyond the facts and make an inference, viz. that something happens at the hospital which does not happen at home. This something was, as far as I could judge, storage of fresh infectious matter in the nostrils as the result of the presence of acute cases in the same ward. It is not intended to deny that the infective element of scarlet fever remains visible in the case discharged from hospital, or that it has lost all power of infectivity, but it is suggested that the strains of infectious material *foreign to the individual*[1] when stored up in his nasal cavities remain less impaired by the action of his tissues than the infective material peculiar to himself.

Professor Simpson in his report to the M.A.B. appears to have taken a similar view, as he concluded that "long detention in infective wards will not reduce the percentage of return cases."

Precautionary action based on the views expressed in the

[1] Italics not in original.

above quotation was taken in various towns. Acute cases were separated from convalescent cases, complicated from uncomplicated cases, and, in my own and other hospitals, patients after bathing were often kept a few days in an isolated discharge room before being sent home. No certain reduction in return cases was experienced.

The view reached by me after anxious study of many cases during several years is given in my paper to the Royal Medico-Chirurgical Society in 1904, in which illustrative cases of protracted and recurrent infection are given in full detail.

I concluded that in a small minority of cases—not enough to impugn the utility of isolation hospitals—a special condition exists, which

> must be either a condition of the mucous membrane enabling the scarlatinal germs to continue to live and propagate, or the presence of a race of germs capable of exceptional length of life. It is more in accordance with the clinical facts to suppose that the scarlatinal germs multiplying and collecting in the patient's own mucous membrane will be in larger numbers and will be more efficient to produce secondary infection than the relatively small number which can obtain ingress from without.

I further pointed out that protracted infection occurred in typhoid fever in circumstances in which no question arose of extraneous infection from other patients; and that in the gall bladder and in periosteal abscesses typhoid germs have continued to live and multiply for many months in exceptional instances.

Relapses in both scarlet fever and typhoid fever, I added, showed that secondary attacks (in this instance in the same patient) occur when external reinfection from other patients is excluded. Furthermore, protracted infection is well known to occur in home-treated cases of diphtheria, a closely analogous disease.

As illustrative of my view, I referred to ringworm. In most instances of tinea, as in diphtheria and scarlet fever, infection ceases after treatment. But tinea capitis (except when certain modern methods of treatment are adopted) is an exception. The tinea spores can be destroyed as they reach the surface of the scalp, but with the growth and reappearance of hairs from the follicles tinea also emerges. The suggestion was that in like manner the scarlatinal organisms persist in the deeper tissues, remain latent, and multiply and resume activity under the influence of a chill or catarrh or some unknown factor. This factor of prolonged latency with protracted infectivity is in reality an effort, occasionally successful, of the micro-organism to survive and thus thwart the efforts of sanitary officials! It is unnecessary to exaggerate the total importance of these cases, but one wishes that a more general immunity against attack could be built up. In a rough and ready and not satisfactory manner it is going on, by means of the sub-clinical infections now occurring.

CONTRIBUTIONS

The Utility of Isolation Hospitals in Diminishing the Spread of Scarlet Fever, considered from an Epidemiological Standpoint (*Journal of Hygiene*, Vol. I, No. 1, January 1901).

The Epidemiology of Scarlet Fever in Relation to the Utility of Isolation Hospitals (*Transactions Epidemiological Society*, Vol. XX, 1901).

The Role of "Missed" Cases in the Spread of Infectious Diseases. A Lecture at Victoria University Public Health Laboratory, March 1904 (Sherratt and Hughes, Manchester).

Protracted and Recrudescent Infection in Diphtheria and Scarlet Fever. A paper read before the Medico-Chirurgical Society, London, March 28, 1904 (*Medico-Chirurgical Transactions*, Vol. 87).

CHAPTER XXIV

THE CONTROL OF DIPHTHERIA

The difficulty of controlling respiratory infection—Stages in investigation—Behring and Roux—Artificial immunity—Causation of pandemics

THE epidemiology of diphtheria illustrates as clearly as that of typhoid fever (Chapter XXV and earlier chapters) what a marvellous change in the control of a specific infectious disease can occur during the lifetime of a single observer. But there are great differences in the natural history of these two diseases, and so also in the methods by which they have in varying degree been brought under control.

These differences lead to the conclusion that typhoid and paratyphoid infections, as well as the epidemic diarrhœa of young children, will continue to decline almost to the vanishing point, assuming, as we reasonably may, that hygiene, personal and communal, will continue to be observed with increasing accuracy by an increasing proportion of the total population on the lines indicated in Chapters XXV and XXXVIII. And we can be confident that the decline will continue even though in the past these diseases have always prevailed excessively in hot and dry years.

No such complete confidence can be entertained with regard to diphtheria. Given steady progress in sanitation and in personal hygiene, and in completeness of such measures as disinfection and isolation for every known case of diphtheria, we cannot anticipate—through these measures alone—the dramatic decline manifested by the intestinal diseases. Diphtheria occurs at irregular intervals in great epidemics, even in countries or districts in which a smaller number of cases are always endemic; and against these epidemic waves past experience has proved that we have been relatively helpless when all the ordinary measures of modern sanitation are vigorously adopted. I have shown that these epidemics occur especially when a series of dry warm years are experienced, although there is also much endemic disease; and such measures as have succeeded for typhoid and other intestinal diseases, combined with measures of segregation of the sick and disinfection, have failed to prevent recurrences of diphtheria. The reason is not far to seek. The limited channels of infection by which intestinal infections are spread can be blocked with ease and success. Diphtheria is spread by personal contact, and by such acts as coughing and sneezing. This disease, in fact, is a typical illustration of the greater difficulty of preventing the spread of infection when the infective material is ejected by coughing and like acts. This explains the failure to control not only diphtheria but also influenza and (until recently) measles, which for long have been the despair of health officials and parents. The lesson appears to be that, so far as we yet know, respiratory infections can only be prevented by producing artificial immunity in the exposed persons; whereas typhoid and its congeners can be prevented by blocking the sources of infection. The production of artificial immunity against typhoid (which happily is practicable) is only called for when the external sanitation needed to prevent infection cannot be adopted.

MEDIÆVAL DARKNESS

During my lifetime the history of diphtheria has passed through three phases. In the earlier decades we were almost completely helpless, and epidemics wore themselves out, influenced but little by the preventive or curative treatment we could apply.

When I was in general medical practice tracheotomy was often needed to relieve patients with laryngeal diphtheria, but a high proportion of patients, although temporarily relieved, died from subsequent cardiac paralysis. As already indicated (p. 139), most of us were possessed by the notion that defective drainage was responsible for the disease, and thus our preventive energies were largely misdirected. This did not continue indefinitely, as is shown by the following extract from a letter sent to me on February 26, 1898, by Sir Samuel Wilks, the distinguished pathologist, formerly President of the Royal College of Physicians, in acknowledgment of my brochure on *Pandemic Diphtheria* (p. 194).

I remember that when Huxley denounced the parish authorities at Kilburn on account of the bad drainage which he considered to be at the root of the prevailing diphtheria, I wrote to say that Jenner[1] many years ago had stated his strong conviction that this disease had nothing to do with insanitary conditions, but was *caught*, and I myself have said the same.

Sir Samuel then quoted from a lecture of his, published in 1873 in the *Guy's Hospital Gazette*, in which he described the introduction of the disease into England in 1855. He went on to refer to a more recent paper by Dr. George Johnson in the Proceedings of the Medico-Chirurgical Society, in which from personal observations it was maintained that diphtheria was always associated with bad drainage.

THE DAWN

The first ray of light on this darkness was shed when Klebs in 1883 identified the diphtheria bacillus. In 1884 Loeffler proved its causal relation to diphtheria, and thus it became possible to recognise the disease in cases clinically doubtful, and to determine the period of infectivity; also to recognise those "carriers" of infection who harboured the bacillus, although there was no clinical evidence of disease. The significance of this discovery (as of that of the tubercle bacillus) was only gradually realised. Loeffler in a paper read to the International Congress of Hygiene, Berlin, 1890, summarised the then state of knowledge. He had already shown that the specific bacilli of diphtheria remain localised in the lesions in the throat or elsewhere, that they do not invade the circulation, and that the serious secondary symptoms of

[1] Sir William Jenner, not Edward Jenner.

diphtheria are due to a toxin absorbed into the blood from the local lesions. He then gave particulars showing the duration of persistence of the bacilli in the local lesions.

Perhaps the earliest public health authority to adopt routine examination of "swabs" from throat and nasal secretions in cases of suspected diphtheria was that of New York, led by their astute health officer, the late Dr. Hermann Biggs. This application of bacteriology to public health in a municipal laboratory began in 1894. Similar measures were adopted in England. Professor Delepine began the examination of diphtheria "swabs" for the City of Manchester in 1894, and similar action was taken by Dr. (now Sir John) Robertson in St. Helens in 1895.[1] It may be said, therefore, that the period of latency between a scientific discovery and its application in the practice of medicine was not, in this instance, inordinately long.

After attending the International Congress on Hygiene and Demography at Budapest in 1894, I reported to the Town Council of Brighton that

> the most important papers and discussions at the Congress were on the subject of diphtheria. . . . With improved sanitation typhoid fever has rapidly declined, but diphtheria has not shown itself amenable in the same way to sanitary measures. . . . One of the reasons why it spreads . . . is the difficulty of recognising slight cases.

I then quoted from "the important paper on this subject by Dr. W. H. Welch" of Baltimore, in which the new methods of bacteriological diagnosis adopted in New York and some other centres were described; and I recommended the starting of such a laboratory in Brighton. I had already prepared myself for this work in a laboratory at the University of Heidelberg. But it was not until 1897 that I obtained the necessary funds for the full working of this help in diagnosis for the practitioners of Brighton.

This improved means of diagnosis in doubtful cases, although of value in preventing spread of the disease, was also sometimes

[1] These particulars are taken from the Hermann Biggs Memorial Lecture, prepared by me for delivery in New York in 1932.

responsible for serious delay in administering antitoxin to the patient; for some practitioners waited for a bacteriological report before beginning antitoxin treatment. Investigation on the toxin of diphtheria led to the discovery that animals to whom large doses of diphtheria bacilli had been given were immune to further large doses of diphtheria, and that their blood serum administered subcutaneously stopped the diphtheria process in animals already suffering from diphtheria, thus immensely increasing their prospect of recovery. This was followed quickly by the application of the new knowledge to the treatment of human diphtheria patients. In 1887 Roux and Yersin in Paris, and almost simultaneously Behring in Berlin, arrived at the above results in experimental animals, and in 1891 the first child desperately ill with diphtheria was successfully treated with antitoxin in a Berlin hospital.

Roux was mainly responsible for bringing the subject from the experimental to the practical stage. The general adoption of the antitoxin treatment of diphtheria followed rapidly on a contribution to the International Congress on Hygiene and Demography at Budapest in 1894. After this meeting, Dr. Roux gave me a copy of his paper, which I translated in full, and in October 1894 it appeared in *Public Health*, the official journal of the Society of Medical Officers of Health, of which I was then the editor.

To the enthusiastic audience whom he addressed in Budapest Roux was able to announce that the case-mortality in children suffering from diphtheria in the Paris Children's Hospital had already been reduced from 52 to 25 per cent.

A few further notes may be made respecting Emil Roux. I came into personal touch with him in Budapest in 1894, and again in Cannes in 1919. One could not fail to be impressed by his habits of a recluse, and by his total absorption in his life-work. He died in November 1933 at the age of 80, after having suffered from chronic pulmonary disease for thirty years. The Nobel prize for the discovery of diphtheria antitoxin was awarded to him along with Behring. Roux and Martin were the first to employ horses for the preparation of antitoxin, thus making it widely available in treatment. Roux and

Yersin in collaboration worked out the conditions under which the diphtheria toxin is produced, and demonstrated the occurrence of diphtheritic paralysis in laboratory animals that had survived large doses of toxin. In his later years Roux did much to stimulate more effective public health work in France.

In 1929 I visited a health centre at Vannes, a few miles out of Paris, which was named after Roux; and as its chief told me, its marching orders given by Roux included the injunction to proceed "with the good will of the people and the local practitioners" (see p. 103, Vol. II, *International Studies*, Milbank Fund).

The photograph of Dr. Hermann Biggs of New York is shown on p. 245. That of Professor Delepine of Manchester, who was also a pioneer in applying bacteriological diagnosis to epidemic diseases and especially to diphtheria is shown here, along with that of Sir John Robertson.

But although the administration of large doses of antitoxin has reduced the fatality among diphtheria patients to a remark able extent, it has done but little to prevent the spread of epidemic diphtheria. This is so even although the administration of antitoxin gives partial temporary immunity to attack.

In order to complete the history of the potential triumph over diphtheria, I must be permitted to escape from the tyranny of chronology and to narrate progress made beyond the time-limit of this volume.

In 1913 Von Behring found that injection of neutralised diphtheria toxin into an animal served as a prophylactic against attack by diphtheria, and in 1913 Schick of Vienna discovered that by the introduction of a measured quantity of diluted toxin under the skin a local redness and infiltration was produced in persons who had no natural antitoxin in the blood. Schick's test when positive served to show, at least partially, that there was an absence of immunity against a clinical attack. This test has been employed on a large scale, and especially so in New York—where Dr. Park has been the

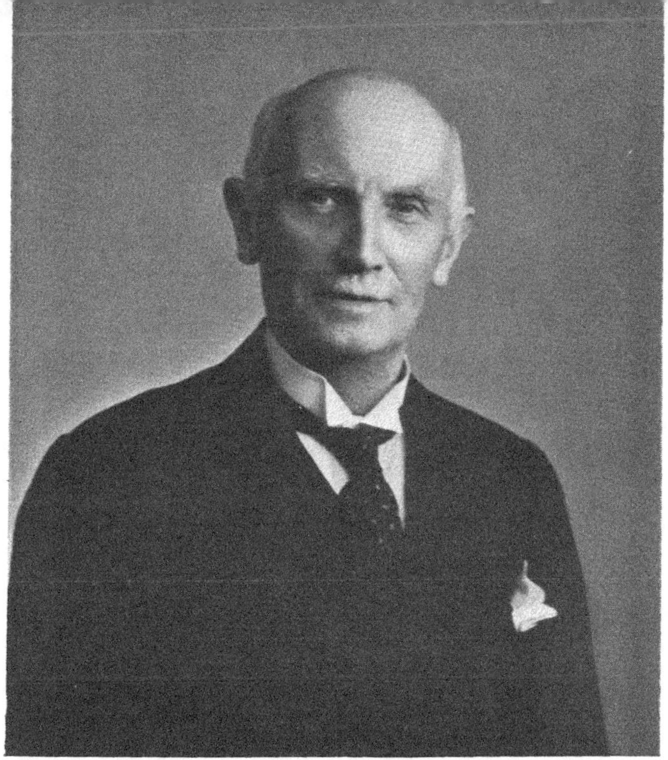

SIR JOHN ROBERTSON

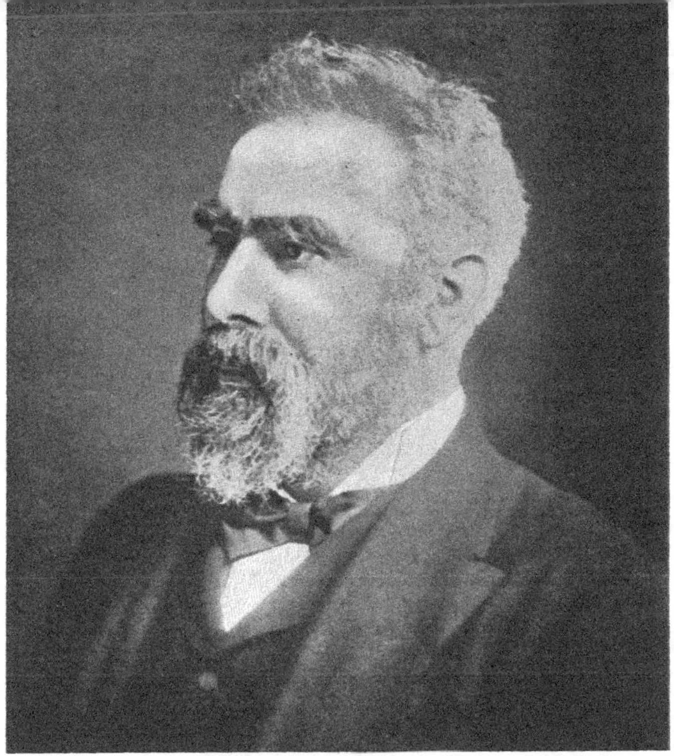

PROFESSOR DELEPINE

pioneer in this work—and on the results of the Schick test it can be decided whether children shall be immunised artificially by means of a mixture of toxin and antitoxin. This mixture obviates the risk to life involved in giving diphtheria toxin alone. It is found that a mixture in which the toxicity has been reduced by formalin, and known as toxoid-antitoxin, is safe and successful.

Towards adolescence a natural partial immunity against diphtheria appears to be established. The chief danger of death from diphtheria is in childhood, and the administration of toxoid-antitoxin protects during this period of danger. Although I refrain from quoting figures illustrating the remarkable success that has been achieved in some American cities, it can be stated without exaggeration that the prophylactic administration of toxoid-antitoxin has been a phenomenal triumph of preventive medicine, which can be placed side by side with vaccination in the prevention of smallpox.

In my *Story of Modern Preventive Medicine* (Baillière, 1929) I remarked:

> It is too early to give complete statistical proof of the protection afforded a community against diphtheria by general immunisation of children by toxoid-antitoxin. The unknown factors of epidemicity may break through local defences in future years if active immunisation has not been universal, or if its effect has worn out with time.

In this statement, which does not detract from the immensely valuable protection secured by young children by immunisation —I had in mind the natural history of diphtheria, in the study of which I spent several years. This study showed how "epidemic influences" at irregular intervals had leaped over the fences raised against this disease; and it was suggested that this might again occur unless a large portion of the young population everywhere was actively immunised. The need for immunisation of each successive "crop" of children is evident. Great gain comes from immunisation of even a minority of children. The gap between successive patients is widened, and transmission is thus rendered less likely. How far this will be counterbalanced by immune children becoming "carriers" remains to be seen.

The results of a protracted personal study of diphtheria were embodied in a brochure of 196 pages, published by Allen & Unwin in 1898, under the title of *Epidemic Diphtheria. A Research on the Origin and Spread of the Disease from an International Standpoint.*

As this volume is but little known, I propose at this point to indicate some of its main facts and then to comment on the conclusions at which I then arrived.

I may claim some slight originality in insisting in this investigation on the importance of dealing with annual death-rates from diphtheria (yearly case-rates were unavailable) and eschewing death-rates for groups of years. This appears to me to be an essential condition of the study of any disease if we are to ascertain the true height and depth of the curve of its incidence. Even then we fail to avoid the minor fallacy involved in the fact that an infectious disease may vary not only in prevalence but also in virulence.

I also claimed that by the use of diagrams it was unnecessary (except for reference) to burden one's pages with detailed tables. From the multitude of diagrams given in the brochure I drew two main conclusions: (*a*) that diphtheria spreads from town to town and from country to country, the means of spread being almost certainly personal infection; and (*b*) that certain climatic conditions are required for the development of diphtheria as an epidemic, and still more for its development on a pandemic scale. Both these conclusions are, I still think, sound (see also p. 226).

In the following diagram I reproduce a statement of the death-rates from diphtheria in New York (1867–95) and London (1869–96) respectively. I omit the parts of each diagram which originally gave also the death-rates from croup (chiefly laryngeal diphtheria), as this would not materially affect the comparison between the two cities.

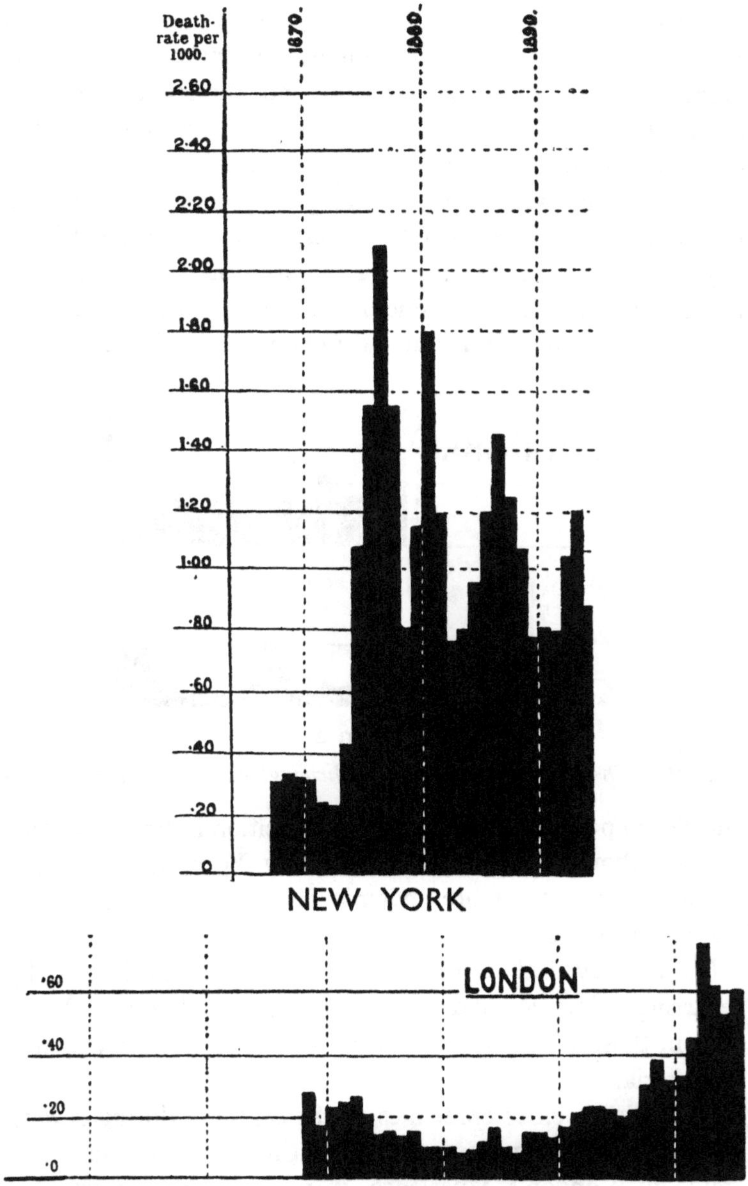

Diagram I

Annual Death-rate from Diphtheria in New York (1867–95) and in London (1869–96)

For further comparisons I give corresponding rates for two provincial English towns, Birmingham (1871–96) and Leeds (1871–96) and for Berlin (1868–96) and Budapest (1868–96) among European cities. These and other curves given in the original brochure demonstrate several points:

(1) Not only were there recurring epidemics of diphtheria in the countries investigated, but in towns and especially in large continental cities there was a large mass of diphtheria constantly endemic. The amount of endemic diphtheria was least in the United Kingdom and in New Zealand, while Paris

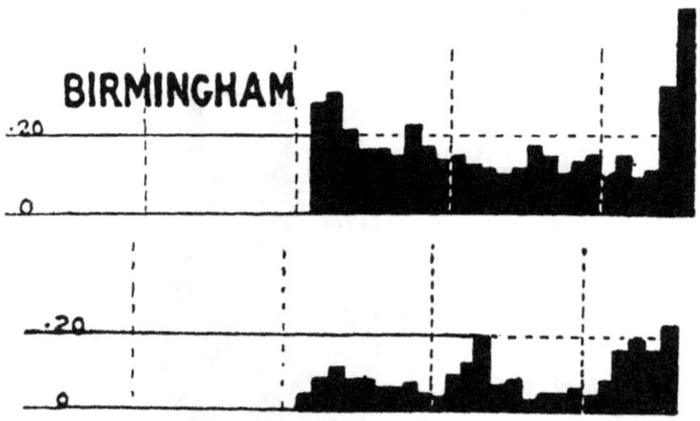

Diagram 2

Annual Death-rate from Diphtheria in Birmingham and Leeds (1871–96)

and Berlin occupied a supremely bad position in Europe in this respect, though probably Boston, New York, Chicago, and Montreal had even more endemic diphtheria than these two European capitals.

(2) The cyclical character of diphtheria, evidenced by recurring epidemics and pandemics, was much more clearly seen in those communities which had relatively little endemic diphtheria.

(3) In large cities epidemics might continue during several years; but the "true inwardness" of this statement was illustrated by London's experience, in which it was shown that diphtheria gradually spread from one district of London to another, and that "in the course of the one great epidemic the

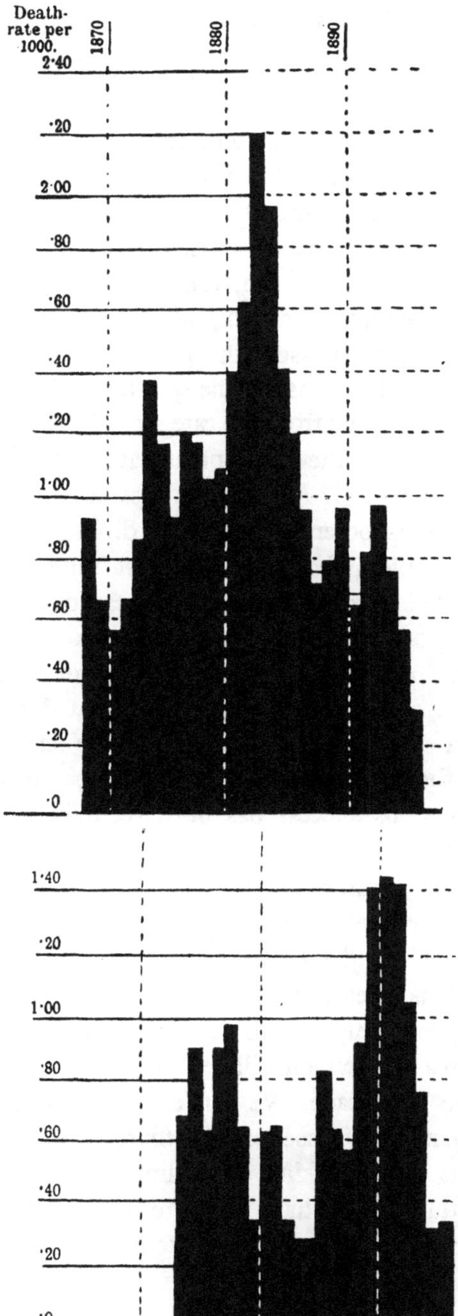

Diagram 3

Annual Death-rate from Diphtheria in Berlin and Budapest (1868–96)

same district in a great city may suffer epidemically more than once."

(4) When the statistics for a sufficiently long series of years were obtainable, it became "clear that there is more diphtheria in urban than in rural communities."

In Chapter XV, I have discussed briefly the climatic factors additional to infection which appear to be required for the development of pandemic diphtheria. Whether or not these secondary factors possess the importance attributed to them, we are now able to answer the question, Has diphtheria or has it not been removed from the category of those diseases—influenza, for instance—the development and spread of which is still beyond our control? And we can answer this question in the affirmative. This potential escape of diphtheria from the list of uncontrollable infections is a great milestone in the history of medicine. Already humanity had escaped from intestinal infections potentially and in large measure practically, but the extension of such a possibility to diphtheria—a disease belonging to the group which are communicated by contact or by expiration—represents an inroad into the last and most recalcitrant of the infectious diseases of temperate climates. This new momentous success has been secured, not by the institution of environmental precautions, but by the artificial production of active immunity.

In another respiratory disease—measles—probably a similar success may be achieved by means of the serum of patients recovered from this disease. But to secure permanent abolition of diphtheria by immunisation there is implied continuance in immunisation on a scale which will be difficult to secure year by year and decade by decade. We can encourage ourselves by remembering that every case of diphtheria prevented from occurring means the breaking of a link in the numerous chains of infection which have hitherto barred our way to complete control of this still too prevalent and fatal disease.

CHAPTER XXV

THE CONTROL OF TYPHOID FEVER

Rapid decline—Serum diagnosis—Specific prophylaxis—Relation to water supplies and sanitation—Manchester, Nottingham, and Leicester—First reports on oyster infection—Attempt to secure powers of control—Personal episodes—A logical difficulty—The missing link—Carrier cases

LIKE the rest of the country, Brighton experienced a striking reduction in the incidence of enteric or typhoid fever. In 1892, the first year for which the number of notified cases as well as of deaths in Brighton can be given, the number of cases was 54 per 100,000 of population. The number varied from year to year: in 1899 it was 148, but since then there has been an uninterrupted decline. Beginning with the year 1900 and ending with the year 1907 the annual number of cases per 100,000 of population in Brighton was:

67, 37, 52, 31, 27, 27, 17, 19.

In more recent years typhoid fever has declined almost to the vanishing point, and I notice that in the annual reports of the M.O.H., Dr. Forbes, for 1931 and 1932, no paragraph is devoted to this disease.

This record is probably matched broadly in most parts of England. It is a signal triumph of the Public Health Service: and its story is perhaps the most outstanding feature in our sanitary history. As I have been a worker myself and an interested onlooker on the sanitary work of others, it is appropriate here to name the chief factors concerned in this marvellous saving of life and health.

As already noted, Eberth in 1880 first discovered the *Bacillus typhosus* in the organs of a typhoid patient, and in 1884 Gaffky grew this organism in pure culture. For some years afterwards it was thought that the *Bac. Coli communis*, an intestinal organism found in healthy animals, might in special circumstances possibly become the *Bac. typhosus* by evolution. The view that the two organisms could not be distinguished was held as late as 1890. But this view was untenable on epidemiological grounds: and more recent serum tests have made it possible to distinguish between the typhoid or Eberth bacillus and others likely to be mistaken for it.

Bordet in 1895 made the first serum experiments on cholera, and Durham in 1896 pursued a similar investigation on the serum of patients who had recovered from typhoid fever. These experiments showed that the serum from a patient recovered from this disease agglutinated and immobilised typhoid bacilli contained in a broth culture. Widal took the matter a step further, showing that the agglutinating reaction occurs also during an attack of typhoid fever. Thus the agglutination of suspensions of typhoid bacilli by appropriate dilutions of the serum of a patient who has been suffering from typhoid for not less than ten days gives valuable help in diagnosing a doubtful case of typhoid fever and in distinguishing it from paratyphoid or undulant fever.

The late Dr. D. S. Davies, M.O.H. of Bristol, was, I believe, the first in England to utilise this test in investigating an outbreak of enteric fever, and to show its importance in discovering overlooked cases of the disease, and thus completing the links of causation. It is now the routine to use the agglutination (Widal-Durham) test to determine the suspected source of an outbreak; and with suitable refinements (absorption, etc.) the test similarly can be utilised in detecting cases of paratyphoid, of Gaertner infection, and of undulant fever, suspensions of the bacilli of those diseases being employed against the blood serum of the suspected patient.

Thus bacteriology helps in the discovery of doubtful cases of typhoid fever. It has proved valuable also in rendering available a method of vaccination against this disease. The method is based on the work of Haffkine on cholera. He showed that inoculation of dead cultures of the spirillum of cholera led to the appearance of a specific anti-bacterial substance in the blood serum and to the protection of the individual against the infection of cholera.

A. E. Wright in 1896 made preliminary observations showing that dead cultures of the typhoid bacillus could be used to protect against an attack of typhoid fever; and this method was employed partially during the Boer War (1899), though its full measure of success was disguised by the fact that the paratyphoid group of infections had not then been distinguished from typhoid. In the Great War (1914–18) mixed cultures of typhoid and paratyphoid were successfully employed as a prophylactic against attack by these diseases; and American experience has shown the efficiency of this method of protection when exposure to infection cannot be avoided. This points to the obvious limitation of the employment of prophylactic injections in civilian practice. It is useful in controlling and preventing spread of the disease where the source of infection cannot be traced, or in backward countries where the immediate provision of proper environmental sanitation is beyond the resources of the community. But it should never be regarded as a substitute for sanitary improvements, including satisfactory disposal of excretal matters, a pure water supply, and protection of foods, which render inoculation unnecessary.

But although modern bacteriology has played an important role in tracing suspected cases, in early recognition of cases already under observation, and in the detection of carriers, the application of bacteriology has only been a minor factor in the earlier stages of the marvellous reduction of typhoid fever which has been experienced in most civilised countries.

First and foremost are two factors which can scarcely be thought of apart: (*a*) The provision of communal water supplies adequately protected from pollution, and (*b*) the prompt and complete removal of all liquid and solid excremental matter from dwellings and from their vicinity, including the carriage and ultimate disposal of sewage in such manner as to preclude the possibility of contamination of water supplies or foods such as milk and oysters and mussels.

If (*a*) can be separated in practice completely from (*b*) it may be regarded as the supreme preventive measure; but oft-times this cannot be done. I have known districts in which for long years insanitary domestic conditions, including leaking cesspools, have continued, and no typhoid fever has broken out. These districts were provided with drinking water coming from a distant and safe source. As a rare exception to the general experience, I may cite the case in which a village with some 2,000 inhabitants abutting on a borough (population 15,000) was persuaded to abandon its water supply from local wells and to receive the supply distributed to the 15,000, which was derived from deep wells in the chalk, with adits running from them to intercept the subterranean water on its way to the sea. But soon after the change was effected, the adits of the urban water supply were extended, and one of the workers employed, suffering from an unrecognised slight typhoid attack, appears to have defœcated while at work underground. Several hundred cases of typhoid fever followed, and the villagers suffered equally with the town dwellers from the sudden calamity. The moral of this experience is not that shallow wells are superior to a municipal water supply but that every possible safeguard against pollution must be maintained, especially pollution which may result from human frailty.

Apart from "accidents" such as the one indicated above, communal supplies under adequate supervision and control are always safer than small local supplies in which safeguards are apt to be casual and precarious.

It is not always possible to supply large communities with water which is pure when collected, and many great towns like London drink water from rivers which have received more or less contamination by sewage higher up the river than the point at which water is abstracted. For many years these communities have been protected from infection by carefully controlled sand filtration, preceded by storage of the collected water in reservoirs which allow sedimentation and some self-purification to occur. In recent years this method of protection has been supplemented by chlorination of the water as an additional precaution. By these and allied measures—among which adequate supervision and protection from contamination of the streams and gathering-grounds furnishing the water are especially important—it may now be said that the water supplied in large towns both in this and in other western countries, can nearly everywhere be drunk with confidence in its salubrity.

But when drinking water has been eliminated as a vehicle of typhoid fever, organic filth may continue to spread this disease; and it can do this not only by contaminating milk supplies or such foods as oysters or mussels, but also by direct conveyance of the filth to human beings from hands which have been in contact with this filth, from bare feet or shoes which bring it into the dwelling, from the dust of dried dejecta blown on to food or directly into the mouth, and by flies which have flitted from the filth to various foods. Hence an essential means of preventing typhoid consists in organic cleanliness of dwellings and their surroundings. The sanitary history of England is full of illustrations of this general statement. I will only give two of these.

The city of Manchester in 1871 had 38,132, in 1881 only 1,233 privy middens, and in 1883 only 606, while new pail-closets in substitution for these greatest of all forms of sanitary barbarism were 696 in 1873, and had become 63,267 in 1881.

In later years these were gradually replaced by water-closets.

Privy middens were an evil-smelling abomination in themselves. Their infrequent emptying necessitated dumping of their contents in the backyard and then shovelling it into carts. Satisfactory cleansing after this process was almost impracticable; spillings occurred, and commonly filth was trodden on and carried indoors, while children's hands were liable to be smeared with similar filth. These privy middens were suitable places for keeping typhoid and diarrhœal organisms alive, and there were hosts of flies to convey them and to pollute liquid and solid foods therewith.

The substitution of pail-closets for privies was a step forward in sanitary civilisation: but their contents required systematic removal, a process liable to spillings, apart from the occasional over-filling of the pails. Then began a systematic replacement of pails by water-closets. In terms of the death-rate (per 1,000 living) from typhoid fever the corresponding story is as follows:

Manchester

1871–75	1876–80	1881–85	1886–90	1910–14
0·43	0·29	0·20	0·30	0·07

The second instance of association of excessive disease, especially typhoid fever, with persistence in the use of privies or pail-closets instead of the modern water-closet, is taken from my report as Medical Officer to the Local Government Board 1908–9. It narrates the experience of the late Dr. P. Boobbyer, the M.O.H. of Nottingham, comparing it with the parallel experience of Dr. Millard at Leicester. Leicester formerly had the highest diarrhœal mortality among the great English towns, and, like Nottingham, an excessive amount of typhoid fever. The population of each town was about a quarter of a million. In 1896 both were generally in an unsatisfactory sanitary condition, but Leicester already had 20,000 water-closets, Nottingham only 7,200. In 1896 Leicester had approximately 7,000 pails and 2,000 middens, while Nottingham had 40,225 pails and 440 middens.

Leicester completed in a few years a scheme of conversion of all its middens and pails into water-closets, while in 1908 Nottingham still had 100 middens and 36,531 pails, as compared with its 26,729 water-closets. The correlative experience of the two towns in respect of typhoid fever is significant. Comparing the five years 1889–93 with the five years 1904–8, the typhoid mortality in Leicester declined from 100 to 22, that of Nottingham only from 100 to 57 (see also p. 353). The moral drawn in my report in 1908–9 was as follows:

A gigantic experiment has been performed on these two communities in circumstances which enable fairly trustworthy comparison to be made . . . in Nottingham a large number of deaths from diarrhœa and from typhoid fever are occurring year by year, which would cease to occur were this city to adopt, like Leicester, a more cleanly system of disposal of excremental matter.

It is clear that the reduction of typhoid fever varied in rapidity in different areas in England, in accordance with the measure of their adoption of sanitary measures. On this I may quote some further figures derived from later years. In 1912 the notified cases of this disease per 100,000 of popula-

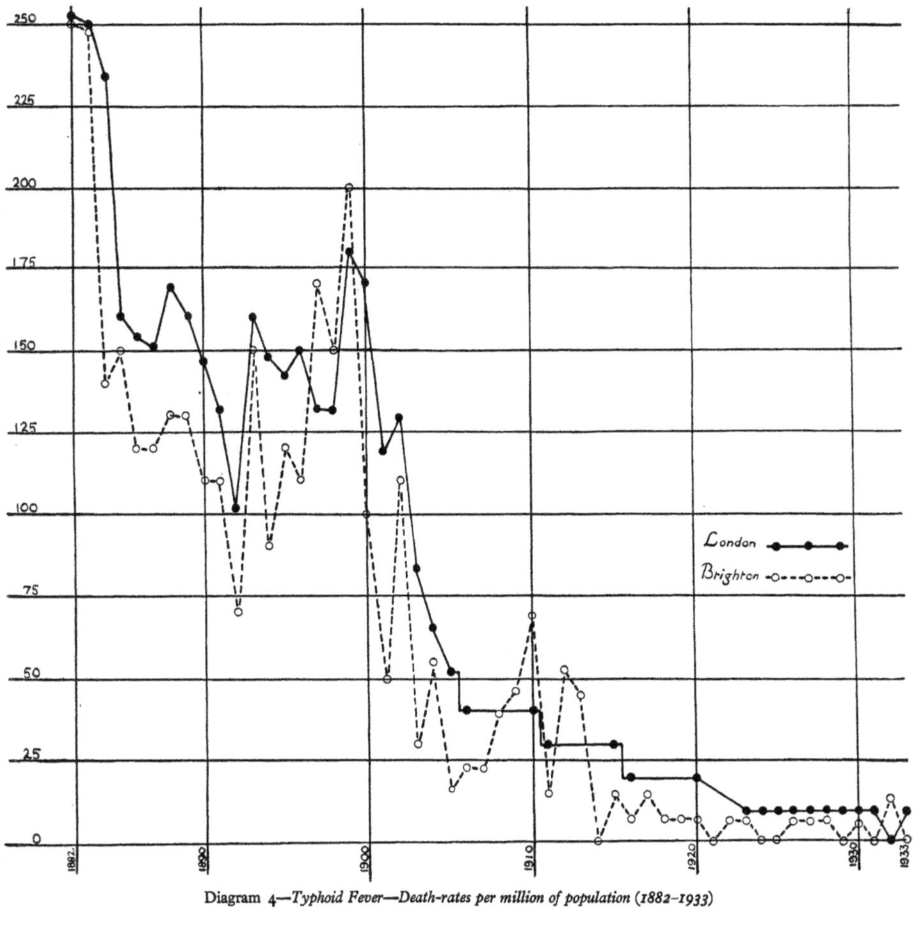

Diagram 4—*Typhoid Fever—Death-rates per million of population (1882–1933)*

tion were 89 in Bradford, 82 in Wigan and 59 in Stoke-on-Trent, while in London the case-rate was only 16. Notwithstanding these variations the abolition of typhoid fever had in 1912 come nearer to realisation than a sanitarian writing in 1870 or even 1880 would have regarded as possible.

Having shown how intimately inter-related and inter-dependent are a pure water supply and elementary domestic and municipal sanitation in protecting against typhoid fever, two other factors remain, the discovery of which in recent years has enabled us almost completely to control the incidence of enteric fever.

This is illustrated by the more recent experience of Brighton and London.

The accompanying curves show the course of events in London and Brighton for a long series of years. The diagram is copied from my annual report for Brighton, 1906, extended to include more recent years; and these curves may be regarded as fairly representative of the course of events in the more sanitary parts of England. It will be noted that a marked decline in the death-rate from typhoid occurred between 1871–75 and 1886–90. This was the cumulative effect of the sanitary improvements of these years and of the preceding decade. From thence onwards for fifteen years, although the death-rate showed yearly oscillations, no evidence of improvement emerged. During the whole period 1875–1930, both Brighton and London had water supplies which can be absolved from the suspicion that they contributed to typhoid infection, and during the same period domestic sanitation was steadily improving. Neither in London nor in Brighton were there privies or pail-closets to disseminate typhoid infection. During the same period in both London and London-by-the-Sea cases of typhoid fever were usually treated in hospitals, and personal infection from patient to relative or nurse was not a large source of additional cases, though in cases treated at home it sometimes occurred.

New light in causation was needed if the large amount of

residual typhoid was to be attacked and eliminated, and this new light was forthcoming. It consisted in two discoveries; first, that the consumption of shell-fish was largely concerned in producing the sporadic cases of typhoid which still occurred; and second, some years later, the discovery that sporadic cases and also outbreaks in groups of cases might be infected by a chronic "carrier" of typhoid infection. Action based on this second factor can hardly be regarded as in substantial existence in the years 1895–1908, though the increased rapidity of the fall since 1908 is ascribable in very large part to the action rendered possible by the wide attention given to Koch when in 1902 he emphasised, and through the Typhoid Institutes in the south-west of Germany demonstrated, the importance of the carrier as a source of spread of typhoid fever (see also p. 214).

The general recognition of carriers dates only from 1906–8, and the sharp fall shown in earlier years by the curves on page 205, must be traceable to some other factor than action based on this knowledge. This new factor was the discovery that shell-fish (uncooked) often are the vehicle of typhoid fever.

And at this point I am obliged to appear egotistical, for I believe I was the first person in England to publish detailed circumstantial evidence of this source of typhoid fever and to make repeated persistent urgent representations concerning it not only to the sanitary authority which I served, but also to the Local Government Board as the central department of health. My first cases ascribable to oysters were reported by me officially in March 1894. I learnt many years later that at the 48th Annual Meeting of the British Medical Association, held in 1880, Sir Charles A. Cameron read a paper on "Sewage in Oysters," of which the only account appears to be the short summary given in the *British Medical Journal* for September 18, 1880. He pointed out that the oysters on the north side of Dublin Bay, at low tide, were literally bathed in sewage, and he suggested that if typhoid could be transmitted through the media of potable water and milk, it was at least as likely that oysters, taken raw, might be the vehicle of the *materies morbi* of typhoid fever, or other disease. "It was clear," he added, "that oyster beds should not be laid down at any point on or close to the mouth of a sewer."

In September 1893, I reported to the Town Council of Brighton that in view of the possibility of importation of Cholera, the condition of Shoreham Harbour (near Brighton) was a serious menace to the inhabitants of Brighton.

In March 1894, as stated above, I reported eight cases of typhoid fever which appeared to be caused, some by mussels and some by oysters, derived from Shoreham Harbour.

I give here from this report the particulars of the first three of the eight cases reported in March 1894, as they illustrate the usual history of such cases.

1. On March 4, 1894, a fishmonger's errand boy, aged 13 years, developed typhoid fever. There were in the same house eight other persons, five children under 10 years of age and three adults, who all, including the father and mother, remained well. About seventeen days before the onset of his illness the boy remembers that the foreman of the shop gave him three oysters. The drainage of this house was perfect. There were no other cases of typhoid fever in connection with the same milk supply. No other members of this household took oysters.

2. On March 14, 1894, a girl aged 13 years developed typhoid fever. She and her mother ate oysters frequently before the onset of the girl's illness. The mother had an attack of diarrhœa at the time of onset of her child's fever, but did not keep to her bed. Drainage of this house was fairly good, and did not pass under the house. There were no other cases of typhoid fever in connection with the same milk supply.

3. On March 17, 1894, a man aged 37, an invalid attendant, began with typhoid fever. On February 28th he bought fifteen oysters from a barrow in the street. His wife declined to join in eating these. The man ate them all himself. The wife and one other adult living in the house have remained quite well. The drainage of this house was bad. The wife had lived in this house alone, her husband living at Havant until the day on which he had the oysters.

The histories in these and similar cases came under one of four categories.

(*a*) The only person eating the oysters was the only person acquiring typhoid fever.

(*b*) Other persons taking oysters at the same time as the typhoid patient may have had an illness within a day or two of taking the oysters. In some of these cases typhoid fever also developed ten or fourteen days later.

(*c*) In other cases defective house drainage was found as well as a history of eating oysters, and in the then stage of sanitary opinion one had an alternative choice of possible causes.

(*d*) Sometimes only one person out of many eating oysters acquired typhoid fever.

At intervals during the same year I reported further cases to the Town Council of Brighton.

The oysters which I regarded as responsible for most of these cases in Brighton were derived from ponds at Southwick in Shoreham harbour, and it was shown that the untreated sewage from a very considerable population discharged in dangerous proximity to these ponds.

On April 20, 1894, I consulted Mr. (later Sir William H.) Power, then the assistant medical officer of the Local Government Board, as to possible lines of action against this source of infection.

On December 5th in the same year a deputation of the Brighton Town Council, consisting of the Town Clerk, Sir Joseph Ewart (Chairman of its Sanitary Committee), and the medical officer of health, waited on the Local Government Board. They were received by Sir Walter Foster (afterwards Lord Ilkeston), who was then parliamentary secretary to the Board, Sir Hugh Owen (permanent secretary) and Sir Richard Thorne (principal medical officer). Sympathy with the Brighton corporation was expressed, and the advice was given that oysters from this source should be seized under the same powers as are given in respect of diseased meat. It was pointed out, however, that this procedure was impracticable, for reasons that will be obvious to administrators in public health.

On January 30, 1895, the medical officer of health visited the oyster ponds in question, along with Dr. H. T. Bulstrode, of the medical staff of the Local Government Board. This visit was paid in connection with the "decision of the Board, made early in 1895, that the medical department should undertake a comprehensive inquiry into the circumstances under which molluscs were cultivated and stored along our coasts."

Dr. Bulstrode's comprehensive report "On Oyster Culture in Relation to Disease" was issued near the end of the year 1896, and on my instruction in 1911 as principal medical officer of the Local Government Board it was followed by a further report prepared by Dr. Bulstrode, giving similar evidence as to shell-fish other than oysters.

In 1893 sporadic cases of cholera occurred in several places in England, and these formed the subject of a report issued by the Local Government Board towards the end of 1894 entitled, "Report on Cholera in England in 1893." The facts elicited were not published before the end of 1894, but the investigations on cholera embodied in it were made in the autumn of 1893. The reports on a few groups of cases of cholera in Grimsby, Cleethorpes, and a few other places led Sir Richard Thorne "to express the conviction that shell-fish from these places must, in some cases, remain under suspicion as having contributed to the diffusion of the disease" (Preface to Dr. Bulstrode's Report).

In May 1896 the corporation of Brighton sought parliamentary powers to inspect suspected oyster layings and ponds and other places in which shell-fish might be exposed to sewage when the medical officer of health was of opinion that infectious disease had been derived from these shell-fish, and to prohibit their supply within the borough if this was found to be necessary in the public interest. The parliamentary committee which considered the application, advised by a Government department, threw out the bill, and it was not until 1908 that the corporation of Blackburn secured similar local powers. More general powers of control have followed.

My evidence before the parliamentary committee was to the effect that approximately one-third of our local cases of enteric fever resulted from the eating of shell-fish; that in another third other sources could be traced, or the cases of typhoid were imported, and that the source of a third of the total cases could not be traced. It was on this last third that a distinguished member of the parliamentary committee (Mr. Reginald McKenna) fastened. Might not the unknown cause or causes of these cases have been responsible for the third of total cases attributed to shell-fish?

In my evidence I emphasised the circumstantial evidence as to the relation of shell-fish with the disease:

1. Members of the same family who did not eat oysters escaped.
2. While it was true that many eating these oysters escaped it was unreasonable to expect that every oyster would be specifically contaminated.
3. Many eating oysters, while escaping enteric fever, suffered from acute diarrhœa and vomiting within a few hours after their contaminated meal.
4. Others first had this attack of diarrhœa, etc., and ten to fourteen days later started with enteric fever.

A considerable number of former victims gave evidence illustrating the above points, but the parliamentary committee in its wisdom rejected the bill.

Late in 1894 the distinguished physician Sir William Broadbent wrote to *The Times* stating that he had recently had several cases of typhoid fever, which in his opinion were caused by oysters. This did much to impress public opinion. My own experience in agitating on the problem had some interesting episodes.

The logical difficulty raised in Mr. McKenna's question (p. 210) is interesting. The question suggested that, inasmuch as known sources of infection or the eating or drinking of sewage-contaminated food did not explain every case of typhoid fever, there remained some unknown cause or causes of this disease which might also explain the cases attributed by me to eating contaminated oysters or mussels.

There was at that time such an unknown or at least undetermined cause of typhoid fever, the existence of carrier cases, but this did not justify the rejection of the strong circumstantial evidence advanced on behalf of Brighton's contentions.

First, the circumstantial evidence adduced in the Brighton hearing was as conclusive as it could be in the then state of medical science. Secondly, in the practice of public health it is incumbent to act when the evidence satisfies common-sense deduction, even although it stops short of complete demonstration.

A further point could not be urged in 1896, but can now be stated. The history of enteric fever, as shown in the experience of Brighton and England since 1894, proves that the discovery of the importance of contaminated shell-fish and of unrecognised carrier cases—other sources of infection having been in large measure eliminated—has been a supremely important factor in the rapid diminution of this disease, amounting almost to its impending disappearance from most communities. This and other aspects of the shell-fish problem are discussed more fully in the contributions, the titles of which appear at the end of this chapter.

PERSONAL EPISODES

1. The fishermen of Southwick warned me of the physical risks I should incur if I visited their foreshore again.
2. In the second year of the persistent local agitation for which I was responsible, a lawyer, a member of the Town Council, gave an oyster supper to a party of about a dozen friends. He and several members of the public health committee, including its chairman (one of his guests at the supper), had been derisive in a friendly way of my oyster and mussel "fad." The supper was an oyster and champagne feast. Care had been exercised to obtain the oysters from a known safe source; but they ran short, and others were sent for from "round the corner." Within the next sixteen days three cases of

enteric fever were notified from guests of this supper-party. One of them, my chairman, was my patient in the Fever hospital; and no further opposition to my shell-fish recommendations was experienced in Brighton.

3. A London comic paper had a cartoon which was instructive and amusing.

When parliamentary powers to control the sale of shell-fish were refused, the only course open to us was publicity, which unfortunately might harm the vendors of good oysters as well as those who sold shell-fish known to be dangerous. Conspicuous boards were erected on the sea-beach at intervals with the inscription shown in the cartoon opposite. This cartoon depicts a disconsolate vendor of oysters, with his barrow stationed under one of these notices, wondering why trade was so bad! The inscription on the cartoon points out the disadvantage of not being able to read.

A large trade in shell-fish had been carried on from barrows on the beach; and it was not infrequent for me to receive letters from the M.O.H.s of distant parts of England giving particulars of typhoid fever cases apparently acquired in Brighton.

4. One evening I arrived early at a Masonic Lodge, the chaplain of which was the much respected Jewish Rabbi of the town; and as I knew that a lady who the previous week had died of typhoid fever was a member of his synagogue, I mentioned the case.

"Ah!" he remarked, "had she been a conforming Jew it would not have happened." I asked, "How is that?" He then took me to the Master's desk of the Lodge, and opened the Bible at Leviticus xi. 10–13, in which it is stated:

> whatsoever hath no fins nor scales in the water, that is an abomination unto you . . . ye shall not eat of their flesh.

WHY WAS BUSINESS SO SLACK?

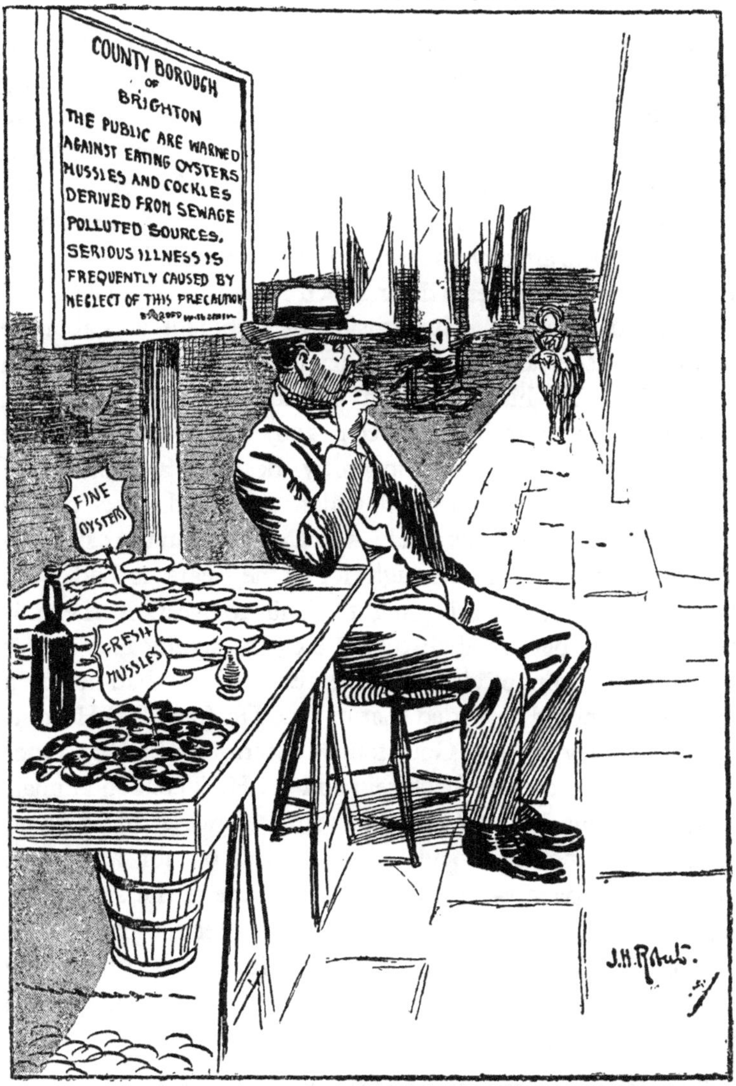
COUNTY BOROUGH
OF
BRIGHTON
THE PUBLIC ARE WARNED AGAINST EATING OYSTERS MUSSLES AND COCKLES DERIVED FROM SEWAGE POLLUTED SOURCES.
SERIOUS ILLNESS IS FREQUENTLY CAUSED BY NEGLECT OF THIS PRECAUTION
FINE OYSTERS
FRESH MUSSLES

A knowledge of reading is essential to all commercial enterprise. Our friend here depicted would never have taken up his present position if he had been able to read.

Diagram 5

Cartoon from a London weekly journal (name unknown)

CARRIER CASES

It is convenient to summarise the facts as to carriers at this point, although realisation of their importance in the history of typhoid fever belongs mainly to more recent years than 1908. Already the importance of apparently healthy carriers of infection in scarlet fever and diphtheria had been realised (p. 185); but R. Koch in 1902 first emphasised the importance not only of the already appreciated need for disinfection of the excreta of enteric patients during their illness and convalescence (p. 95), but also of the supervision of ambulant and abortive cases, and especially of those anomalous types often met with in children. At his suggestion bacteriological stations were instituted in various districts (see p. 206), and by the systematic examination of persons apparently healthy, a number of carrier cases were discovered which explained cases of the disease of unknown source. This was a new fact in the causation of enteric fever; for although for some years it had been known that typhoid bacilli might remain for years in the gall-bladder, or in periosteal abscesses, etc., the significance of this fact from the point of view of preventive medicine had not been realised. It should be added that in 1900 Dr. (now Sir) Horton-Smith Hartley in his Goulstonian Lectures (*Lancet*, 1900) quoted experiments of Blackstein and W. H. Welch on animals (*Johns Hopkins Hospital Bulletin*, 1891), showing that typhoid bacilli intravenously inoculated might live on for at least a hundred and twenty-eight days. An instance of the survival of the bacilli in a bone abscess for six years after the patient had recovered from an attack of enteric fever was quoted by H. S. Hartley, who also emphasised the frequency of typhoid bacilluria, and very appositely remarked as follows:

Truly no longer can we say with Dr. Budd (in *Typhoid Fever*, 1873, p. 100) that "by destroying the infectious powers of the intestinal discharges the disease may be in time extinguished." So far, indeed, from the stools being the only agents by means of which the disease is spread, they are but one of a series of agents. So far, too, from the patient ceasing to be a source of danger after his restoration to seeming health he may carry about in himself the seeds of infection for months or even years.

But these important facts were unknown or unappreciated, until Koch and his collaborators by amplifying them and by proving their value in field-work on a large scale brought the routine search for carriers into public health work, especially into such work for the prevention of typhoid fever. At the present time the search for a carrier—not only in typhoid but also in cases of food poisoning—is a routine procedure as soon as more obvious sources of infection have been eliminated.

Once wide attention was drawn to the chronic "carrier," and it was realised that he was not only a storehouse or reservoir but also a breeding-ground for the typhoid bacillus, doubts already felt as to the possibility of the typhoid bacillus living a prolonged life outside the human body increased, and it was generally accepted that although, as Delepine had shown, typhoid bacilli could be found in middens, for instance, for long periods, they did not multiply in the soil or in organic filth at ordinary temperatures. It was found that some human carriers were transitory vehicles of infection, others chronic; and that sometimes they infected single patients or families, and sometimes large groups of persons, through their handling of food and especially of milk. The histories of some outbreaks, as of that caused by a Strasburg baker's wife (reported in 1906) and of "Typhoid Mary" in New York (reported in 1907), are well known.

The story of the successive stages in the history of administrative control of typhoid fever is, I think, the most complete in the history of the application of preventive medicine in this country, additional knowledge acquired from careful field-work and from the laboratory bringing additional means for control within the reach of administrators.

The ultimate issue is that, except for "accidents" due to

oversight or carelessness, enteric fever has ceased to be an epidemic disease in England.

CONTRIBUTIONS

The Spread of Enteric Fever by Means of Sewage-Contaminated Shell-Fish (*Journal of the Sanitary Institute*, Vol. XVII, Part III, 1896).

The Spread of Enteric Fever and other Forms of Illness by Sewage-Polluted Shell-Fish. Contribution to section of State Medicine, B.M.A. meeting, Swansea, 1903 (*British Medical Journal*, August 8, 1903).

CHAPTER XXVI

THE NATURAL HISTORY OF RHEUMATIC FEVER

International investigation of prevalence—Separateness from "Rheumatism"—Epidemic years are years of small rainfall —Non-relation to dampness—Relation to soil conditions— Ground-water levels as an index

THE subject of rheumatic fever has intrigued me from my student days when (p. 44) I witnessed the dramatic curtailment of its clinical duration in patients treated by salicylate of soda. Then cases of rheumatic fever formed a considerable proportion of the patients in hospital wards; now they are relatively few; and while this change is due in part to rheumatic fever being treated at home with rapid success, it cannot be doubted, I think, that there has been a reduction in the prevalence of this disease in its typical form, namely that in which there is multiple arthritis.

Some preliminary investigations led me to propose this subject for four Milroy Lectures to the Royal College of Physicians in 1895. Had I known that my proposal would mean ten months of the hardest work ever experienced by me, I should have hesitated. The plan I outlined necessitated collecting statistics of the number of cases of rheumatic fever in hospitals in every part of the United Kingdom, and in every country of the world from which they were obtainable for a considerable series of years. This meant an immense correspondence; as I write I have before me the statistical returns sent me from the medical officers of these institutions in many countries as well as in Great Britain; and I cannot adequately express my obligations to so many confrères who were personally unknown to me. Cases of rheumatic fever are required to be notified weekly in Scandinavia, and by visiting the countries comprised in this name I was able to obtain returns of the incidence of this disease in the general population during a long series of years.

I may be permitted, in passing, to express regret that most of this valuable epidemiological statistical information remains unprinted. The *Lancet* published a full abstract of my lectures, and I could not expect more from a medical journal; but I think that now material valuable to epidemiological students would not be allowed to remain unavailable for future use.

It may interest a few to state that the sheet sent out by me asked for information as follows:

PLACE............................ NAME OF HOSPITAL....................

Year	Number of Cases of Acute and Sub-acute Rheumatism admitted to the Hospital	Total Number of Medical Cases (all Diseases) admitted to the Hospital

Figures were requested for all years from 1865 onwards. For some hospitals these were given, for most of them only for a shorter series of years. From the yearly medical reports of the metropolitan voluntary hospitals I was able to collect returns personally. Incidentally I realised the lack, still continuing, of a central controlling power which would enforce uniform methods of medical tabulation, though, of course, leaving complete freedom for unlimited extension of the minimum uniformity.

It will be noted that I obtained a return not only of cases of rheumatic fever, but also of the total number of medical cases admitted during each year. The proportion between these two was assumed by me to be fairly representative of the incidence of rheumatic fever each year, a not improbable assumption; at the least any discrepancies in this relation could scarcely obliterate evidence showing special epidemic years.

Even though, in consequence, this chapter may become unduly long, I propose to give some details of my Milroy Lectures, and of discussions in medical societies which followed.

The first need was a definition of rheumatic fever, and I deprecated the use of the words "acute" and "sub-acute rheumatism" as an alternative, although (to avoid omissions) I had been obliged to use the alternative form in soliciting statistical returns. The term "acute rheumatism" appears to suggest—a suggestion not based on clinical experience—that "chronic rheumatism" is the same disease which has become chronically persistent. A like objection holds to the term "rheumatic diseases." It would be a gain to medicine if we could erase the name "rheumatism" from all chronic forms of articular, muscular, and fibrous inflammation, which, so far as I know, are unrelated to articular rheumatic fever or to the cardiac lesions attributable to the virus of rheumatic fever. Although cases of rheumatic polyarthritis are now less frequent, there is still a vast amount of cardiac and pericardial inflammation which owes its origin, almost certainly, to the same virus, and these must continue to have a place in our picture of the syndrome of rheumatic fever. Including these the rheumatic virus still causes a vast amount of disabling disease.

In my Milroy Lectures, after preliminary definitions and a sketch of recorded epidemics of rheumatic fever, I drew attention to Dr. G. B. Longstaff's paper (*Trans. Epidem. Society*, 1880) in which he had shown the occurrence of four periods of excessive mortality from scarlet fever in England and Wales, associated more or less with a similar excess of "rheumatism accompanied with heart affection," erysipelas, pyæmia and puerperal fever. But hitherto there had been so far as I knew, "no wide and comprehensive investigation of the epidemiology of rheumatic fever." I then described the results of my own inquiries.

Dealing first with death-rates in England and Wales, I showed that the death-rate from rheumatism

In 1855	was	15	per cent	higher
in 1859	„	18	„	„
in 1869 and 1870	„	18	„	„
and in 1875	„	52	„	„

than in the respective years of minimum mortality next preceding each of the above years. This was preliminary evidence of cyclical prevalence. I then detailed the more trustworthy figures of cases derived from hospital experience. They are more reliable than death-returns because the case-mortality of rheumatic fever is low. In various hospitals its case-mortality has varied from 1 to nearly 4 per cent, being highest in children. I need not repeat here the argument used by me to justify hospital statistics of varying degrees of accuracy (see *Lancet*, March 9, 1895). Curves of annual cases treated in metropolitan hospitals showed a decreasing number of hospital cases proportional to total cases of sickness in these hospitals in the more recent years. Part of this I regarded as due to the easier and quicker cure in the more recent years by salicylates, facilitating home treatment. But this, as I pointed out, "did not invalidate conclusions drawn from the oscillations displayed by the downward curve."

Combining the picture from various metropolitan voluntary hospitals, it was clear that there were definite epidemics and inter-epidemic periods in London. The returns from provincial hospitals gave similar results, and were consistent with the returns from Scotland and Ireland.

In Scandinavia, practitioners, who are chiefly in the public service, are required to report periodically the nature of the cases of illness under their charge. The following diagram taken from a contribution to the *Royal Statistical Society's Transactions* (Vol. LIX, 1896) shows the course of events in Norway. Cases for each year have been calculated per 1,000 of population; and then, to make the curves more easily

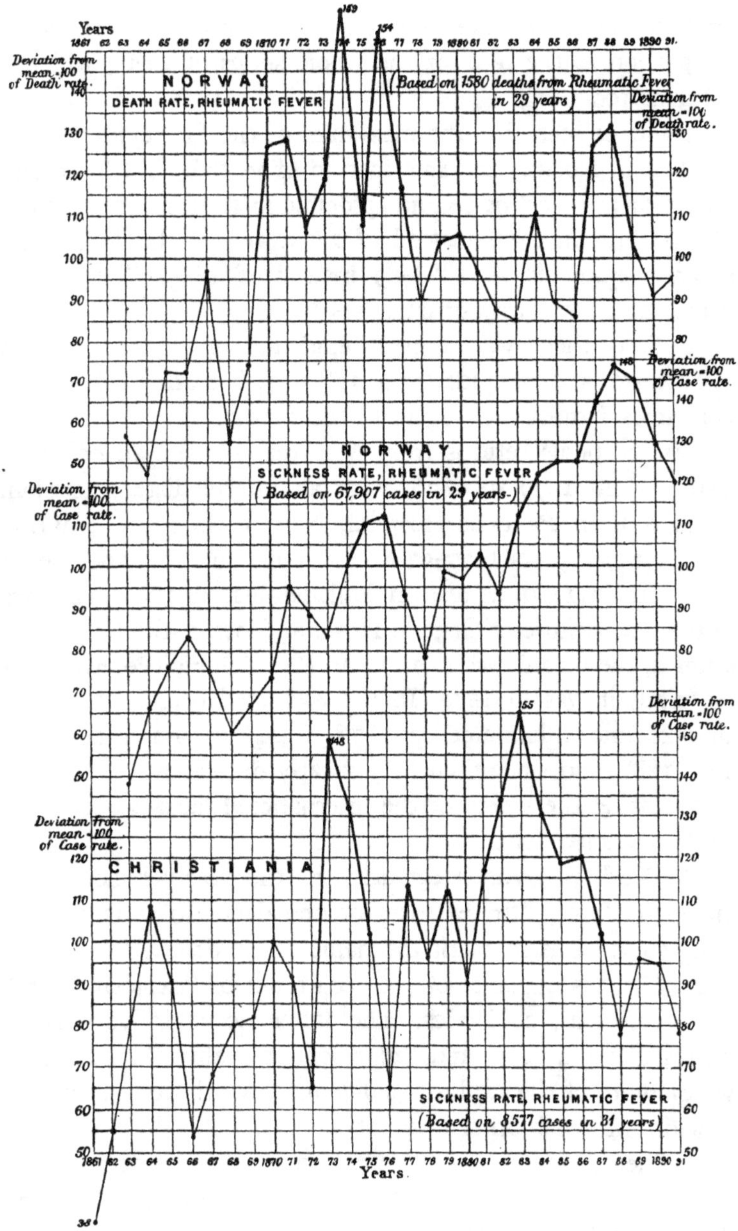

Diagram 6

Showing Yearly Incidence of Cases of Rheumatic Fever in Norway and Oslo (1861–91)

comparable, death-rates and case-rates have been stated in proportion to the rate for the whole series of years, which is taken as 100.

It will be seen that the maximum of the first epidemic was reached in Norway in 1866, instead of in 1864, in Christiania, its capital; that of the second epidemic in 1871 instead of 1870, of the third in 1876 instead of 1875, and of the fourth and greatest epidemic in 1888–89 instead of 1885. (See *Lancet*, March 1895, for further particulars.)

In Paris there was a great epidemic of rheumatic fever in 1874–76, and an epidemic in 1880–82. For other continental epidemics I must refer again to the *Lancet*.

Two hospitals returns from Montreal showed an epidemic lasting from 1870 to 1876, with an intermediate remission. Returns from Bellevue Hospital, New York, showed during the seventeen years 1877–93 a high point in 1877, and then a minimum in 1880, as also in Philadelphia. In the experience of the Massachusetts General Hospital, Boston, the first maximum in the record was in 1871. In Philadelphia (Pennsylvania Hospital) it was in 1870. In the Sydney Hospital (1874–92) an epidemic culminated in 1876. Cases remained excessive until 1881, and since then they greatly decreased.

Reviewing the whole of the international facts collected by me I concluded that:

(1) There is great irregularity in the yearly incidence of rheumatic fever, "the excesses of prevalence in certain years being so great as to merit the name of 'epidemic.'"

(2) There is evidence of the occurrence of "explosive" and of "protracted" epidemics. The latter occur in very large centres of population, and "represent in reality the fusion of two or more of the explosive epidemics, which do not exactly coincide with each other in point of time."

(3) There are certain favourite years for epidemics. In England these were 1855–56, 1859, 1864–65, 1868–71, 1874–76, 1884–85, 1888, and 1893. In other countries the same years are frequently characterised by epidemics, but in some instances

there is an anticipation or lagging behind the years of epidemic rheumatic fever in England.

The argument as to the infective character of rheumatic fever was summarised as follows:

(1) The clinical features of the disease and its analogy with recognised specific febrile diseases indicate that it belongs to the same group. The mode of onset, the frequent occurrence of preliminary sore throat, and the course of the fever point in this direction. It shares its tendency to relapse with such diseases as influenza, enteric fever, scarlet fever, and diphtheria.

(2) The liability to second and later attacks does not preclude this conception of the disease. There is among diseases admittedly infective a regular scale of immunity following a first attack, ranging from smallpox, in which it is nearly absolute, through enteric fever and scarlet fever, in which it is feebler, to diphtheria, in which immunity is evanescent, and down to erysipelas, in which one attack appears to predispose to further attacks. Rheumatic fever comes at this end of the scale.

(3) Nor can it be said that the liability to family inheritance argues against the infective character of rheumatic fever. A special proclivity in certain families to diphtheria, enteric fever, and scarlet fever is probable. That a special proclivity is required to develop the virus of rheumatic fever when it has gained entrance may be agreed, but this does not preclude its infective character, any more than in the analogous case of erysipelas.

(4) The apparent absence of infection from patient to patient is explicable by the fact that the contagion is buried in the infected joints. Direct personal infection is relatively rare in typhoid fever and cholera, in which diseases the contagion has exit from the patient. It is likely that the majority of the micro-organisms causing rheumatic fever pay for their hardihood in invading the closed synovial cavities by securing a sepulture in their cells.

(5) The fact that the joints are the common seat of the trouble favours the infective theory. As Dr. J. F. Payne has put it, the

"vessels of the synovia of the joints appear to have some special proclivity to form a nidus for the wandering germs of disease."

(6) The therapeutics of the disease confirms the same view. The almost specific power of salicin in rheumatic fever is comparable to that of quinine in malaria and of mercury in syphilis.

My investigations showed that although rheumatic fever appears to be almost ubiquitous in temperate countries, it varies greatly in extent in different countries. I made an estimate as to the average annual number of cases of rheumatic fever in London, basing the estimate on the known case-mortality in metropolitan hospitals and the death-rate from rheumatic fever in the general population. On this basis there were on average 3·5 cases per 1,000 of population in each year, a figure regarded by me as an under-estimate. The data showed also that rheumatic fever is more an urban than a rural disease.

DAMPNESS AND RHEUMATIC FEVER

That dampness of air and of soil and excessive prevalence of rheumatism are related is so generally accepted that most textbooks of medicine and hygiene have enshrined and endorsed it. And yet the statistical evidence contradicts the view that the prevalence of rheumatic fever is favoured by these conditions. The evidence I collected in Great Britain and in foreign countries all confirms the conclusion that a heavy annual rainfall is usually associated with a low amount of rheumatic fever, and a small rainfall with an excessive amount of rheumatic fever, though no exact proportion between the two factors can be predicated. It is certain, however, that two or three years of deficient or excessive rainfall are more potent than a single year. I have arrived at a somewhat similar conclusion with regard to diphtheria. These data, during the period investigated, represented actual facts in the natural history of these diseases. There are minor differences between the two diseases. Thus comparison of the Christiania curve of annual rainfall with those of the annual sickness rates from diphtheria and rheumatic fever appears to show that a longer series of dry years is required to produce a great epidemic of diphtheria than of rheumatic fever. The latter disease becomes more regularly and more quickly epidemic than the former in cycles of dry years.

It may be that the supposed analogy between malaria and rheumatic fever has been in part responsible for the common notion that wetness is a cause of rheumatic fever. But the miasmatic view of the causation of malaria has disappeared, since we have known that infected mosquitoes are solely responsible for its spread; and there is even less justification for retaining a miasmatic conception of the causation of rheumatic fever. The confusion introduced by giving the same name to the chronic forms of "rheumatism" and rheumatic fever is probably the chief cause of this serious error. The mental evolution of the idea that "damp" produces or aggravates rheumatism may be illustrated and perhaps partially explained in the words of the old familiar rhyme enumerating the signs of on-coming rain:

> The distant hills are seeming nigh,
>
> . . . .
>
> Low o'er the grass the swallow wings.

Some lines lower the rhyme gives the pathological sign that

> Old Betty's joints are on the rack.

The reasoning would be as follows:

With changes of weather joints become painful.
These pains are "rheumatic" in character.
Hence damp and wet favour the onset of "rheumatism."

The inference would proceed:

But rheumatic fever is simply an acute form of "rheumatism."
Hence rheumatic fever must be favoured by wet weather.

It is but a step further in this growth of a doctrine to suppose that inasmuch as dampness favours rheumatism, a damp soil must have the same effect, and that, for instance, a clay soil is more conducive to attacks of rheumatic fever than a gravel soil.

The primary error consists in assuming that there is any pathological or etiological relationship between the heterogeneous diseases known as chronic rheumatism and the specific febrile disease, rheumatic fever.

THE INFLUENCE OF SOIL CONDITIONS

My investigation showed that epidemics of rheumatic fever occur in years of minimum rainfall. Thus they occur in years in which the soil is exceptionally dry and the ground-water exceptionally low. It is open to doubt whether rainfall or level of ground-water forms the better index for forecasting the amount of rheumatic fever which may be anticipated. The effect of deficient rainfall is not produced immediately. It takes time to develop, and in my Milroy Lectures I concluded that "the influence of deficient rainfall is exerted chiefly as the result of its effect on the subsoil, this effect usually showing itself by a marked lowering of the ground-water." Low ground-water was regarded by me as leading to excessive rheumatic fever, *not by any essential causative relationship between the two.* The low ground-water, it was held, was an indication of certain conditions of dryness and temperature of the subsoil, which greatly favoured the life-history of the contagium of rheumatic fever.

This being so, it is conceivable that low ground-water, when through collateral circumstances it is unassociated with the required conditions of temperature, etc., may not be accompanied by an increase of rheumatic fever, though, on the contrary, a high ground-water is not accompanied by excessive rheumatic fever.[1]

In discussing my lectures the constancy of the seasonal curve was considered by Dr. (afterwards Sir William) Church "to be opposed to the theory advanced by Dr. Newsholme of a connection between the prevalence of rheumatic fever and of

[1] Milroy Lecture, 1885, *Lancet*, March 16, 1895, p. 661.

a low level of ground-water. I cannot think that London, where the bulk of the rain that falls runs off on the surface, and where the subsoil is drained by railway tunnels, and cuttings, and sewers, can have any great variations in the level of the ground-water; or that for twenty-one years it should vary so uniformly."

In reply to these comments I pointed out that rheumatic fever shares its fairly regular seasonal incidence with other diseases, like diphtheria, scarlet fever, and enteric fever, the prevalence of which also is favoured by dry years, associated with relatively dry and warm subsoil and low ground-water. But it was not intended to imply that level of subsoil water is the only factor at work. Thus I showed that in Munich the steady lowering of the ground-water caused by the sewerage, etc., had not been followed by an increase of rheumatic fever. Furthermore, in certain soils, e.g. at Christiania, there is no continuous ground-water.

The level of the ground-water is simply a convenient index, and in my view probably the best index, when it can be ascertained, of certain conditions of the soil favouring the extra-corporeal life[1] of the hypothetical microbe of rheumatic fever.

In the Milroy Lectures I speculated as to how and why dry years favour the causation of epidemic rheumatic fever as follows: Direct infection from patient to patient is rare, if it occurs.

It seems most feasible to regard rheumatic fever as essentially a soil disease, due to a saprophytic soil organism, which is "drowned out" in wet years, multiplies rapidly in dry years, and is transferred to the human recipient by unknown means. Possibly dust convection accounts for a large proportion of the cases. In dry years the number of contagious particles is probably increased, and the facility with which they are communicated to the human subject is similarly increased. In the light of our recently acquired knowledge of the methods of infection in malaria, it is not, perhaps, too far-fetched to

---

[1] I should not now dogmatise on the extra-corporeal life of the virus of rheumatic fever. It may be that the external conditions named above affect the intra-corporeal vitality of this virus.

surmise that inoculation of the contagium of rheumatic fever may be caused by domestic vermin, or that the house-fly may convey it to milk or other foods. Perhaps bacteriology in a few years will throw important light on what, for want of more accurate knowledge, can at present be only guessed at.

The influence of soil conditions on disease has been further discussed in Chapter XIV, but I may here give some miscellaneous notes of discussions on the causation of rheumatic fever which followed the Milroy Lectures in 1895.

At the annual meeting of the British Medical Association in July 1895, Dr. W. B. Cheadle, then Physician to St. Mary's Hospital, London, in a thoughtful paper introduced a discussion on Rheumatic Fever. He drew attention to the statistics given in my Milroy Lectures which showed in hospital experience a remarkable similarity in the seasonal and annual curves of chorea and rheumatic fever, and in the fact that both are preponderantly urban diseases. He added:

> Dr. Newsholme's researches bring out another curious fact, namely, that acute rheumatism is most prevalent in dry seasons when the rainfall is exceptionally scanty, the ground-water at its lowest. So that a dry, hot season, and if two follow in succession, the second, is the most productive of acute rheumatism; negativing the popular association of it with damp and cold, and in this respect the general canon that a persistently low ground-water is healthy, a persistently high ground-water unhealthy. This, however, is not incompatible with the view that chill is a factor of the disease. It is under such conditions of dry air that rapid cooling of the surface of the body by evaporation occurs, especially on free perspiration after exercise.

Reference has already been made to Dr. G. B. Longstaff's data (1880). In 1905 he read a further article "A Contribution to the Etiology of Rheumatic Fever" (*Transactions of the Epidemiological Society*, N.S., Vol. XXIV, 1904–5), which was followed by an interesting discussion. Dr. Longstaff drew attention to the fact that the annual mortality from rheumatic fever, as well as of scarlet fever, erysipelas, and puerperal fever, all showed a downward tendency, and gave no support to the old idea that rheumatic fever "is mainly caused by cold, wet, or chills." He concluded that most of the diseases just enumerated "show a rough inverse relationship to rainfall."

In my personal contribution to this discussion, I once more drew attention to the possible error involved in attempting to determine the epidemiology of rheumatic fever from deaths alone, in view of the fact that the fatality (case-mortality) of this disease commonly is only 1 to 2 per cent. I also indicated the fallacies involved in stating average death-rates for a series of years or for an entire country or county. "Such a method," I said, "tends to behead the peaks of the epidemics, and to elevate the valleys, and generally to conceal the true incidence of the disease."

Referring once more to the relation of soil moisture to prevalence of rheumatic fever, and the criticism that in cities modern drainage, etc., had made it improbable that any inverse causal relation could exist between these, I remarked:

> My contention is that the level of the subsoil water is merely an index, and I believe the most satisfactory index, we have; much more so than the inverse rainfall. The same conditions may obtain in the absence of the subsoil water as in its presence: just as the works of a clock may still go on even if the hands are removed. The hands of the clock are represented by the subsoil water, which is a very convenient index; but the dry and warm condition of the soil favouring rheumatic fever may be there, even in the absence of the index.
>
> . . . . .
>
> Of course, both Longstaff's and my own investigations deal only with secondary causes—the real cause being microbic. But in getting at the facts which will enable us to prevent the spread of a disease, it sometimes happens that we are able to discover and counteract the general conditions which favour the prevalence of the disease more easily than to prevent the action of the micro-organism itself. Moreover, we cannot be said to know the natural history of any disease until we know not only the *causa causans*, but also those efficient causes, such as climatic conditions, in the absence of which the disease does not become epidemic.

So far as I know no great advance has been made in recent years in our knowledge of the essential causation of rheumatic fever. In its typical clinical form it has declined to a remarkable extent, and thus it comes within the category of diminishing diseases, of the cause of whose decrease we have no exact or complete knowledge.

The decline of some diseases we can reasonably attribute to improved personal and communal hygiene. This is especially true of epidemic diarrhœa and typhoid fever; and probably the decline of erysipelas is explicable by the practice of Listerism in surgery and to some extent in domestic life.

There may be reasonable differences of opinion as to the cause of the great reduction in the death-rate from scarlet fever. Although other factors are also concerned, it is probable that cyclical changes in virulence of its contagium are a chief factor; and it may be that the same is true concerning rheumatic fever in its typical manifestations. But I cannot personally doubt that increased attention to the hygiene and surgical care of the naso-pharynx and of the teeth has borne an important share in producing this important effect on the rheumatic virus, and also in improving health conditions in many other respects.

CONTRIBUTIONS

The Milroy Lectures to the Royal College of Physicians on the Natural History and Affinities of Rheumatic Fever: A Study in Epidemiology (*Lancet*, March 9 and 15, 1895).

Rheumatic Fever: Contribution to the Discussion in *Transactions of the Epiidemological Society* (Vol. XXIV, 1904–5).

CHAPTER XXVII

MAN AND ANIMAL DISEASES

Review of history of prevention—Glanders—Hydrophobia—Tetanus—Anthrax—Undulant Fever

REVIEW OF HISTORY OF PREVENTION

Communicable diseases, as has already been urged, still remain one of the chief concerns of public health workers; and of these, diseases communicated to man by animals have much importance.

There is an impression shared by some hygienists that direct prevention of the communication of infection is subordinate, for many diseases, to hygienic measures for increasing the powers of resistance to pathogenic microbes. This may become true in the future. Even now the recently acquired power to prevent rickets, and to a large extent dental defects, by affording to the expectant mother and her infant adequate sunlight and air with an improved dietary, are illustrations of possible vast future extensions of prevention of disease and improvement in the standard of health, aside from any prevention of infection.

But, writing in 1934, it can be said that such success as has hitherto been experienced in the prevention of disease has been predominantly by blocking the channels of infection from man to man or from animals to man.

The triumphs of Listerism over septic infections form the greatest example of this; and further striking examples are afforded by the disappearance of cholera and typhus from Western countries, and by the obsolescence of typhoid and diarrhœal infections.

Respiratory infections form the sad exception to success in blocking infection. Measles, by the prophylactic use of serum from a former measles patient, may ere long be removed from the list of exceptions; diphtheria already has disappeared, at least potentially, from the list; but among acute febrile diseases, influenza and allied acute catarrhal infections remain almost uncontrolled, and their spread appears likely to continue uncontrolled, except by the adoption of personal precautions which few of us are willing or able to carry out efficiently.

In following chapters I shall give considerations on one of the two most formidable chronic infectious diseases, syphilis and tuberculosis, of Britain, which still remain only partially controlled. Both these diseases may persist for years before they end in recovery or death. The discussion on syphilis must be postponed to a later volume, as the chief public health struggle against it belongs to years more recent than 1908. So, likewise, I must postpone the more recent efforts to control tuberculosis. In this chapter I give a few notes on other animal-derived human diseases which in my lifetime have come partially or entirely under control.

Glanders has never been a serious cause of human deaths in England; in the earlier years of my professional life it was occasionally transmitted to man. During the ten years 1919–28 only four deaths were registered in England and Wales as due to this disease, and it has now disappeared. Horses have ceased to be a chief means of transport, and the use of mallein (corresponding to tuberculin) in diagnosis has also been an important factor in bringing about the disappearance of this disease.

Hydrophobia has become extinct in this country. I have only seen one case of this terrible disease, which was being treated in St. Thomas's Hospital when I was a medical student. In 1881 hydrophobia was responsible for thirty-four and in 1885 for sixty deaths in England and Wales. Since 1903 its column in the Registrar-General's statistics remains an annual blank, and for this magnificent demonstration of successful blocking of infection Mr. Walter (later Lord) Long has the credit. The action taken was the Muzzling Order in 1896, rigidly enforced during that year, and in that year and continuously since, the enforcement of a six months' quarantine for any dog introduced into Britain from overseas. Human hydrophobia disappeared from the British Isles; and only two or three cases of the corresponding disease, rabies, in dogs have occurred, due to the smuggling of dogs into the country by aeroplane. Against this disease there is a double line of defence; the first is indicated above. On the second, prophylactic vaccination, as developed by Pasteur, it is unnecessary to enlarge; its importance is much greater in Continental countries than in Great Britain where rigid quarantine of dogs from abroad is practicable.

Tetanus is still a cause of considerable mortality in England and Wales. In the ten years 1919–28, 1,530 deaths were registered from this disease, as compared with 2,250 (for a smaller population) in the ten years 1903–12. Some of this reduction is ascribable to the increasing use of tetanus antitoxin after accidents; and the use of this antitoxin in the Great War, 1914–18, doubtless saved many lives (see also p. 130). The late Sir Thomas Legge (1863–1932) in *Industrial Maladies*, Oxford Medical Publications, 1934, a volume published posthumously, has drawn attention to fatal cases of tetanus, of which eleven occurred in the ten years 1890–99 in Dundee. Five of these worked in jute mills, and in several other cases there was possible dust contact with these mills. Legge had the dust examined, and it was found that "tetanus bacilli must be present in incredible numbers in much of the dust in jute mills." The relation of tetanus and jute is similar to that of anthrax and wool, except that, as Legge pointed out, tetanus "cannot be brought about, like anthrax, by inhalation, nor does it develop, as a rule, in a wound except as a result of mixed infection." Legge recalls the fact that the poison in the poisoned spears of Solomon Islanders is given them by dipping the points into mud which is a pure culture of tetanus bacilli.

The above volume should be widely known. It gives the main results of Legge's life-work in industrial hygiene, a branch of public health work with which medical officers of health are too little associated in their daily work. I recall with pleasure that some of Legge's earliest work in public health work was done in Brighton.

Anthrax, though a declining cause of death, is still a source of anxiety, especially in certain industries. In the ten years 1919–28 it was responsible for 112 deaths in England and Wales, as compared with 170 in 1903–12. The life-history of the anthrax bacillus is a most important part of the history of scientific bacteriology. It was worked out by Robert Koch in the year 1876, when he was a general medical practitioner in East Prussia. In later years I heard the late Dr. William H. Welch (1850–1934) of Baltimore, Maryland, describe how, when he was a student with Cohn, of Breslau, in 1876, Robert Koch, then twenty-three years old, came to the laboratory and demonstrated his new culture methods and the complete life-history of the anthrax bacillus. His discoveries on anthrax not only elucidated the causation of this particular disease, but along with the work of Pasteur on parallel lines, initiated the extension of protective vaccination to a considerable group of diseases.

When my home was in Bradford during 1874–80, "wool-sorters' disease" was a not infrequent cause of fatal pneumonia among those engaged in sorting wool, especially wool coming from Asia Minor and Persia. In 1879 Dr. J. H. Bell of Bradford first proved the identity of anthrax in man and animals, by transmitting anthrax from man to animals. Pneumonic anthrax was due to the inhalation of the spores of anthrax derived from the wool of sheep during the sorting process. With the adoption of disinfection of the wool, and methods of exhaust ventilation, thus removing the dust from the workers' bench, it has nearly disappeared.

The same disease, in the form of malignant pustule, may occur in those handling hides from diseased animals. One case I remember in Brighton. A railway worker was found to have malignant pustule in the neck. Investigation showed he had been carrying on his shoulder trusses of hay, which had travelled in a railway truck still blood-stained from hides previously conveyed in the same truck. This patient had probably been inoculated with a blood-stained spicule of the hay.

In another instance a very competent sanitary inspector on my staff noticed a number of hides, on one of which the blood-stains appeared to be unusually dark and "tarry." Not having an outfit with him, he brought smears of the blood spread on some broken glass to the municipal laboratory, and in them I found anthrax bacilli. The inspector's keen observation led to the discovery of an unnotified outbreak of anthrax on a farm some miles from Brighton.

Once more extending my recollections to a more recent year than 1908, the year ending the story covered by this volume, I may mention the anthrax (malignant pustule) acquired during the Great War by a not inconsiderable number of laymen and soldiers, which was traced to the shaving brushes used by them. Attention was drawn to this possibility by a case of anthrax found in a patient at a metropolitan hospital by Dr. Elworthy (*Lancet*, 1915); and shortly afterwards several cases were reported in soldiers. Altogether nineteen cases among civilians were reported on in 1917 by my colleague, Dr. F. J. H. Coutts, C.B., of the medical staff of the Local Government Board. The malignant pustule in all the cases was on a shaved surface of skin; in one instance it was on the left forearm, which had been used for temporary placing of the lather derived from the man's shave. The shaving brushes from several consignments were examined, and found to contain the spores of anthrax bacilli. The suspicion was entertained by some that the shaving brushes had been deliberately infected by the Germans; for pre-War shaving brushes appeared to be mainly of Teutonic origin. But, in fact, the cases were due to the absence of German shaving brushes! In lieu of these, shaving brushes were being imported from Japan and other countries; and the pigs' and other bristles used for manufacturing the brushes were obtained from countries in which anthrax prevailed, while no adequate disinfection of the bristles had been effected. Once the source of infection was discovered and existing consignments of shaving brushes had been confiscated, anthrax from this source abruptly ceased.

Undulant Fever, perhaps better known as Malta or Mediterranean fever, was formerly a chief cause of invalidism among British soldiers in Malta, and I recall hearing an after-dinner speech by Mr. (later Lord) Haldane to a number of sanitarians, when he was Minister of War, a few years before the Great War. He described how he had recently been present at a ball in a large empty ward of a military hospital in Malta, which in past days was filled with soldiers suffering from this endemic plague of the island. Its prevalence ceased when Bruce, following up W. H. Horrocks' discovery of *Micrococcus melitensis* in the milk of goats demonstrated the same organism in the blood of patients and produced the disease experimentally in animals. As soon as the drinking of uncooked goats' milk ceased the disease disappeared.

It may be added that more recent events show that the same disease prevails in many countries, and that contagious abortion in cattle—also a frequent disease—is due to an almost identical organism. The relationship between these two organisms is being closely investigated.

CHAPTER XXVIII

HUMAN TUBERCULOSIS OF BOVINE ORIGIN

The old controversy as to direct and indirect means of control —Infection from meat and milk—The beneficence of Koch's great error—Past disproportion between prevention of bovine and human sources of infection

THE most important disease transmissible from animals to man is tuberculosis.

From the standpoint of prevention of human disease it is unnecessary to consider tuberculosis of other animals than bovines. When the tubercle bacillus was discovered by Koch in 1882, as Dr. J. S. Fulton put it, "A child of great promise had quickened in the womb of time." How strange that even in this period of relatively advanced modern science Koch's discovery only very slowly led to effective action against a great enemy of mankind! Even now direct action against the bacillus is too often placed in a secondary position, and removal of conditions which "make the bed" for tuberculosis are regarded as being alone essential. In practice the two lines of attack are one and indivisible. When direct attack against the bacillus was advised, greater emphasis was laid during many years on the avoidance of milk and meat from tuberculous cattle than on the prevention of infection from human consumptives. The underlying assumption was that tubercle bacilli producing disease in cattle and in mankind were identical.

In my earlier official life is seen some of the same disproportionate devotion to the prevention of bovine infection. On page 155 I have recounted activities in meat inspection which threatened to end my career as a medical officer of health. In several instances the associated local butchers called in "expert witnesses" in rebuttal of my application to have a carcase of a tuberculous beast condemned; and I found myself faced with contradictory evidence from my seniors in the public health service. One of these seniors, I recall, chewed some of the flesh under adjudication in the presence of the stipendiary magistrate with whom the fate of the carcase rested! Gradually objection to condemnation on account of tuberculosis ceased, especially after the statement of rules given by the first Royal Commission on Tuberculosis, which were published in 1898. I had given evidence before this Commission, and I find on reference to the Report that I answered one hundred and seventeen questions asked by various Commissioners. In reporting to the Town Council of Brighton in May of that year I stated, with what I hope was pardonable self-righteousness:

> I have gone carefully through the official notes of the condition of the carcases in the cases brought before the Brighton magistrates in the past, and am happy to find that we have (in our action) anticipated the recommendations of the Royal Commission.

I went on to express my satisfaction that the local bench of magistrates had acted on the recommendation of the M.O.H. some years before the official standard had been laid down, adding a further expression of satisfaction that "for the last four years it has not been necessary to contest a single case of tuberculous meat before the magistrates."

But it was already realised that the chief risk of tuberculosis from bovines was from the drinking of uncooked cows' milk; and I quoted the Commission's Report as to the futility of the powers then possessed to prevent this. The position is now somewhat improved; but bovine tuberculosis still prevails extensively among our herds of cattle, and—notwithstanding efforts, sometimes having a measure of success at its partial local elimination—I might instance extensive work undertaken in Birmingham and Manchester—the only means of ensuring a safe milk supply at an expenditure within the reach of the mass of the people are by efficient pasteurisation of milk by the farmer or the wholesale agent, by domestic boiling of milk, or by limiting the family supply of milk to desiccated and powdered milk. So fully is this realised that at the time of writing (1934) there is a general consensus of conviction among those who understand the practical difficulties of eliminating bovine tuberculosis that all fresh cows' milk consumed by human beings should be pasteurised, and that there should be a general enactment requiring this.

But is bovine tuberculosis responsible for much human tuberculosis? The almost universal answer to this question was affirmative for many years until Robert Koch delivered his famous address, to which—and the subsequent discussion on it—I listened. This address was given to a crowded audience in London on July 23, 1901, at the meeting of the British Congress on Tuberculosis.

In the earlier part of his address Koch emphasised the lesson, which is now more generally appreciated than it was in 1901, that "it is a great blunder to treat pestilences uniformly"; and having illustrated this from international experience of plague and cholera he proceeded to discuss the problem as to "the transmission of the germ of tuberculosis from tuberculous animals to man . . . [which is] generally regarded nowadays as proved." He then detailed experiments proving that healthy cattle when inoculated with tubercle bacilli from human sputum suffered no ill effect; but that active disease resulted when similar cattle were inoculated with tubercle bacilli derived from the lungs of cattle suffering from tuberculosis. Koch therefore concluded that bovine tuberculosis is not easily transmissible to man, and went on to doubt that the milk of tuberculous cows was dangerous for children. Obviously in testing this contention direct experimental evidence on human beings was inadmissible; but although Koch said "the important question whether man is susceptible to bovine tuberculosis is not yet absolutely decided," he contended that "if such a susceptibility really exists, the infection of human beings is but a very rare occurrence." He then proceeded to emphasise—as we now all agree—that "the only main source of the infection of tuberculosis is the sputum" (we should now add whether in spray during coughing or inhaled in dust) "of consumptive patients." His cogent remarks in developing this dictum will receive further comment (p. 265); but now we may note the reception of his statement that the risk of human infection from bovines by meat or milk was minimal or absent.

The statement produced a profound sensation, and was at once challenged after his address. Lord Lister, in proposing a vote of thanks to Koch, emphasised the debt which humanity owed him. "Thanks to Koch we now know the enemy we have to deal with, while, thanks to Pasteur, we know that this microbe is incapable of originating *de novo* in the human body."

Lord Lister added "that the evidence which Dr. Koch has brought before us, that human tuberculosis cannot be communicated to the bovine species, seems exceedingly conclusive" . . . "the converse proposition that bovine tuberculosis is incapable of development in man is a totally different one," and he agreed with Koch's suggestion that "a matter of such enormous importance should be established by further inquiry." He was followed by Nocard, Bang, and Sims Woodhead, who expressed similar doubts; and the Congress before dispersing passed two resolutions expressing the view that there should be no relaxation of effort to prevent the spread of tuberculosis by milk and meat, and that it was expedient for the British Government to institute an inquiry into the doubts thrown on the identity of human and bovine tuberculosis. The first recommendation was endorsed in a circular of advice to local authorities issued in September 1901 by the Local Government Board, and soon afterwards a Royal Commission was appointed to investigate the relationship between bovine and human tuberculosis. Sir Michael Foster was its first chairman, and on his death Sir William Power, my predecessor at the Local Government Board, succeeded him. To Power's guidance and scientific acumen the experiments made during a series of years on an experimental farm owe much of their value. Theobald Smith in America had already established that human and bovine tubercle bacilli should be classed as separate types or races of one species. I need not particularise the morphological and cultural differences between these types, which were further investigated by the workers of the Royal Commission. As concerns power to produce human disease, it was found both by the Royal Commission and by German and American observers that tubercle bacilli of the bovine type are sometimes responsible for human tuberculosis but very rarely for pulmonary phthisis, the most frequent and most fatal form of tuberculosis in man.

In one series of observations Dr. A. S. Griffith found that in tuberculosis of cervical glands 49 per cent, in lupus 52 per cent, in scrofulodermia 36 per cent, in bone and joints 19 per cent, and in pulmonary cases 2·6 per cent of cases examined had been infected with the bovine type of tubercle bacillus. So that even in the relatively minor forms of death from tuberculosis only a minority had a bovine source.

I confess that when Koch gave his announcement at the London Congress in 1901 I rejoiced; for although it put out of focus the needed precautions against bovine infection, it gave a quietus, badly needed, to the widespread view that preventive medicine should direct its chief attention to infection of bovine source. Some of the previous emphasis on bovine infection may have been unconsciously actuated by fear of those more advanced workers who were agitating in favour of active work to prevent human infection, an agitation which was regarded by the majority of physicians and in Governmental circles as likely to be prejudicial to the interest of consumptives.

Two illustrations can be given. They are taken from the Harben Lectures on "The Administrative Control of Tuberculosis," by Sir R. Thorne Thorne, the distinguished Principal Medical Officer of the Local Government Board (Baillière, 1899). On page 16 Thorne states:

> I am, indeed . . . convinced that the main vehicle by which tubercular infection is conveyed to the digestive tract is to be found in . . . meat and milk.

Even for non-pulmonary forms of tuberculosis this is not strictly correct; but the statement gave accurately the impressions of its date.

On page 72 of the same book allusion is made to a meeting in December 1898, presided over by the then Prince of Wales, to inaugurate the work since done by the National Association for the Prevention of Consumption (see also p. 248). Thorne was struck, he wrote, by the "absolute unanimity" among the speakers at this meeting on two points, namely:

(1) That the greatest danger which man incurs of receiving the tubercular infection lies in the use of milk from tuberculous cows; and
(2) That the best chance of destroying the tubercular infection when once received into the lungs is by treatment in the "open air."

It is clear that in Britain, although Koch's discovery of the tubercle bacilli dated back to 1882, leading medical opinion in 1898–1902 regarded infection from milk as the chief enemy; although others, including the writer, regarded this as of secondary importance and were active propagandists in favour of direct action against pulmonary tuberculosis by administrative measures designed to control the spread of infections from phthisical patients.

In concluding this chapter mention should be made of the possibility that tuberculous cows' milk imbibed in childhood may be the source of pulmonary tuberculosis in adolescent or adult life, the bovine tubercle bacilli losing their racial characteristics and becoming transformed by long habitation in human tissues into the variety or race which is regarded as human. To this problem the English Royal Commission devoted itself, and experiments were made over long years on animals, with consistently negative results. I need not enter into details; but the unavoidable conclusion is that public health officials must concern themselves chiefly—of course not exclusively—with infection from human consumptives, if human tuberculosis is to be brought completely under control. This would be so even were it agreed that the transmutation of tubercle bacilli from the bovine into the human type occurs after long years in the human tissues, for we know that human consumptives are also a source of human infection, and that for practical purposes control of infection of human origin is needed. Happily, universal pasteurisation is a certain preventive of infection from milk, and for infection from human sources it is equally true that the oft-repeated or massive infection required to produce active human tuberculosis in all except perhaps infants and very young children can be and is being increasingly prevented. This is so whatever view may be taken of circumstances auxiliary to infection, of which more will be said hereafter.

I specify "oft-repeated or massive" infection, for all available evidence indicates that the vast majority of mankind in civilised communities possess some measure of natural or acquired immunity against tuberculosis. The degree of this resistance varies in different persons and may vary in the same person from time to time; and the duty of social and medical workers is to minimise infection, so that while nearly all are tuberculised in a minor degree the dosage of infectious material shall not suffice to excite active disease.

Koch's main contention that bovine tuberculosis was not a source of human tuberculosis was an error; but, as I have already suggested, his error was followed by, and I believe was instrumental in leading to, a rapid extension of measures against human sources of infection.

The facts show that the bovine variety can infect man and is responsible for perhaps one-fourth of the human cases of non-pulmonary tuberculosis. These relatively to pulmonary tuberculosis are a minor source of deaths. It cannot be said that the two varieties of tubercle bacillus never mutate. They probably do so; but the evidence is against the hypothesis that this occurs within the short lifetime of a human host.

CHAPTER XXIX

THE NOTIFICATION OF TUBERCULOSIS

Niven and Biggs—Degree of infectivity of tuberculosis—Fear of harm to patient by notification—History repeats itself re *notification—Advocacy of voluntary notification—Official and unofficial obstacles—Action of the Society of* M.O.H.*—Notification only a means to an end—To be adopted if consequential measures practicable—Brighton and Sheffield—Step sof action of Government—Irrelevant postscript: is Parturition a disease?*

THE bibliography at the end of the next chapter shows the extent of my interest in tuberculosis over long years. I cannot hope to give a satisfactory summary of my experience and writings in these chapters, but must refer the reader to my *Prevention of Tuberculosis*, 1908, for a more complete statement. I propose here, frankly, to narrate chiefly the stages of my own share in securing various reforms; and even this only partially, for the main advances occurred after 1908, when I became Principal Medical Officer of the Central Health Authority. An account of these later stages must be reserved.

Although in England chief stress continued to be laid in the years preceding 1908 on the prevention of bovine tuberculosis, this was not so among many medical officers of health in Britain and in America, nor in Germany in which the sanatorium movement had its beginnings on a considerable scale.

Dr. James Niven was an early pioneer in efforts against tuberculosis both bovine and of human sources, and no account of the human side of this work would be complete which did not honour his name. Dr. Hermann Biggs, who held the post of medical officer to the City of New York, also needs to be specially mentioned. His photograph faces this page.

As soon as it became recognised that tuberculosis is a communicable disease, and in that respect resembles the acute infectious diseases, the notification of which after a prolonged

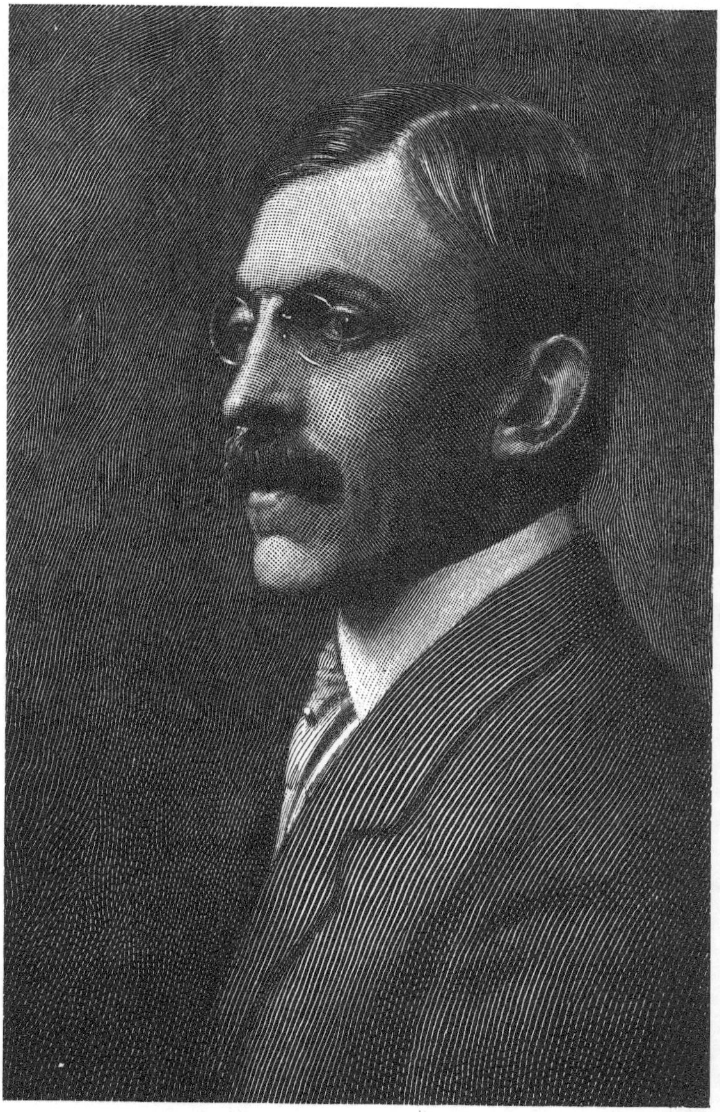

Reproduced by permission] [*From a wood engraving by Timothy Cole*

HERMANN MICHAEL BIGGS

struggle had become obligatory in Britain, the question arose as to whether tuberculosis should not be added to the list of these, and each case on recognition by the attending doctor be notified to the medical officer of health.

It is not surprising that there was long delay before opinion in this direction began to be effective. In the first place, it was not until at least a decade after Koch in 1882 had demonstrated the role of the tubercle bacillus that realisation of the implications of this knowledge had filtered down to the majority of practising doctors, and even then it was with severe limitations that the prevention of infection was regarded as important in the prevention of tuberculosis.

The late Dr. H. T. Bulstrode, a very able medical inspector of the Local Government Board, the author of the exhaustive report on Sanatoria to that Board, in giving the Milroy Lectures (*Lancet*, 1903, Vol. II, p. 75) said:

> While there can be no reasonable doubt that pulmonary tuberculosis is under certain conditions a communicable malady, there can equally be no question that its communicability is of a lower order;

and with this opinion many physicians would, I believe, still agree. I place on record here my own view as stated in a paper to the Epidemiological Society, read in December 1905, though the progress of events has rendered further discussion of the relative share of infection and of other factors lowering resistance in causing tuberculosis almost unnecessary. One thing is certain. In the absence of the tubercle bacillus there can be no tuberculosis, though it may be agreed that protracted or heavy exposure to infection is commonly needed for the insemination of active tuberculosis.

Here is the statement embodying my experience up to 1903, which subsequent experience has continued to confirm:

> Having investigated nearly 1,600 voluntarily notified cases of phthisis, as well as a much larger number of fatal cases of phthisis, from a public health standpoint, I do not conceive it to be possible that any physician having personally done similar work could fail

to realise to the full extent the infectivity of this disease, when exposure to infection is protracted, and the dosage of infection is great: a state of matters which is the common domestic lot of most of the working classes when tubercular infection attacks a member of the household. The evidence convincing one as to this does not lend itself to statistical statement, and when stated in print it may not be convincing; but the steady succession of cases in infected households at intervals of one or two years, or longer, the intercurrent destruction of children by tubercular meningitis or "broncho-pneumonia" while their parents are suffering from chronic phthisis, and other similar evidence, can leave no doubts in the minds of those who come into continuous contact with the actual facts (*Transactions of the Epidemiological Society*, Vol. XXV, p. 70).

The most frequent argument against notification of tuberculosis has been that even when tuberculous patients go promptly to their doctor, they are likely to have been bacilliferous for a considerable time before this, and the mischief is already done. But this argument ignores the undoubted influence of dosage in determining whether infection shall or shall not be efficient in producing disease. As I have put it (*Prevention of Tuberculosis*, p. 339):

The healthy occupants of a tuberculous home may be compared to a city which is the subject of a protracted siege, in which the combined effects of arms, of starvation, and depressing emotions are at work. The inhabitants of such a city may escape with but little damage if the siege is raised at a comparatively early period; but they succumb if it is protracted.

More serious in causing protracted hesitation to agree to notification on the part of an almost solid medical profession has been the fear that the patient would be liable to be "regarded as a leper," and his social and industrial freedom be seriously shackled. I need not traverse this argument; in most cases, as I have often said, the "risk of interference does not exist in practice."

Notwithstanding the approximate consensus of general medical opinion against it, the desirability of notification became gradually recognised.

References to it which in the main were academic may be first mentioned. Koch in his London address in 1901 said: "in the conflict with tuberculosis we cannot dispense with obligatory notification." Dr. Arthur Ransome (*Public Health*, 1894–95, Vol. 7, p. 128) quoted Dr. Arnold Chaplin as advocating extension of the Infectious Disease (Notification) Act to phthisis "with careful limitations." He further quoted Dr. H. Bennett as saying that this would mean that "social relations would be all but disorganised." Burdon Sanderson, in Vol. II of the *Proceedings of the International Congress of Hygiene and Demography*, 1891, considered that "tuberculosis should be included in the Infectious Disease (Notification) Act. . . . We still want information as to the actual prevalence of tuberculosis."

Dr. (now Sir Robert) Philip quotes (*British Medical Journal*, June 23, 1934) from an address in 1890 in which he said that the adoption of compulsory notification of pulmonary tuberculosis in Edinburgh would soon give valuable confirmation of the fact that this disease is communicable and urged this notification. (As to Edinburgh, see also page 250.)

To appreciate the difficulties in securing notification, we need to recall the similar difficulties encountered in securing the compulsory notification of acute infectious diseases, to which the vast majority of doctors were at first opposed. It required a slow conversion of public opinion and especially of medical opinion from opposition to favour or at least to accept this intrusion, in the public interest, into the confidential relationship of the family doctor to his patient.

Prolonged agitation had gone on for many years before the late Dr. Sergeant secured the first local Act for the notification of acute infectious diseases in Bolton, Lancs. Other towns gradually secured the same powers; then in 1889 a more general Act was passed giving local option, and in 1899 an Act of Parliament made compulsion universal in all districts.

A similar history attaches to the enforcement of compulsory notification of births within thirty-six hours. Huddersfield led the way in 1905 by a local Act, other towns followed slowly.

Then a more general permissive Act was passed in 1907, and compulsion became universal in 1915.

A like history holds good for the notification of tuberculosis, though in this instance the difficulties involved in overcoming the opposition of the leaders of the medical profession and of many local authorities were almost immeasurably great, as can be inferred from the general attitude of the medical profession and of the Local Government Board in England.

Before I give some particulars as to the spread of notification throughout Britain so far as I know it, some further mention should be made of the opposition to it or silence concerning it. The inauguration of the National Association for the Prevention of Tuberculosis took place at a meeting in Marlborough House on December 20, 1898, H.R.H. the Prince of Wales (afterwards Edward VII) being in the chair. The chief resolution of the meeting was proposed by the Marquess of Salisbury, who made the following, among other remarks:

> Nothing is more striking in the luminous statement of Sir William Broadbent or in the discussion following than the absence of all desire that the powers of the law should be brought into operation to carry out the objects of the Association. . . . This is a snare which they will carefully avoid. They must be content with preaching the salutary doctrine which they hold, and must not think of applying to the secular arm.

This statement appeared to embody the unanimous view of the Conference, at which the chiefs of the medical and veterinarian professions spoke (see also p. 242).

At the Portsmouth meeting of the British Medical Association reported in the *British Medical Journal*, October 1899, a discussion in which twenty-two speakers joined was introduced by the late Sir Clifford Allbutt on the Preventive and Remedial Treatment of Tuberculosis. Many distinguished speakers—Sir William Broadbent, Dr. (afterwards Sir William) Osler of Baltimore, Sir Douglas Powell, Sir Hugh Beevor, and Dr. Mitchell Bruce took part in the discussion. Of those mentioned above, none mentioned notification. Dr. Ransome mentioned the value of notification with suitable safeguards; Dr. Shingleton Smith of Bristol "hoped that all active steps by health officers would be avoided," while my own contribution was that the chief factor that could be directly attacked was that of the communicability of phthisis, and that for this attack it was imperative to bring the medical officer of health into action. The main discussion turned on diagnosis and sanatoria.

At the meeting of the Sanitary Institute at Southampton in 1899 I introduced a discussion on "Notification of Consumption; its Pros and Cons." It was a large meeting, and in the discussion many medical officers of health took part. My address concluded with the following resolution:

> That this Conference of Medical Officers of Health is strongly of opinion that phthisis . . . is preventible by measures which are completely within the range of personal and public hygiene. That of such measures the disinfection or destruction of the sputa of phthisical patients, and the abatement of insanitary conditions of dwelling-houses and workplaces, especially those associated with overcrowding, hold the first place. That for the carrying out of such measures, notifications of cases of phthisis to the Medical Officer of Health are indispensable, to secure economy of effort and the maximum benefit. That this Conference recommend the notification of phthisis for adoption in all sanitary districts, the question as to whether it be voluntary or compulsory being left to the discretion of Local Sanitary Authorities, and that the Local Government Board be urged by the Council of the Sanitary Institute to take the necessary steps to legalise such notification.

The discussion (Vol. XXI, Part I, *Journal of the Sanitary Institute*) illustrates clearly that most health officials were still opposed to notification.

Dr. Niven seconded my resolution and favoured compulsory notification, which avoided the invidiousness of selection. He was confident that compulsion would follow the voluntary system now established in Manchester and Brighton. The late Dr. S. Marsden (Birkenhead) pressed the usual arguments against notification and evidently did not appreciate the benefit derivable from knowing of houses in which, owing to a case of phthisis, overcrowding or sanitary defects were exceptionally dangerous to healthy occupants.

Dr. E. W. Hope of Liverpool doubted whether compulsory notification would enable him to take more preventive steps than were possible with voluntary notification in respect of housing. The steady decline of phthisis showed that they were already on the right lines.

The late Dr. P. Boobbyer (Nottingham) emphasised the necessity of proceeding slowly with voluntary notification and educational measures, especially by means of the object lesson of sanatorium work. He had no doubt that notification would eventually come.

Baillie Pollard, of Edinburgh, said: "It was needless to go in for notification, until they were in some measure prepared to deal with the state of matters that notification would reveal." Sir Henry Littlejohn, then M.O.H. of Edinburgh, expressed his regret that "the voice of the medical profession in Edinburgh was totally opposed to the notification of phthisis. . . . For him to go against the medical profession would be to commit *felo de se*. . . . Even the most intelligent of our citizens still require to be educated." (On Edinburgh, see also p. 247.) Others joined in the discussion. In view of the prevailing sentiment of the meeting, after obtaining the consent of Dr. Niven, I withdrew my resolution and no vote was taken.

The arguments against compulsory notification have never been more forcefully stated than in Sir R. Thorne's Harben Lectures in 1899. He "felt certain that the compulsory notification of phthisis is calculated to retard the very object which they (its advocates) have in view." Sir William Power, who succeeded Thorne at the Local Government Board, in his introduction to Dr. Bulstrode's report on sanatoria published in 1908, cautiously indicated the possibility of local experimentation in notification. He referred to Sheffield, which, under the leadership of Dr. (now Sir John) Robertson, had already, at the end of 1903, secured the local enactment of compulsory notification of phthisis, associated with powers which "expressly dissociated administratively phthisis and everyday infectious disease." And Sir William mentioned the experience of Brighton "as indicating that where obvious personal advantages accrue to the patient—where he is not harassed in a social sense . . . a system of voluntary notification may yield useful results."

Early in the 'eighties Niven translated for the *Medical Magazine* German articles on tuberculosis, and in 1887 and 1888, when he was M.O.H. of Oldham, he had distributed to every house in that town instructions for the prevention of infection from consumptives. In 1892 Dr. C. E. Paget prepared a memorandum on similar lines for the North-Western Branch of the Society of Medical Officers of Health; and in 1893 (August 4th), at a meeting of the parent Society of Medical Officers of Health, the following resolution which I had drafted and which I proposed was passed unanimously.

That the Society of Medical Officers of Health, while accepting the view that phthisis is an infective disease, in the prevention of which active hygienic measures should be taken, think it premature to recommend the compulsory notification of a chronic disease like phthisis. They are of opinion that it is incumbent on medical officers of health to take such steps as may secure (*a*) the voluntary notification of cases of phthisis by medical officers of institutions and such medical practitioners as agree that precautionary measures are desirable; (*b*) the adoption of such precautionary measures, including the disinfection of rooms, as can be arranged in conjunction with the family practitioner. For this purpose the memorandum prepared by the N.W. Branch of the Society of Medical Officers of Health would give an excellent basis of action.

In my view, we had not then reached the stage at which it appeared judicious to advocate compulsory notification of cases of phthisis.

The reasons which then influenced me, and which continued to influence me in subsequent stages of practical action for which I was responsible, were that notification is not an end, but a means to an end; that it constitutes an intrusion into the relationship between a patient and his doctor, which is only justified if the public good demands it; and that compulsory notification of cases should therefore only be enforced when the Local Sanitary Authority was prepared to take such action, following notification, as would be beneficial both to the public and to the patient. The significance of the last-named condition will be clearer when I compare the relative efficiency of voluntary and compulsory notification in the earlier stages of the practical anti-tuberculosis campaign.

Towards the end of 1893 a scheme of voluntary notification was recommended by Dr. Niven, in Oldham, and was endorsed by the medical profession of that town at a meeting of its Medical Society. The Town Council declined to adopt it. The details of the scheme were published in the *Lancet* (November 18, 1893). In 1894 a voluntary system was begun in New York, and thus Dr. Biggs first initiated the practice of this important additional measure of practical preventive medicine.

At this point I take up the story of my own share in similar work. In 1893 the disinfection of houses in which a death from phthisis had occurred in Brighton was already being practised, and inquiry into the circumstances of the family was made whenever practicable, sanitary defects being made good. In this way something was being effected towards influencing the minds of family doctors in favour of preventive measures. A further step was taken in 1897, when I began to make gratuitous examination of the sputum of patients suspected of tuberculosis for medical practitioners. In 1899 the specimens thus examined numbered 47, and in the year 1908 they had increased to 672 (population of Brighton, 128,000). This was almost tantamount to indirect notification; though it did not authorise systematic visits to the families from whom specimens had come. But it led to much correspondence and interviews with doctors concerning their patients.

Early in 1899 I invited the medical officers of public hospitals and the parochial medical officers to notify cases of phthisis in their care and in the first seven months of that year 68 cases were thus notified. At the end of these months I had obtained the consent of the Town Council to pay the doctor a fee for each notification received from him, and voluntary

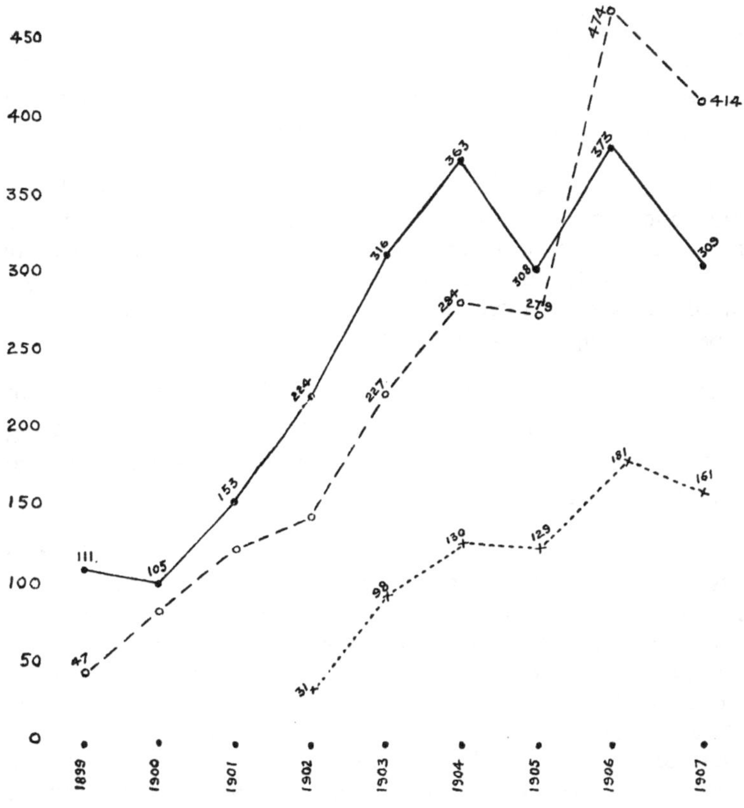

●—●—● No. of new cases of phthisis notified.
o - - o - - o No. of specimens of sputum examined for doctors.
× · · · × · · · × No. of new cases treated in sanatorium.

Diagram 7

Illustrating the close relationship between the number of cases of Pulmonary Tuberculosis notified to the M.O.H. *and the provision of measures for their benefit*

notification of all cases of phthisis was invited from all medical practitioners in Brighton. The number of cases notified steadily rose as will be seen from the diagram above. In 1906 they numbered 373, and were double the number of deaths from phthisis in the same year.

The rapidly increasing strength of the movement towards notification of phthisis began to show itself in various parts of the country. This is evidenced by the following resolution passed unanimously at the final meeting in London of the International Congress on Tuberculosis, 1901:

> That the voluntary notification of cases of phthisis attended with tuberculous expectoration and the increased preventive action which it has rendered practicable has been attended by a promising measure of success, and that the extension of notification should be encouraged in all districts in which efficient sanitary administration renders it possible to adopt the consequential measures.

In reporting on this Congress to the Town Council of Brighton, I commented on the above resolution, representing as it did an under-statement of the desires with which at the Congress I had proposed it:

> From the tone of the large meeting at which this resolution was passed, there is little doubt that a resolution in favour of a modified form of compulsory notification would have been passed with almost equal ease, but it was thought that it was most desirable to advocate the gradual and tentative extension of notification until experience on the subject had accumulated. It is satisfactory that the principle of notification for which Dr. Niven, M.O.H. of Manchester, and we in Brighton have worked for several years past, is now becoming generally admitted, and that the opposition with which the proposal was first received is gradually disappearing.

Brighton was the first town in this country to inaugurate, in January 1899, a practical system of voluntary notification of phthisis by medical practitioners, the payment of fees, 2s. 6d. for each case notified, being authorised by the Town Council in the same year.

It is interesting to compare Brighton's results with those of other towns in which voluntary notifications from all practitioners were invited. In 1899 both Brighton and Manchester adopted this course, Brighton during the entire year, Manchester from September onwards. In 1903 Sheffield, of which Dr. (now Sir John) Robertson was then M.O.H., succeeded in obtaining from Parliament local powers making phthisis compulsorily notifiable by doctors in that town for a period of seven years. To obtain these powers meant receiving the approval of a Parliamentary Committee, and this would scarcely have been given without the approval of the Local Government Board as the central health authority. The utility of this local Act was limited by the following sub-clause of the local Act:

> No provisions contained in any general or local Act of Parliament relating to infectious disease shall apply to tuberculosis of the lung or proceedings relating thereto under this section.

In my volume *Prevention of Tuberculosis*, 1908, I give a table which enables one to compare the extent to which in 1905–6 doctors were notifying cases of phthisis, the proportion between number of cases of phthisis notified and the number of deaths from this disease being adopted as the most accurate measure of the success of notification. In New York (1905) the proportion was 265 notifications to every 100 deaths, in Sheffield it was 155 in 1906. In these towns the notifications were obligatory, in New York not completely so. Under voluntary systems of notification the proportion in 1906 was 126 in Manchester, 149 in Liverpool, and 202 in Brighton. At that time in Brighton a large proportion of total phthisical patients equivalent to twice the annual number of deaths from this disease were being notified and twice this number were being systematically visited. This did not mean that the voluntary system was preferable to an obligatory system of notification. The relatively greater early success in Brighton was ascribable to the fact that all the patients who were willing to enter the Borough Sanatorium were admitted, and received open-air treatment and good feeding for from four to six weeks, besides being carefully trained in a desirable manner of life. Notification was a necessary preliminary to this tempting programme!

In this relative experience I found confirmation of my own view that:

> The success of notification, whether voluntary or compulsory, depends in the main on the extent to which a Local Authority and its officers can be helpful to the notified patients (*Prevention of Tuberculosis*, 1908, p. 347).

Notwithstanding the difficulties and opposition which were encountered, the movement in favour of notification rapidly spread in circles concerned with public health administration. A considerable number of local authorities in England adopted notification of phthisis on a voluntary basis, and two or three towns succeeded in obtaining for a trial period the limited powers already given to Sheffield.

In both Ireland and Scotland there was local activity, and in their national Local Government Boards. As early as 1901 the Irish Board issued a circular of advice on tuberculosis, and the Board's report for 1908 stated "there should be compulsory notification of pulmonary tuberculosis subject to safeguards to avoid unnecessary interference with the liberty of the subject."

The Scottish Local Government Board was also active. Dr. (now Sir Leslie) Mackenzie has summarised Scottish events in a volume by many writers in honour of Sir R. Philip (*The Control and Eradication of Tuberculosis*, 1911). Mackenzie states that as early as 1891 he had proposed the application of the Infectious Disease (Notification) Act to phthisis in Galloway, but central permission had been withheld. In 1903 in the annual report of the Local Government Board for Scotland it was laid down that phthisis is to be regarded as an infectious disease within the meaning of the Public Health (Scotland) Act, 1897. In 1906 the Board issued a circular authorising notification of phthisis, and the dealing with cases of this disease "as they dealt with other infectious diseases." This action would include disinfection, isolation, and treatment. The circular recommended the inclusion in local preventive organisation against tuberculosis of a dispensary, as already initiated

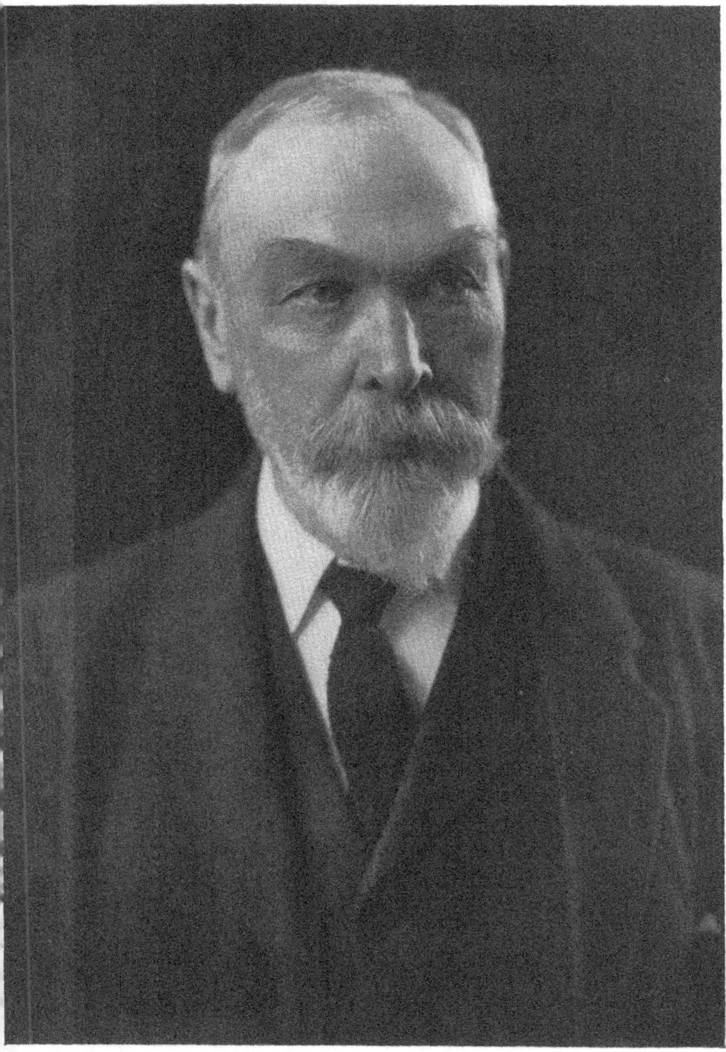

DR. JAMES NIVEN

by Philip in Edinburgh. In 1907 the over-stringency of the principal Act as applied to tuberculosis was modified.

In 1907 out of 313 Scottish local health authorities, eight had applied the Notification Act to phthisis; in 1909 this number had risen to fifty-three. Evidently this course of events differed markedly from the course in England, where only tentative attempts at notification were officially favoured, and then with legal restrictions which did not aid active preventive work.

My own position is stated on page 249, and I had succeeded in getting resolutions passed by great public associations to the effect that notification of tuberculosis was desirable, but only when effective action against tuberculosis could be taken by the Local Authority concerned; this action to be of a character which would benefit the patient as well as the public. In my *Prevention of Tuberculosis*, published in 1908, and written before I became Principal Medical Officer of the Local Government Board, I re-emphasised this view in the words quoted on page 251. And in view of the fact that in many localities this condition could not be fulfilled I stated my view that it would be inopportune and of relatively little use to advise at once the general adoption of compulsory notification of phthisis.

At the Local Government Board I proceeded to make recommendations on the lines just expressed. My own local experience had shown me that a gradual extension of notification was the best procedure, and my first effort was directed to secure the compulsory notification throughout England of cases coming under the medical care of the Poor Law, whether at home or in workhouse infirmaries. These were the most helpless of patients; and they were patients for whose care the Poor Law Authority was responsible in every area. But for some months action was blocked. All the precedents were against bringing pulmonary tuberculosis, a disease oft-times of protracted duration, into the net which was appropriate for acute and definitely limited infectious diseases like smallpox and typhoid fever. The obstacle was serious; but eventually the President of the Board (Mr. John Burns) made a special appeal to the Board's legal adviser (Mr. Adrian) who found an ingenious way out by proposing Regulations enforcing notification of phthisis under Section 130 of the Public Health Act, 1875, which satisfied the legal mind. This clause gives power to the Local Government Board to make Regulations for preventing its spread, "whenever any part of England appears to be threatened with or is affected by any formidable epidemic, endemic, or infectious disease"; and salvation was found in the blessed word "endemic" (see postscript to this chapter). The preamble of the Regulations was catholic enough; for it definitely stated, "Whereas tuberculosis is an endemic disease, and the form of the disease which is known as pulmonary tuberculosis is an infectious disease." And the powers given by the Regulations were satisfactory, for they included "all such measures . . . as are authorised in any case of infectious disease" for cleansing and disinfection; also all measures needed for the prevention of infection from infectious matter. The Regulations became operative January 1, 1909. A copy of the Regulations and of the Memorandum prepared by me on "Administrative Measures against Tuberculosis" is given on pp. 225–39 of my first Annual Report as Medical Officer of the Local Government Board, 1908–9.

In my second Annual Report to the Board (1909–10) I reported that much good work had already been done under the above Order, and advised extension of notification beyond Poor Law cases, "especially in those districts in which means for helping the patients are fairly well developed." I stated that "the early (compulsory) notification of all cases of consumption is desirable." As a further step in this direction I pointed out that the stratum of society above that coming under the Poor Law "consists of the poor, who, especially in towns, resort when sick to charitable hospitals and dispensaries. Many of these drifted in and out of the administration of the Poor Law, and their modes of life were seldom satisfactory from the communal standpoint." In May 1911 compulsory notification was extended to all such hospital and dispensary patients, and the same powers to help were given as in the case of the earlier Order. Very soon compulsory notification was extended to all cases of pulmonary tuberculosis, and this became law from January 1, 1912. This extension was, I reported, favourably received, and "remarkably few instances of individual hardship, resulting from notification, have come to light," which spoke volumes for the tact displayed by the sanitary staffs; for the two more recent Orders had imposed a definite duty on the medical officer of health, after receipt of a notification

> to make such inquiries and take such steps as may appear to him to be necessary for preventing the spread of infection and for removing conditions favourable to infection.

The final step in complete notification of tuberculosis was taken in February 1913, when the Local Government Board extended compulsory notification to cases of all forms of tuberculosis, and consolidated its three preceding Orders. In the National Insurance Act, 1911, a special Sanatorium Benefit was provided, which came into operation in July 1912, and the Finance Act, 1911, provided a capital sum of £1,116,000 for the building of sanatoria in England and Wales. The Treasury also undertook to pay one half of the approved expenditure incurred by local authorities in the treatment and prevention of tuberculosis. It soon became evident that tuberculosis being an infectious disease, provisions for its control under the above provisions could not be limited to insured persons; and vigorous representations to this effect were made by the Local Government Board and Associations of Local Authorities. The (Astor) Departmental Committee on Tuberculosis which reported in April 1912, reported that any scheme for controlling tuberculosis should be available for the whole community; and this was agreed to by Mr. Lloyd George, who at that time represented Treasury Funds and had inaugurated Sickness Insurance.

Reviewing this history of notification of tuberculosis as a means of taking practical action for the prevention of tuberculosis, it will be clear that notification was rapidly extended, as measures for the administrative control of tuberculosis became practicable; and that when financial support from national funds was accorded, the machinery of notification and the local sanitary administration following on it were ready for utilising the new financial resources.

POSTSCRIPT: IS PARTURITION A SICKNESS?

The value of the word "endemic" in a preceding paragraph recalls to my mind a further illustration of the drawbacks of strict legality, which though irrelevant to this chapter, may be given here. The great Public Health Act, 1875, in Section 131 states that "any local authority may provide for the use of the inhabitants of their district hospitals or temporary places *for the reception of the sick*"; and the Town Council of a large town, having found the need of a Lying-in Hospital, applied to the Local Government Board for consent to provide it. Consent was refused, because it was held that parturition is a physiological process and that the mother, even though "in sorrow she brings forth" her child, is not sick.

Soon after I came on the staff of the Board a similar application was made; and I recall the joy with which I read Dr. Franklin Parsons' minute in the earlier case to the effect that were it practicable for the legal advisers of the Board to undergo the pains of normal childbearing their legal opinions might be profoundly changed. I endorsed the previous medical opinion, but a few further years elapsed before this embargo on rate-provided institutions for lying-in women was removed. This was in 1914, when child welfare work was interpreted as including the welfare of the mother in its scope. Then the obstacle was removed by the process, of which politicians are supposed to be masters: look a difficulty straight in the face and pass on.

CHAPTER XXX

THE EARLIER ADMINISTRATIVE CONTROL OF TUBERCULOSIS

Measures of social usefulness following on notification—Treatment of consumption in fever hospitals—Difficulties as to lateness of notification—Value of infirmaries for advanced cases

In the last chapter I have exceeded the time limit, 1908, in order to complete the story of the slow but steady steps needed before notification could be made everywhere an effective aid in the administrative control of tuberculosis. In the present chapter I propose to adhere more strictly to the time limit, leaving for later description a statement of the measures rendered possible by the grant in 1912 of 50 per cent of authorised local expenditure on tuberculosis from the Treasury, and by the giving of large capital grants for the construction of sanatoria. To describe the various forms of social usefulness, and of helpfulness to the patient and his family which naturally follow on notification of his illness to the M.O.H., would mean traversing familiar ground. They comprised preventive measures which were scarcely practicable to the patient's own doctor, even when he had time for such help and was willing to give it. They included also the detection of previously undiagnosed cases in the family, which was gradually developed, the adoption of precautions in coughing and spitting, the provision for separate sleeping, and scrupulous cleanliness—all of them measures conducing to prevent further cases of phthisis or of acute tuberculosis and meningitis, which, failing these measures, occur in the family of a patient with untreated chronic phthisis.

EDUCATIVE SANATORIUM TREATMENT

It was in preventing this sequence of infection that I became strongly convinced of the value of a short stay in the Borough sanatorium. It not only secured temporary improvement of the patient, but he became convinced of the importance of a separate bedroom, of good nutrition, and of the elementary hygiene which his condition required him to practise if risks to his family were to be minimised. I regard this part of my Brighton experience as having special importance; and I regret that when in 1912 the Sanatorium Benefit was made the most popular item in the National (Health) Insurance Act, it was not specified as being chiefly of this character, with more protracted sanatorium treatment for carefully and judicially selected cases. Had this been done vast sums of public money would have been saved, and every tuberculous patient might have been satisfactorily educated in the necessary hygiene of his condition.

TREATMENT OF PHTHISIS IN FEVER HOSPITALS

A few details may be given of the Brighton method of sanatorium treatment. It was undertaken at the fever hospital. The various blocks of the fever hospital are on the usual plan of detached pavilions, and one of these intended for typhoid fever was usually empty, or the odd cases of this disease needing to be treated could be placed in small rooms attached to other pavilions. In 1902 I secured the consent of the Town Council to treat consumptives in the pavilion thus freed. Some two hundred to three hundred cases were thus treated in the course of a year, the duration of treatment being from four to six weeks. Much astonishment was expressed that no cross-infection from the scarlet fever and diphtheria wards occurred, although all nurses had a common dining-room. It did not occur in a single instance. The experiment began in 1902 and was extended in 1904, the beds available being increased from ten to twenty-five. A private bequest left in 1903 made the interest on £20,000 available for help to the patients, and patients under this bequest in any stage of disease were kept in the sanatorium sometimes for more lengthy periods. They also received monetary aid at home when necessary. The benefits claimed under our procedure were summarised as follows in my Annual Report for 1907:

(1) The patient himself is benefited and enabled to start afresh with an improved prospect of recovery.
(2) While he is in the sanatorium his house is cleansed and purified, and his wife and family have a holiday in the sense of being free from repeated attacks by tubercle bacilli.
(3) The patient when sent home has been taught to so manage his coughing and expectoration that he need no longer be a source of risk to his family and to those with whom he works.

My experience was that patients discharged after their month's treatment "were without exception ardent advocates for the fresh-air regime."

At that time there was no official tuberculosis clinical consultant, and members of the family who were out of health were urged to consult a doctor. In the last complete year, 1907, of my official work in Brighton, 182 deaths from phthisis were registered, and 161 new cases of this disease were treated temporarily in the Borough sanatorium. A still larger number were treated in what was then the Poor Law Infirmary, most of them for protracted periods.

As bearing on this last-named point, which will need to be expanded in a later volume, I may record here (Annual Report, 1901) some early observations. In this report I outlined the German system of sickness insurance, which had been inaugurated in 1891. At the date of this report there were already forty-nine sanatoria in Germany for the poor and many others in preparation, and I quoted Burdon Sanderson's plea for similar help for consumptives in this country. I then detailed what was done for the special treatment of consumptives in this country, before making my proposals for Brighton, which have already been described. I faced in this report the problem as to whether sanatorium treatment could be permanently successful, and expressed doubt as to whether we could expect more than a temporary stay of the disease in view of "the conditions to which the patient is exposed after leaving the sanatorium." My remarks of a later date on the supposed choice, so often alleged, between better housing and sanatorium treatment are quoted on page 304.

I then showed what a large proportion of the life of advanced or acute cases of phthisis was lived in the Poor Law Infirmary. For 211 consecutive patients, whose records I analysed, the average number of days of institutional segregation was 316 for each consumptive. A large proportion of the cases were under repeated treatment in the Infirmary.

Like other workers in the same field I had to admit that many cases were not recognised until, quoting my Annual Report for 1905,

> the disease has become fatally established, and until much mischief has been done among fellow-workmen. If a skilled overhauling of each patient with persistent and repeated cough could be secured, much earlier diagnosis would be practicable. As matters now stand, large numbers of consumptives are treated winter after winter for "bronchitis," examination of the chest being exceptional and rare in certain classes of practice, and specimens of sputum being seldom submitted for examination.

Inquiries into deaths from non-pulmonary forms of tuberculosis led me to connect many of them with some unrecognised source of infection, a patient with phthisis who was still living. From an Annual Report as early as 1895 I extract the two following illustrations:

> A woman aged 34 died in August 1894 from phthisis. Her son died in May 1893 from tubercular meningitis.
>
> On January 19, 1894, a boy aged 8 died of phthisis, a sister having died from the same disease in December 1891. On January 14, 1894, a lodger's child, aged 12 months, who had lived in this house since birth, died of tubercular meningitis.

In September 1903 (in a paper read at the International Congress of Hygiene and Demography, Brussels, September

1903) I ventured on a forecast and an expression of opinion as to the relative value of various anti-tuberculous measures, which I may quote as still held by me, although I had not then completely convinced myself of the supreme value of prolonged segregation of acute and advanced consumptive patients:

Two ends are aimed at, and there need be no quibbling as to their relative importance. The first is to fortify each member of the community to resist the invasion of the tubercle bacillus. The second is to protect each member of the community against the invasion of the tubercle bacillus. I have already indicated my belief that many of the reforms which are supposed to have operated in the first direction, especially improvements in housing and cleanliness, have operated still more in the second direction. A difference of opinion as to the *modus operandi* need not prevent combined action in the struggle against tuberculosis in both directions. Sanatorium treatment and training are ideal in this respect (outdoor life, improved nutrition, general hygiene, and the special hygiene of the patient's condition). It is easy to foresee that with the general adoption of the wider measures now practicable a reduction of tuberculosis will occur at a rate more rapid and extensive than has hitherto been secured. There is more hope of the almost complete extermination of tuberculosis than of any of the acute infectious diseases, with the possible exception of typhus, typhoid, and smallpox.[1]

In the same address I quoted Koch's statement at the meeting of the British Congress on tuberculosis in 1901 to the effect that:

The only country that possesses a considerable number of special hospitals for tubercular patients is England, and there can be no doubt that the diminution of tuberculosis in England, which is much greater than in any other country, is greatly due to this circumstance.

I commented that although this statement was incorrect as regards special hospitals, if it were applied also to the vast numbers treated in general hospitals and still more in poor law infirmaries "there is good reason for attaching a high importance to the removal of these patients from their relatives

[1] Specific prophylaxis of diphtheria was then unknown.

and to the nursing of them under conditions in which personal infection is greatly limited in extent." I then quoted the Brighton figures referred to on page 263.

A fuller discussion of this subject and of the further development in the administrative control of tuberculosis is reserved to a subsequent volume. I reserve also for this later volume discussion of the relation of poverty and of housing to tuberculosis, and of the relative value of various factors in producing the decline in tuberculosis, a decline which is still proceeding with unabated speed.

CONTRIBUTIONS

The Prevention of Tuberculosis. Address to the Association of Sanitary Inspectors (*Sanitary Inspectors' Journal*, 1895).

The Causes of Tuberculosis and the Means for Stamping it Out. Address to Brighton Dairymen's Association (January 1897).

The Prevention of Phthisis, with Special Reference to its Notification to the Medical Officer of Health. A Paper read before the Society of Medical Officers of Health (*Public Health*, February 1899).

Notification of Consumption: Its Pros and Cons. Opening a Discussion at the Southampton Congress of the Sanitary Institute (*Journal of Sanitary Institute*, Vol. XXI, Part I, 1899).

The Influence of Soil on the Prevalence of Pulmonary Phthisis (*Practitioner*, February 1901).

The Notification of Phthisis Pulmonalis (*Practitioner*, July 1901).

The Administrative Prevention of Tuberculosis. Introduction to a Discussion in Section of Public Medicine, Manchester Meeting, British Medical Association, 1902 (*British Medical Journal*, August 16, 1902).

The Intervention of Public Authorities in the Struggle against Tuberculosis (International Congress of Hygiene and Demography, Brussels, 1903).

Public Health Authorities in Relation to the Struggle against Tuberculosis in England. Paper read at the Meeting of the International Congress on Hygiene and Demography, Brussels, September 1903 (*Journal of Hygiene*, Vol. III, No. 4, 1903).

Four and a Half Years' Experience of the Voluntary Notification of Pulmonary Tuberculosis (*Journal of Sanitary Institute*, Vol. XXIV, Part III, 1903).

The Relation of the Medical Practitioner to Preventive Measures against Tuberculosis. Post-Graduate Address (*Lancet*, January 30, 1904).

A Study of the Relation between the Treatment of Tuberculous Patients in General Institutions and the Reduction in the Death-rate from Tuberculosis (*Trans. Congrès International de la Tuberculosis*, Paris, 1905).

The Relative Importance of the Constituent Factors involved in the Control of Pulmonary Tuberculosis (*Transactions of Epidemiological Society*, Vol. XXV, 1905–6).

The School in Relation to Tuberculosis (*Transactions Second International Congress on School Hygiene*, 1906).

Poverty and Disease, As Illustrated by the Course of Typhus Fever and Phthisis in Ireland. Presidential Address, Epidemiological Section of the Royal Society of Medicine (*Journal Royal Society of Medicine*, October 1907).

The Voluntary Notification of Phthisis in Brighton: including a Comparison with results obtained in other Towns. Paper read at a Sessional Meeting of the Royal Sanitary Institute (*Journal of Royal Sanitary Institute*, Vol. XXVIII, 1907).

The Causes of the Past Decline in Tuberculosis and the Light thrown by History on Preventive Measures for the Immediate Future. Special Lecture at the International Congress on Tuberculosis (Washington, September 1908).

The Prevention of Tuberculosis (pp. 429, Methuen & Co., 1908).

PART V

VITAL STATISTICS AS A BASIS OF PUBLIC HEALTH WORK. SPECIAL STUDIES IN VITAL STATISTICS

CHAPTER XXXI

VITAL STATISTICS

Three special guides in public health work—Bacteriology, Epidemiology, and Vital Statistics—The method of surveys—Farr's work—Failure to utilise vital statistics fully

ADVANCE in medicine in large measure is dependent on the application of scientific methods and knowledge, and preventive medicine even more than clinical medicine is now based chiefly on exact knowledge of pathology and physiology.

I do not discuss in this chapter epidemiological work as bearing on public health progress. Illustrations of such work occur in several chapters in this volume. Modern epidemiology has been profoundly modified during the last sixty years by the advances in bacteriology, and illustrations of this also are given throughout this volume. But to vital statistics I must devote several chapters, as the study of sickness and death returns and their immediate bearing on preventive medicine has filled my working years.

The history of sanitary reform as illustrated in previous chapters shows the importance of the three methods of investigation mentioned above. But this history shows also that even when all of them were lacking or only available to a limited extent, investigation leading to sanitary reform was already being actively pursued under the leadership of Edwin Chadwick.

THE METHOD OF SKILLED SURVEYS

This was effected by painstaking surveys of areas in which epidemic diseases were rampant, the surveys being conducted by physicians of wide experience. They utilised such imperfect records of sickness and mortality as were available; and they utilised even more a full statement of the sanitary abominations found in their peregrinations as demonstrating the need for repentance and reform. This method of surveys has continued to be a mainstay of sanitary work. In more recent years it has been carried through by a civilian army of medical and lay inspectors of the Central Government and of local authorities; and a vast amount of disease, especially of intestinal disease, has been prevented as the result of their investigations and of action taken thereon. As records of sickness and of deaths became more fully available, the utility of surveys was enhanced; the surveys themselves have continued to be essential in the campaign against disease.

VITAL STATISTICS

Vital statistics are concerned with whatever affects health and welfare. This implies that problems of wages and poverty and of housing come within the range of vital statistics. They cannot indeed be excluded if all the factors bearing on life and death are to receive consideration. But more ordinarily one includes in vital statistics (*a*) statistics of births and deaths and of the causes of death which relate to the beginning and end of life; and (*b*) statistics of sickness which relate to intermediate experience.

Statistics of births and deaths were first utilised; and long before special sickness statistics became generally available the more or less accurate statement of number and causes of death embodied in official records formed a chief impetus to the sanitary reforms carried out in Great Britain during the nineteenth century.

In the chapter dealing with William Farr's life I have outlined the chief facts as to the initiation of registration of births and deaths in England, and the primary utilities of this registration, and of the publication of collective experience based on it.

These compilations and the comments in Farr's reports thereon furnished a searchlight compelling public attention to the evils revealed in the figures. They showed vast difference in the experience of sanitary and insanitary areas and districts, thus specifying and stigmatising the areas in which sanitary reform was most urgently needed. These reports, furthermore, went a long way towards demonstrating the source of certain diseases.

These benefits were summarised in a paper read by me before the Royal Statistical Society in March 1896 in the following words:

> The Office of Registrar-General of Births, Deaths, and Marriages in England was created in 1836. The first report of the Registrar-General was published in 1839, and to this report Dr. W. Farr contributed the first of that long series of essays which have been the basis of the science of vital statistics in this country. It is not too much to say that the system of death-certification and registration in this country is the foundation on which the great sanitary ameliorations already achieved have been built. The mortality of every district throughout the country has been the subject of analysis. The attention of local authorities has been compelled to any special incidence of deaths in their districts. Medical officers of health have been created throughout the country, one of whose chief duties is to draw forcible attention to the local incidence of deaths, and recommend measures tending to decrease sickness and death-rates. Where the local supervision has been lax, or the medical officer's recommendations have not been carried out, the Registrar-General's periodical returns have enabled the medical staff of the Local Government Board to intervene and investigate any local outbreak of fatal disease. The publicity given to the Registrar-General's weekly, quarterly, and annual reports has evoked a spirit of inquisitiveness and even of emulation throughout the country; and although the comparison of death-rates of great towns with each other, particularly for short periods, is fraught with fallacies, the general result of the publicity secured and of the consequent efforts on the part of local authorities has been an immense improvement in the public health of the community.

As soon as I became a M.O.H. (p. 136), I was called on to edit the statistical reports of the six medical officers of health of the Wandsworth district, and they, and especially Dr. Nicholas, soon made me familiar with the methods of correcting death-rates for institutions within and without their districts, which included inmates or deaths needing to be transferred to or from the vital statistics of each district, if a correct account of its experience was to be given.

I became a student of the Registrar-General's reports containing Farr's classical contributions, and made myself familiar with the many problems of public health as embodied in vital statistics. When in 1887 I moved to Brighton, these studies were extended in various directions, and their substance was embodied in the first edition of the *Elements of Vital Statistics*, which was published in 1889. In 1885 the Royal Sanitary Institute had published a volume of extracts from Farr's reports, edited by Mr. Noel Humphreys, of the General Register Office, a former colleague of Farr. In the Preface to my elementary guide to vital statistics I referred to this volume, and remarked that while it was invaluable as a book of reference, it did not meet the need of students and junior medical officers of health, who, as I had found, needed guidance in their daily statistical work and in studying the periodical reports of the Registrar-General.

This may be illustrated by the absence of explanation of the method of correction (or standardisation) of death-rates for age and sex-distribution. Factors for correction of the recorded death-rates in twenty-eight towns of England and Wales had been published in the Annual Summary of the Registrar-General for 1883, but no explanation was given of the method employed in obtaining these factors. However, I succeeded in reproducing the method, and on the eve of publication of my volume I sent the pages describing it for confirmation to Mr. Noel Humphreys, along with the table of contents of the new volume. He courteously replied confirming my description, and at the same time said that he had been commissioned to write a textbook similar to mine, but in view of my forthcoming volume his book would be postponed or abandoned. It has not since appeared, but Mr. Humphreys' Farr Memorial Volume, and his special contributions to the Proceedings of the Royal Statistical Society, are among the classics of vital statistics.

My *Elements of Vital Statistics* was not a complete guide to statistical methods, and more recent advances in biometrics comprise processes required for more elaborate investigations. But without the aid of higher mathematics the study of current vital statistics can unfold a vast amount of valuable knowledge, and is competent to point the way to promising fields of preventive work, and thus to further the progress of medicine. The contributions to the Registrar-General's reports by Dr. T. H. C. Stevenson during the years 1908–31 are among the best illustrations of how much can be accomplished by the methods of statistics described in my *Elements* to illuminate the problems of medicine and public health when pursued with a strict regard to accuracy, while avoiding fallacies of reasoning or method, and especially avoiding the most common error of all, the use of heterogeneous or untrustworthy figures as if they were homogenous and accurate.

It is lamentable that so few medical officers of health and other social workers study the publications of the Registrar-General and possess themselves of the riches which can be delved from them. It is scarcely less sorrowful that in so many annual reports of medical officers of health, while the statistical tables required for each sanitary area by the central health authority are given—which standing alone are necessarily dull and uninspiring—the local figures of life and death have not been fully utilised in initiating investigation of life-saving value.

My work in vital statistics brought me many friends and much correspondence in both Europe and America. I had no intention of attempting to revise, almost rewriting, the *Elements of Vital Statistics*, which had already been several times republished, but in 1923 I undertook this task as I was assured by the publishers that although the last edition, written in 1899, had long been out of print, there was a steady purchase at enhanced prices of old copies. I may be forgiven if I mention two illustrations of pleasant relationships due to *Elements*. I was one of the secretaries of the demography division of the Seventh International Congress of Hygiene and Demography, 1891, and called on Korösi, the distinguished statistician of Budapest, at his London hotel. I found him at a desk in his room, on which was my book, which he informed me always travelled with him. Subsequently we often corresponded on points of mutual interest. This Congress was attended by some 2,700 members. Francis Galton, who first used the word "Eugenics," was president of its demography division.

In 1928 I was in Budapest on a second visit, engaged in an investigation, the results of which are embodied in my volumes on *International Relations between Public and Private Medicine*, and I called on Dr. Georg Gortvag, the Sectional Councillor of the Institute of Social Hygiene. He was a stranger and of a younger generation than myself: I stated my object, and explained my mission and the fact that mine was an unofficial inquiry. He stopped me and said: "I am engaged in a conference for a short time; may I suggest that the book I will hand to you may interest you." The book in question was the 1923 edition of my book, which on its title-page more fully indicates than did earlier editions its main object: "The Elements of Vital Statistics in their bearing on Social and Public Health Problems."

CONTRIBUTIONS

The Elements of Vital Statistics (George Allen & Unwin). First published 1889 (pp. 326). Revised edition 1899 (pp. 353). Rewritten and published 1923 (pp. 622).

CHAPTER XXXII

THE REGISTRATION OF SICKNESS AND ITS UTILISATION

Information the basis of action—Information of sickness as well as of deaths—Earlier efforts to secure notification of general sickness—Notification of infectious diseases—Notification of suspected communicable diseases

WORK in preventive medicine, and especially the work of the M.O.H. and his colleagues, is based "on information received." This information even now is often not easily forthcoming; and the feature of the work of the M.O.H., which notably distinguishes it from that of the family physician, is that it is his duty to search out the facts on which his preventive work can be based. Much has been accomplished with information which was incomplete and belated; while in the course of the last sixty years successive efforts have been made to secure additional information of sickness, thus supporting and extending the preventive work which can be based on field work, i.e. by actual surveys in each sanitary area.

We still wait for that complete registration of sickness which earlier reformers sighed for and attempted to secure; and it is almost scandalous that so little has been done in England to secure and to publish more complete information concerning general sickness in the third of the total population who are compulsorily insured in the State system of sickness insurance.

Of the value of mortality statistics in throwing light on health problems we have no doubt. But knowledge of the initial and terminal ends of life, of every birth and of every death, does not suffice for the worker intent on the solution of social problems. This is so in the study of disease.

It is true that the study of mortality, of its local incidence, its relation to occupation and to housing, and the varying incidence of deaths from different diseases in varying circumstances, has been most fruitful in compelling sanitary and social reforms. This is abundantly shown in a study of the Registrar-General's reports, and of the reports of many local and central health officers and other social workers. The study of infant diarrhœa (Chapter XXXVIII) is in point.

But not all disease is fatal. A vast amount of incapacitating illness does not end in death. Mortality statistics ignore everything that precedes the close of life, and when a medical officer of health knows only the fatal cases of a preventible disease, he may, in part at least, be reduced to the position of a mere recorder of events. In regard to communicable diseases, especially, it is evident that registration of sickness when it is prompt gives invaluable help in "telling us of the coming storms, and enabling us to trim our vessels to meet them."

The need for information of sickness was realised by early social workers, among whom Charles Dickens deserves an honoured place. In the fourth volume of *All the Year Round* (p. 227) he said:

> It concerns a man more to know the risk of the fifty illnesses that may throw him on his back than the possible date of the one death that must come. We must have a list of killed and *of the wounded too*.

In 1896, in a paper read before the Royal Statistical Society, I gave an account of various attempts already made to secure records of sickness, and of the success attained in this direction in several European countries. It would occupy too much space to repeat this account here. Many early leaders in preventive medicine took part in the promotion of endeavours to secure the registration of sickness. Among these the name of Dr. Rumsey deserves special mention. His *Essays and Papers on some Fallacies of Vital Statistics*, 1875, are still worth reading. He was an acute but fair critic of some of the Registrar-General's statistical methods, and did effective work in promoting public health advance. His influence was great in securing the appointment of the Royal Sanitary Commission of 1869–71, the report of which led to the passing of the great Public Health Acts of 1872 and 1875. As early as 1844, in giving evidence before the Medical Poor Relief Committee of the House of Commons, he had proposed a comprehensive plan for the uniform registration of the sickness which affects the poorer classes. This was adopted in various districts; as early as 1848 in Whitechapel, Dr. Liddle proposed the utilisation of these returns in general sanitary inquiries. Simon in his work in the City of London (1848–55) utilised similar returns: and in later years, while I was M.O.H. of Clapham, I called every week at the Public Relief Offices to extract similar information from the official records of the district (poor law) medical officer. These records were made available in every sanitary area by order of the Local Government Board.

B. W. Richardson did splendid work for a series of years from 1855 onward by collating and publishing in the *Journal of Public Health and Sanitary Review* sickness statistics collected from many parts of England. Other efforts were made in London, which included voluntary returns from many hospitals; but they collapsed in 1858, the second year of publication of the data. In 1860 a more successful attempt was organised by the Sanitary Association of Manchester and Salford, Dr. Arthur Ransome being the moving spirit in this movement. Other efforts followed, and the British Medical Association at Dr. Ransome's instance formed a committee which did much to promote more active interest in the project.

In answering a deputation of the Association, which in 1870 pressed for the general registration of disease, Mr. Goschen, the President of the Poor Law Board, was "in spirit heartily with the deputation," but remarked that "care should be taken not to impose additional labour upon the poor law official." This was just before the formation of the Local Government Board.

The reception of this deputation has present-day bearing on the fact that in 1934 there exist unutilised though available medical data as to the amount and duration and forms of sickness in the third of the total population of Great Britain who are insured under the National Health Insurance Acts; and, with a few relatively insignificant exceptions, we thus remain unable to compare the incidence of sickness generally and of special sicknesses in various localities in different occupations and in the two sexes. This statement, which seems incredible, is nevertheless lamentably true.

Although the British Medical Association, actively led by Mr. Ernest Hart, the enterprising editor of its Journal, continued their efforts, these were unsuccessful in obtaining governmental co-operation, and gradually the towns contributing to existing voluntary notification schemes fell out by the way. This failure to influence the official mind persisted, notwithstanding Farr's eloquent statement of the value of the proposed system in the Thirty-fifth Annual Report of the Registrar-General.

> The thing to aim at ultimately is a return of the cases of sickness in the civil population as complete as is now procured from the army in England. It will be an invaluable contribution to therapeutics as well as to hygiene. . . . The national returns of cases and of causes of death will be an arsenal which the genius of English healers cannot fail to turn to account.

The leaven of the protracted agitation was, however, at work. As stated in my paper to the Royal Statistical Society (1896):

> Medical officers of health in various parts of the country complained that their preventive measures were belated, owing to the fact that epidemic diseases had obtained a firm foothold before the occurrence of fatal cases brought them under their cognisance. Gradually the idea of compulsory notification of infectious diseases —the first step, we hope, towards a more general notification of sickness—became actual fact in a characteristically British fashion. The experiment was allowed to be made by those towns desiring to make it. In September 1877, the first local Act for enforcing the compulsory notification of the chief infectious diseases came into operation in Bolton, Lancashire. This example was followed by other towns, and the adoptive enactment of the Infectious Diseases

(Notification) Act in 1889 was followed by a rapid adoption of the Act by urban and rural Sanitary Authorities throughout England.

Eventually, the majority of local authorities having secured local powers to secure the compulsory notification of the chief infectious diseases by the doctor in attendance, Parliament in 1899 made this duty universally obligatory.

In 1888, when thirty-three large towns had already fairly complete knowledge of their infectious cases by notification, Dr. J. F. W. Tatham, then M.O.H. of Manchester, arranged for a weekly exchange of returns of these cases between the thirty-three towns. In 1889 the Local Government Board took over this task. The advantages of this scheme were obvious: the returns facilitated the making of forecasts and the taking of precautions against the importation and spread of disease, and they promoted the interchange of more detailed information.

In 1908, when I became medical officer to the Local Government Board, it was my agreeable task to organise an obligatory system for the whole country. It became the duty of every M.O.H. to make a weekly return of cases of notifiable infectious disease; these were rapidly tabulated along with similar returns from all areas, and on Thursday of each week, every M.O.H. had posted to him a printed return acquainting him with the experience of every other district in the country in the preceding week. These statistics are now published in the weekly returns of the Registrar-General, and are circulated on the Friday of each week, along with particulars of deaths in the week. The telephone is now utilised in sending more urgent data.

Even if the compulsory notification of infectious diseases had not proved—as it has done—an indispensable part of our machinery for control of the notified diseases, it would still be an essential means for the advance of the science of epidemiology. By its means we are, as I said in 1896,

> gradually accumulating a mass of information as to the seasonal, annual, epidemic, and cyclical prevalence of the chief infectious diseases such as has never previously been possessed by epidemiologists;

and as a knowledge of the natural history of a disease is a condition of success in its prevention, new vistas of prevention are opened out by this increased knowledge.

In other chapters of this book, the value of notification in public health medical practice is illustrated as regards scarlet fever, diphtheria, and enteric fever.

The cost of notification—a fee being paid to the practitioner performing this public duty for each case notified—is sometimes objected to; and I was criticised because, in the paper already quoted, I doubted the policy of paying a fee, even of only two shillings and sixpence, for this act. On reviewing the point after thirty-eight years, I am still unrepentant. Great Britain alone in the world—I believe—pays for such notifications.

I argued that every citizen is required, when called on, to perform public duties without payment: he must, if not a medical man, for instance, serve on a jury, while medical practitioners are exempted from this irksome duty. No payment, furthermore, is made by the State for a certificate of the cause of death required by the State from the doctor who has attended the deceased. It may be argued that this is another instance of injustice; but the performance of this duty may, not unreasonably, be regarded as a partial return to the State for the privilege and monopoly (far from complete, I know) accorded by it to practitioners to give medical care to the sick. I leave the point as it stands; except to state that so far as concerns the insured third of the general population the case in favour of State requirement of notification and periodical returns (say weekly) of the cases of sickness attended by insurance doctors appears to me to be overwhelming (see also p. 277).

In the paper (1896) already mentioned, I described foreign systems of notification of sickness. For the purposes of this paper I had visited and made an elaborate examination of systems then in operation in Scandinavia and in Germany. In these countries the information officially available was more extensive than in England. Their hospitals were chiefly State and municipal institutions, and admirable hospital statistics were usually kept. In Scandinavia, furthermore, domestic medical work was chiefly done by official district medical officers; and there was an essentially sound system requiring daily notification of a limited list of diseases and weekly returns of a larger list, including not only infectious cases but also rheumatic fever, acute respiratory diseases, and some others. The methods employed were more elastic and more calculated to be useful than ours. I have reproduced on page 221 a diagram taken from my 1896 paper, showing how returns then available for a series of years illustrated the epidemicity of rheumatic fever.

VALUE OF NOTIFICATION

Action to prevent the onset or the continuance or extension of disease being dependent on knowledge—prompt, if possible—of its occurrence, and the M.O.H. being the statutory officer entrusted with the task of prevention, we may ask the question whether notifications of sickness have led to more successful control of communicable diseases. An answer can be given without hesitation, though with some reserve. For smallpox the notification of cases, aided by vaccination of contacts, has made the detective work of public health officials strikingly successful. Outbreaks of typhoid fever, scarlet fever, and diphtheria, due to a common infection (water, shell-fish, milk, etc.) have repeatedly been cut short by action based on prompt notification. When, however, the prevalence of an infectious disease (e.g. scarlet fever or diphtheria) is due to direct human infection a less completely satisfactory answer must be given. The human element often fails—the parent or the doctor may not have recognised the disease or may neglect to act, even when diagnosis and action could reasonably be expected. Much more does this occur in an atypical case or when a person apparently in good health is a potential "carrier" of infection to others. These cases still constitute a problem, which in practice is only partially solved. The solution may come in part by the occurrence of sub-infections, short of clinical attack, which as childhood passes appear to protect many children from scarlet fever and diphtheria; and by the artificial production of immunity when this has become practicable for scarlet fever, as it is already for diphtheria and measles.

In view of the difficulties indicated above, I advocated, in my 1896 paper and on several occasions, a system of free medical visitation for diagnosis of school children, who were absent from school with illness of doubtful nature. I pointed out that this system, if adopted, would remove the parents' excuse for not calling in medical aid, and that the fees paid to family practitioners for carrying out this duty would "probably be more than recouped" by the diminution in the prevalence of infectious diseases and in the cost of maintenance of patients in isolation hospitals. No definite action has been taken in this direction. School doctors in the ordinary discharge of their duties evidently do not meet the need, or only meet it very partially.

A further suggestion was made by me at the Eastbourne Congress of the Royal Institute of Public Health (*Journal of State Medicine*, 1901) as an aid in securing more complete information:

> The time is ripe, I think, for asking for the compulsory notification of all cases in which there is reasonable ground for suspecting the existence of an infectious disease.

I pointed out that this obligation already existed for farmers in respect of foot and mouth disease and glanders.

Co-operation between private practitioners and medical officers of health has now become closer than it was: the latter welcome consultations, and laboratory help is always gratuitously available. But there is still need for more universal co-operation in regard to notifiable diseases.

This is urgently needed for diseases at present not compulsorily notifiable, especially for occurrences of food poisoning, producing acute gastro-intestinal illness, for instance, after a public meal, of which many have partaken. The patients may be attended by many doctors, and the M.O.H. may only learn of the outbreak when scientific investigation of its source has become unnecessarily difficult.

A particularly glaring instance of this was detailed in my Eastbourne paper. In 1900 there was a widespread epidemic of peripheral neuritis in Manchester and Salford, the source of which was only discovered after Dr. E. S. Reynolds (*Lancet*, January 19, 1901) had noticed in his hospital patients an unusual number of patients with skin eruptions, latterly associated with "quite an extraordinary number of cases of so-called 'alcoholic paralysis.' " Similar observations had been made by others during a period of some twelve months.

The conclusion was reached that these cases were due to arsenical poisoning: and official attention having been drawn to these cases, Dr. Tattersall, M.O.H. Salford, and Dr. Niven, M.O.H. Manchester, aided by Professor Delepine's laboratory investigations, were soon able to establish conclusively that all the sufferers were beer-drinkers, that the beer from a particular brewery was concerned, and that this beer contained considerable quantities of arsenic derived from the artificial sucrose used in its manufacture. Many deaths had occurred before this conclusion was reached. In my paper I remarked:

> The question arises whether a large proportion of these lives might not have been saved had a system of notification of preventible disease been in operation at the time. . . .
>
> The public interest demands that the M.O.H., who is the chief guardian of the public health, should receive information as to all cases of sickness which in the opinion of each medical practitioner are due to conditions of a preventible character. . . . This is the minimum of requirement. It would be easy to base on this epidemic of arsenic poisoning a reasonable demand for such information as to any form of sickness showing excessive prevalence even though its preventible character were not obvious.

The history of the gradual steps taken to secure the notification of tuberculosis are detailed in Chapter XXIX; and the discussion as to whether a similar obligation of notification should be extended to venereal diseases is postponed to my second volume.

In other chapters in this volume the essential part in public health progress played by the study of returns of sickness and death has been displayed. Can it be said that all that is possible has been derived from this source? It is clear that this is not so. In many areas comparisons of death-rates at different ages, from specific causes of death and in different localities and occupations have not been utilised to more than a scanty extent in unveiling removable causes of death, especially deaths in infancy and in the working years of life. There are also vast records of sickness which remain almost entirely wasted as stimuli towards preventive medicine, and as pointers to the paths in which preventive work will be likely to be more effective.

The medical care of every member of the community cannot be regarded as satisfactory until every medical practitioner has studied each case of illness that is entrusted to his care in its preventive aspects, and until he instructs his patient on the strength of a preventive inquiry into his life. In other words the ideal will be attained when the attendant on the sick becomes a M.O.H. within the range of his own medical practice.

This ideal goes much further than the notification of certain specified diseases to the M.O.H., even though this be extended to illnesses merely suspected of an origin common to other illnesses. It means that every doctor, while retaining his freedom as a family doctor, should be an essential part of the public health organisation of the State.

CONTRIBUTIONS

A National System of Notification and Registration of Sickness (*Journal of Royal Statistical Society*, Vol. LIX, March 1896).

The Notification of Infectious Diseases. Paper read before the Southern Branch of the Society of Medical Officers of Health (*Public Health*, March 1898).

Possible Medical Extensions of Public Health Work. Presidential Sectional Address, Congress of the Royal Institute of Public Health (Eastbourne, 1901).

CHAPTER XXXIII

EXCURSIONS IN STATISTICS

LIFE TABLES

Some fallacies of vital statistics—Construction of Life Tables—Does a larger number of survivors mean lowered average health?—Is there over-pressure in modern life?

HAVING emphasised the importance of accurate and complete returns of communal sickness and mortality, always associated with the detailed information given by sanitary inspections and surveys, I may next outline some special investigations in vital statistics undertaken by me while M.O.H. of Brighton.

Soon after I became its M.O.H. I imposed on the Town Council—I now wonder at their tolerance—a long report "On Some Fallacies of Vital Statistics, especially as Applicable to Brighton."

This report included a criticism of statistics by B. W. Richardson and Edwin Chadwick.

Richardson in a report on the health conditions of Brighton made to the Town Council in 1882, had remarked that:

> No town in the kingdom is so subject to residence of persons of advanced and worn-out lives; and it is fair to assume an increase of at least 1 per 1,000 in the annual mortality of Brighton from this cause alone.

In my report (dated November 1888) I had the temerity to demonstrate that the above statement, however agreeable to the city fathers, was erroneous, inasmuch as (1) the total death-rate is the resultant of the death-rates at each successive quinquennium or decennium of life; (2) at ages under 5 and over 55 the death-rate per 1,000 living is higher than all intermediate ages; and (3) in Brighton, although there was a somewhat larger proportion of people aged 55 and over, this was more than counterbalanced by the smaller number of children under 5.

The general conclusion was inevitable that Richardson's statement, however reasonable in appearance, was misleading.

Much daring, in the same report I challenged the inference drawn from a statement made by Chadwick in a recent address at Brighton, to the effect that:

> the average age at death of the well-to-do was 63 years, while that of the wage-earning class was only 28·8 years.

The statement of fact was correct, but no inference from it as to the relative healthiness of the two classes was permissible. It might merely mean that older people have a higher proportion of deaths to the number living than have younger people.

The fallacy of an allied statement made by Chadwick in the same address was pointed out. Among the poor in Brighton, he found that deaths under 5 years of age were 35·2 per cent of the total deaths, while among the well-to-do they were only 8·9 per cent. But this might have been due to the larger number of children among the poor, apart from any differences in sanitary and social conditions. To discover the excessive mortality of the poor due to social and sanitary conditions it is necessary to give death-rates per 1,000 living at ages under 5.

LIFE TABLES

My efforts to avoid fallacies and to provide standardised or corrected death-rates (p. 274) were followed in 1893 by the publication of the first Brighton Life Table, which was based on the mortality of the ten years 1881–90. In the preface I explained that a life table furnished the most trustworthy measure of the vital conditions of a community. It gives the average experience of duration of life of the community, and it states for each age the expectation of life which a person of that age may on the average anticipate. It embraces in this statement the experience of those who die prematurely and of those who live to advanced age: and the summation thus obtained can be compared easily and accurately with a similar summation in other communities, or in the same community at an earlier or a later period of time.

The great merit of a life table over a statement of the death-rate at each successive period of life per 1,000 living of the same age period, say 0–5, 5–10, 10–15, 15–20, 20–25 . . . up to old age, is that while the latter only gives the definite experience at a given age period, the life table sums up also the experience at that age and at all subsequent years of life. For most purposes, death-rates according to age give all that is necessary. Too often, however, we are contented with the gross death-rate at all ages, and thus miss the special indications for research and reform which are concealed in this conglomerate rate.

The graphic method was employed in constructing this life table for 1881–90 and my second life table for Brighton, which dealt with the experience of 1891–1900. It was the first of its kind constructed for public health work. I was instructed personally in the use of the graphic method by my friend Mr. George King, F.I.A., who had discovered that Milne in the construction of the famous Carlisle Table of Mortality had used this method (*Journal Institute of Actuaries*, 1883, Vol. XXIV, p. 186). Previously Milne's method had puzzled successive generations of actuaries.

I need not detail here the processes employed; they eliminated the need of algebraic methods. They have been described in a joint paper by Dr. T. H. C. Stevenson and myself in the *Journal of Hygiene* (Vol. III, No. 3, 1903). The method, if carefully employed, gives results substantially as accurate as the analytical methods.

Given trustworthiness of the data and of the method employed, my interest in the life table lay chiefly in the inferences to be drawn from it.

The national experience in 1871–80 had shown that the duration of life as compared with earlier years had not improved for males aged 20 years and over. Why at these higher ages had there been no improvement? And at this point I traversed the explanation that, owing to the saving of life from acute infectious diseases and tuberculosis, "there had been a larger number of weakly survivors, who would under the former regime have been carried off by these diseases."

I stated:

> This argument assumes that weakly children are more prone to attack by infectious diseases than robust children, an assumption which experience does not confirm. . . . It may reasonably be expected, that with a decrease in the total deaths from infectious diseases, there will have been at least a corresponding decrease in the number of those who are left maimed by an attack of one of these diseases to survive to adult life.

I added:

> The case for deterioration of the race by survival of patients who would formerly have died in early life from phthisis and other tubercular diseases, appears to be a stronger one. Probably a larger proportion of phthisical patients are cured than formerly, and perhaps many children with a strong tendency to phthisis, or even suffering from its earlier symptoms are now prevented from developing the disease, and survive to adult life. . . . But this need not cause any serious apprehension; for tendencies to phthisis only act in presence of the tubercle bacillus co-operating with favourable predisposing conditions. . . . Furthermore, if more phthisical patients survive than formerly, is it not equally true that fewer persons *become* phthisical than formerly? . . . It is, therefore, reasonable to suppose that much at least of the deteriorating effect of survival of tuberculous persons is counterbalanced by the large number of persons who are *prevented by improved sanitary and social circumstances from becoming tubercular*.

Were I now to indicate the favourable factors indicated above, my comment would be still more optimistic.

In a later paragraph I derided a fallacy still too current. Did the increased stress of modern life explain the stationary or increased death-rate in adults? I even doubted the existence of this increased strain "in the community as a whole," though it might exist in certain small sections of the population.

For adults generally I remarked:

> Each adult as he becomes year by year more deeply involved in the battle of life, comes to the conclusion that the general strain of life in the community is increasing, forgetting that the same causes operated as life advanced in previous generations. There is reason for thinking with Dr. P. H. Pye-Smith, F.R.S., that much of the evil ascribed to "over-pressure" is really due to over-feeding and drinking.

In the last paragraph of the first Brighton life table I forecasted that the explanation of the increased death-rate at the higher ages shown in England would be made clear at the end of another twenty years when "the improved conditions of life have endured sufficiently long to enable their full force and value to be determined."

In the construction of the second Brighton life table for 1891–1900 by the graphic method, I had the collaboration of Dr. T. H. C. Stevenson, then my assistant medical officer, who subsequently held Farr's post from 1908 to 1931. This second life table showed that, in Brighton, males now enjoyed an increased expectation of life at birth of a year and a third more than in the preceding decade; and, what is more important, it showed that the expectation of life had increased at all ages up to 75 and not merely at lower ages. I then resumed the discussion of the persistently alleged physical degeneration of the nation, and was in a stronger position to deny it so far as duration of life is an index. It was possible to compare the life table experience of England and Wales as a whole in 1881–90 with that of 1871–80 and this comparison proved that in 1881–90 in England expectation of life had increased up to the age of 44. A special life table of English experience prepared by Dr. T. E. Hayward showed, furthermore, that in 1891–1900 the expectation had become *higher at all ages* except 65–75. In Brighton a detailed comparison of death-rates showed that they were lower in 1891–1900 at all ages, except 20–25 (increase of 3·9 per cent) and 55–65 (increase of 1·7 per cent). In discussing the problems involved, after emphasising the importance of "increased wealth and resulting comfort of our population, and the immense improvements in sanitation during the last thirty years," I added a quotation from the first Brighton life table as follows:

> Men now (i.e. 1881–90) 40 years of age were born in the pre-sanitary period; and the first twenty years of their life were spent under more unhygienic conditions than those now holding good. This fact would go far towards explaining a stationary death-rate at the higher ages;

and then made the following final comment on this point:

> At the end of another ten years, it is still true that persons now 40 or 50 years of age were born under conditions less favourable to health and longevity than the present conditions. It is also true that greater wealth and comfort have brought increased dangers to those of mature years. Alcoholism and gluttony are common even in those who would be indignant at the suggestion of the slightest offence in these directions. These vices, and the equally fatal diseases due to sexual immorality, are the chief reasons why adult life has only shared to a relatively slight extent in the improved prospects of survival shown in the first half of life.

The prospects of continued life had in fact been enhanced right up to old age; and this being so the very dubious proposition that this has been associated with a lower average standard of health may be summarily rejected, failing valid evidence in its favour; at present there is none.

CONTRIBUTIONS

The Brighton Life Table, Based on the Mortality of 1881–90 (Brighton, 1893).

The Second Brighton Life Table, Based on the Mortality Experience of 1891–1900, by A. Newsholme and T. H. C. Stevenson (1903).

The Graphic Method of Constructing a Life Table illustrated by the Brighton Life Table, 1891–1900, by A. Newsholme and T. H. C. Stevenson (*Journal of Hygiene*, July 1903).

Vital Statistics. Article in Vol. XIII, *Encyclopædia Medica*.

The Relation of Vital Statistics to Sanitary Reform. An Address at the Jubilee Conference of the Manchester and Salford Sanitary Association (April 1902).

CHAPTER XXXIV

EXCURSIONS IN STATISTICS

CORRECTED OR STANDARDISED BIRTH-RATES

Arithmetical corrections needed—Distinction from physiological and pathological causes of reduction—Reduced birth-rate an index of desire for comfort—Is the reduction dysgenic?—The Calvinism of eugenists

The study of methods for calculating standardised death-rates (p. 274) led naturally to a similar consideration of birth-rates. By means of factors of correction it had been found possible to eliminate differences in death-rates caused merely by varying proportions, in the populations compared, of persons living at ages at which the rate of mortality deviated from the average rate for all ages. Could not a similar process be applied to birth-rates per 1,000 of the total population, thus eliminating variations caused by differences in the proportion of married women of child-bearing ages (say fifteen to forty-five) in populations under comparison?

If this could be done, then in studying the reduction of the birth-rate in this and other countries, it would be possible to determine the exact share which change in the fertility of married women had borne in the reduced birth-rate.

It was evident that a statement of births (legitimate) per 1,000 married women aged fifteen to forty-five would make comparisons more accurate than comparisons of the crude birth-rate (births per 1,000 of total population). But as Stevenson and I showed in our first joint paper (p. 298) this correction would only be partial, inasmuch as in communities in which there in no practice of contraception, younger are more fertile than older married women within the thirty years of fertility. By using Swedish figures, which gave fertility-rates per 100 wives at each age-period, we were able to obtain a factor of correction for age of married women in the child-bearing years of life which is analogous to the factor of correction used in correcting death-rates for unusual age and sex distribution of populations. But a further correction similarly obtained was needed for the varying proportion of women who are wives at the ages fifteen to forty-five in different populations. It is unnecessary to describe here the methods employed: but we obtained corrected fertility-rates by means of which accurate comparison of true fertility in different populations became possible. By true fertility I mean the number of births occurring in a given population in which arithmetical causes of difference (varying number of married women and number of those at child-bearing ages) have been eliminated.

In a detailed international study using this more accurate process we were able to give important data as to the decline of human fertility in a large number of countries, as well as a more detailed study of this decline in different parts of the United Kingdom. This formed the subject of a contribution to the Royal Statistical Society, December 1905. Although still greater decline of fertility has occurred in more recent years, the comparative data we collected for periods 1861–1901 for England, and for many other countries for 1880–1900 or 1901, have a high historical value, for they throw light on the stages and progress in decline of fertility in different countries. The advantage of use of the arithmetical factors employed to secure *une vue tout ensemble* of relative fertilities in married life is especially well shown in such an international comparison. Note always that the factors calculated in our paper corrected the birth-rates for variations both in the *ages* and in the *number* of wives in each thousand of the populations under comparison. By this means we eliminated *arithmetical* causes of decline in the birth-rate, and left for consideration only those causes which, following the late Dr. Jacques Bertillon, the head of the Statistical Bureau of Paris, I called the *pathological* causes of decline in the birth-rate. The arithmetical factor is irrelevant in a study of true fertility; the non-arithmetical factor is concerned with intentional prevention of pregnancy by mechanical or chemical contraceptive agents, or with its unintentional prevention by maternal or paternal disease.

A short summary of some of the results obtained may be given. To avoid more complex figures the fertility in Sweden in 1891 was taken as 100, and other fertility-rates were stated as related to this standard. In 1881 New Zealand reached this standard, Ireland was 99, Italy 96, England and Wales 94, and France only 65 (all these are relative figures). Most English counties were not far from the standard, but the West Riding of Yorkshire was 89 and Worcestershire 87. Among towns, Aberdeen and West Ham were 99, while Halifax 84, Hull 83, Bradford 81, and Berlin 81 were all from 15 to 20 per cent below the Swedish standard. Paris was 47.

The figures for the later period 1901–3 showed a much greater falling off from the chosen standard. Prussia and Austria were 94, Scotland 91, Italy 89, Belgium 83, New Zealand 82, and selected rural counties of England and Wales 80. France was 55, while England and Wales as a whole was 78.

Few towns were now near the standard, but Dublin was 99, Glasgow 86, and Liverpool 85; while Portsmouth was 69, Bradford 60, and Melbourne 64, Berlin was 53, and Paris 34.

Many detailed comparisons are given in the original paper, and it contains a discussion of the causes of the decline in the birth-rates. Reasons were given for regarding it as not due to increase in the number of sterile marriages, but rather to smaller families. The decline was found to be "associated with a general raising of the standard of comfort, and to be an expression of the determination of the people to secure this greater comfort." In England it had received a great impetus from the notorious trial in 1877 of Bradlaugh and Besant for publishing a pamphlet on contraceptiyes. That the decline and the trial were closely associated in time is shown in Fig. 10, page 329. The following further extracts from our paper (for which I alone was responsible) gave my opinion of two social problems involved in the lowered birth-rate.

The gospel of comfort has been widely adopted, and is becoming the practical ethical standard of a rapidly increasing number of civilised communities. Halifax and Bradford began early. The selected rural counties in England have now approximated to the urban counties. Prussia has not yet overtaken Berlin, but it is following its example. We have no hope that any nation—in the absence of strong and overwhelming moral influence to the contrary—will be permanently left behind in this race to decimate the race. . . . And with this we must look for a lower standard of moral outlook, a lowering of the ideal of married life, and a consequent deterioration of the moral, if not also of the physical, nature of mankind.

Referring to the differential reduction of the birth-rate I remarked:

The facts indicate that the population is now being replenished in a higher proportion than formerly from the lower strata of society. Whether this means that the less fit are now contributing a greater share to the general population than in the past is by no means certain. Very few would venture to assert that the line of intellectual ability or of physical endurance is horizontal and not oblique, or possibly almost perpendicular in relation to social position.

Although I should now make the two comments quoted above with somewhat altered emphasis, I must add that after many more years of study of these subjects I do not think I need to make any substantial change in them.

The policy of so-called "birth-control" has widely extended during the years following 1908, with consequences which are likely to alter the course of Western civilisation. In an early edition of the *Encyclopædia Britannica* James Mill, following Malthus, stated that "the grand political problem is to find the means of limiting the number of births." The teaching that the pressure of population on means of subsistence, unless counteracted, necessarily implies eventual starvation for a large section of the people was accepted as axiomatic; and it only wanted the publication and wide adoption of fairly efficient contraceptive devices to make these popular. The pamphlet *Fruits of*

Philosophy met this need. It had been published by a Massachusetts physician named Knowlton fifty years before 1877, and had a small sale. Its English publisher in that year was prosecuted, the charge being one of obscenity by giving advice as to the limitation of families. The stock and plates of his book were ordered to be destroyed.

Charles Bradlaugh and Mrs. Annie Besant, acting as partners, took over and advertised the publication of *Fruits of Philosophy*. They were tried before the Lord Chief Justice and a special jury, and although the judge summed up favourably to them, the jury found that the book was calculated to deprave public morals. The indictment was quashed on appeal. In the next three years 185,000 copies of the book were sold, and the book was followed by others. A glance at the diagram on page 329 shows how the national birth-rate moved in harmony with this popularising of "birth-control" information. It should be added that Mrs. Annie Besant in 1890, having meantime changed her views, withdrew her book from circulation and destroyed its plates, as being inconsistent with theosophical ideals of man as a spiritual being.

In recent years restriction of births has become increasingly general. It is now common in nearly all stations of life, except the poorest, and to this extent its possible dysgenic effects are being eliminated. It is now being realised that if decline in the birth-rate continues we shall very shortly have a stationary population, which will then begin to decrease.

We are menaced with under-population instead of the over-population which some still regard as a national danger. And this is occurring at a time when man, having learned to restrict conception, has learnt also to increase vastly the productivity of animals and plants and thus abolish the danger of food shortage, even were the world's population to increase indefinitely. The position of those who advocate the continuance and extension of the practice of contraception needs to be re-considered in the light of these facts. Their advocacy of differential breeding is based on "facts" which do not satisfy the scientific mind (see pp. 290 and 402). The "ultra-calvinistic attitude of Galton and his disciples" is not confirmed. As Hogben states (*Nature and Nurture*, p. 121):

> The application of statistical technique in the study of human inheritance is beset with pitfalls. . . . There is the danger of concealing assumptions which have no factual bases behind an impressive façade of flawless algebra.

CONTRIBUTIONS

The Decline of Human Fertility in the United Kingdom and other Countries as shown by Corrected Birth-rates, by A. Newsholme and T. H. C. Stevenson (*Journal Royal Statistical Society*, Vol. LXIX, 1906).

Health Problems in Organised Society: Studies in the Social Aspects of Public Health, by A. Newsholme (P. S. King & Son, 1927, pp. 253 *et seq.*).

CHAPTER XXXV

EXCURSIONS IN STATISTICS

DENSITY OF POPULATION AS INFLUENCING HEALTH AND LIFE

Peabody Buildings—Corrections for migration—Slum dwellings and phthisis—Hospitals in aid of housing

THE discussion of housing problems in Chapter XXI needs to be supplemented by the summary given in this chapter of investigations on density of population and by the remarks on the increasing "hospitalisation" (treatment in hospitals) of the sick (Chapter XXXV) and on the relation between housing and tuberculosis (p. 302).

Very early I had interested myself in the problem of density of population as affecting the death-rate (p. 139); and in 1891 I read a paper before the Royal Statistical Society on "The Vital Statistics of Peabody Buildings . . ." embodying my conclusions. In prefacing this contribution I explained that I had undertaken to write on "the relation between density of population and mortality," and to review Farr's almost axiomatic statement on this relation, explained on page 301. For this purpose I had obtained the statistics of the Peabody Buildings as an extreme instance of a dense population, "an instance which did not exist at the time when Dr. Farr first showed the close relationship then existing between density of population and mortality, and evolved his formula from it."

The statistics obtained concerning the Peabody Buildings were so complete and so valuable as an example of improved housing for the poor that the paper was chiefly devoted to them.

At that time the Peabody Buildings consisted of eighteen blocks of dwellings in various parts of Central London, having a population of 20,462. They were occupied by working people paying weekly rentals which varied from 2s. and 2s. 6d. for a single room to 6s. or a little higher for three rooms. I was able to obtain an exact age and sex census of this population, and of the deaths which had occurred among them in the two years 1888–89. These deaths were stated to include all the deaths of inhabitants of the Buildings that occurred in infirmaries and hospitals. Some doubt was subsequently expressed on this point, but the figures were as completely corrected in this respect as is humanly practicable. There is one correction that it is impossible to make in such comparative death statistics. A family may leave a Peabody building (or a given district) and members of the family subsequently die from disease acquired while in their previous home. The converse may also occur; and it is assumed in all vital statistics that these two opposing influences cancel. This is not always the case.

Parenthetically, one may expand this point. In the condemnation of insanitary areas in a town, the M.O.H. states its unfavourable vital statistics. He is on safe ground in instancing excessive infant mortality, which being stated in terms of births relates entirely to recent experience. But it is otherwise when he quotes the general death-rate and the death-rate from tuberculosis. Pulmonary tuberculosis, for instance, may have been acquired elsewhere, and the patient, unable to pay the higher rent of a satisfactory home, drifts into the insanitary area and eventually helps to swell its death-rate. It is impracticable to distinguish exactly between the share which the slum dwelling and the earlier dwelling of the deceased may have had in causing or at least favouring his death; but accepting the facts as indicated above, the insanitary dwelling is not free from heavy responsibility. It is possible, however, that facts such as the above may have led to some under-statement of the mortality in the Peabody Buildings.

Another objection raised in discussion of my paper was that comparison should not have been made with the statistics of London as a whole, but with groups of small houses similarly circumstanced, except that the people did not dwell in block dwellings. This criticism was just; but a comparison with small dwellings in Central London would undoubtedly have made the comparative rates of the Peabody population even more favourable than they were.

The data mentioned above having been secured, it was possible to obtain the death-rates for each sex at successive age-periods, and to calculate a factor of correction enabling one to give the standardised death-rate at all ages in the Buildings and compare it with the standardised rate for London. This eliminated any selection due to age and sex distribution of population; but of course, as in the discussion on my contribution I agreed, "it cannot be denied that there is selection of a kind." Certain rules were enforced. "The dirty and dissolute, even if admitted, will be discharged when their failings are detected."

In the five years 1881–85 the average corrected death-rate for London was 21·93, for the Peabody Buildings 19·34 per 1,000.

Infant mortality was persistently lower in the Buildings than for London as a whole, and I regarded infants "as forming a very delicate index of the character of the environment of the individual." On the other hand the death-rate in the Buildings at the age-period one to five was higher than that of London, diseases due to direct infection, especially whooping-cough and measles, being more serious than in London as a whole.

FARR'S AXIOM

The main interest in my paper was in relation to Farr's formula, which stated that general mortality increases with the density of the population, but not in direct proportion to these densities but as their sixth root (see p. 280 of my *Elements of Vital Statistics*, 1923 edition). Later, Farr substituted 0·11998 in his formula. In his earlier writings, Farr suggested that in any sanitary inquiry the influence of density should first be discovered by means of the formula, and that the effect of other influences above or below this should then be investigated. It was even said that "the formula thus eliminates the element of density from the analysis of the causes of insalubrity." But in his later reports Farr deprecated the idea that this relationship was inevitable; and in the discussion on my paper Mr. Noel Humphreys, of Farr's old department, while pointing out that during the thirty years ending with 1870, on which Farr's calculations were based, "the relation between density and mortality was constant in a remarkably continuous degree, the Public Health Acts of 1872 and 1875 may be said to have repealed Farr's law of density."

My own conclusion was as follows:

> The number of rooms occupied by each family is of much greater importance in relation to health than the number of persons living on a given acre, as this fact throws important light on the state of each tenement as regards overcrowding. . . . So far as our knowledge goes, we can maintain that, given houses properly constructed and drained, and given cleanly habits on the part of the tenants, increased aggregation of population on a given area has no influence in raising the death-rate, except in so far as it is accompanied by *overcrowding in individual rooms*, an event which is by no means necessary in the circumstances named. In other words, there is no causal relationship between density of population *per se* and a high mortality.

Closeness of human contact, *when it increases the amount of social intercourse*, and only then, inevitably means increased prevalence of such diseases as measles and diphtheria, and we remain dependent on the production of artificial personal immunity for their prevention. This is not so for intestinal diseases (epidemic diarrhœa and enteric fever) in which sanitation is especially concerned, including domestic precautions in the feeding of infants. Nor is it so in regard to typhus in which the freedom from body vermin, now fairly general, has led to the disappearance of this disease (see also p. 120).

DENSITY OF POPULATION AND TUBERCULOSIS

When we consider tuberculosis we are faced by a more complex social problem. Its communicability is dependent largely on intimate and prolonged personal contact between a patient suffering from "open" phthisis and susceptible persons, especially children. We should expect it to be more prevalent in towns than in country districts, and in crowded districts than in those more sparsely peopled. In recent years the death-rate from phthisis in towns has approximated to that in rural areas, and if the experience of towns taken in their entirety is compared there is no constant relation between the proportion of the total population "living more than two in one room" and the phthisis death-rate per 1,000 of the total population. And yet the phthisis death-rate in a given town is always highest among dwellers in the smaller tenements. Doubtless several factors are involved. (*a*) Impoverished and sick members of the community drift into the lowest stratum of society. (*b*) Persons who become consumptive cannot earn good wages and drift into less satisfactory dwellings. (*c*) They also cease to be well nourished. (*d*) The inferior houses increase the mischief, and especially they mean greater exposure to intensified infection.

The anomalies indicated above can be partially explained when we consider what is the most remarkable social amelioration of the last sixty years—the *increased hospitalisation of the sick.*

This has provided most valuable supplementary housing combined with skilled attendance during illness, not otherwise attainable. The amount and quality of the general and special hospital provision of a community ranks next to good and adequate housing as a measure of its social and hygienic position among communities. This does not imply that the prevention of disease is less important than its successful treatment. Pure water supplies and other means of preventing typhoid infection rank higher than hospital provision for individual cases of typhoid fever, though unskilled nursing of a single case of typhoid fever at home may lead to a group of new cases or even to a wide outbreak of the same disease. Nor in the diminution of infant mortality can hospital treatment claim a considerable share. In this instance parental personal hygiene in domestic life has its immediate reward. But in the prevention of chronic infective diseases like tuberculosis and syphilis, treatment, which often must be institutional to be satisfactory, forms an indispensable element. A not inconsiderable share of the lowered death-rate at ages beyond infancy in recent decades must be attributed to the triumphs of modern surgery, especially in hospital practice.

The extent of increase in institutional provision can be measured in part by the increase in the proportion of total deaths which occur in hospitals not including nursing-homes. In 1870 in England and Wales it was 8·3 per cent, and in 1930 it had become 15·5 per cent. In London in 1930 the proportion was 18·4 per cent. Such facts led me (*American Addresses on Public Health and Insurance*, Johns Hopkins Press, 1920) to write of

HOSPITALS AS A PARTIAL SOLUTION OF HOUSING DIFFICULTIES

After discussing the value of hospitals in reducing the duration and fatality of diseases, and in diminishing their incidence, I added:

The aggregation during the last hundred years of a steadily increasing proportion of our population in crowded towns has meant the introduction on a gigantic scale of elements inimical to health. Smoke and obscuration of sunlight, dust and noise, the replacement of outdoor by indoor occupations, the difficulties of milk supply for children, and, above all, inferior (more cramped) housing with associated increased facilities for infection, have combined to render healthy life in towns difficult of attainment. Nor must we omit from the adverse side of the balance sheet the greater essential loneliness of family life in towns, the diminution in neighbourliness, and the failure of public social opinion to procure the wholesome effect on conduct which it exercises in village life. And yet, notwithstanding these factors, urban death-rates and especially tuberculosis death-rates have declined more than rural death-rates, and in parts of some countries urban is even lower than rural mortality.

And I then asked, Why is this? Even though it necessitates repetition I quote the answer :

Our hospitals provide the key to the mystery. Parturition is freer from risks in town than in remote country districts; the means for the prevention of infection are better organised, and accident and disease are more promptly and more efficiently treated. The poor in towns, when admitted into hospitals, receive as a matter of course better treatment gratuitiously or at a low charge than king or president could command thirty years ago. The relief to housing deficiency given by hospitals comes when most needed, in the emergencies of child-bearing and of sickness; and the net result of this and of better sanitary supervision is that although room-accommodation for families is much more restricted in towns than in country districts, the town-dwellers have a large share of their urban handicap removed by their superiority over country people in medical treatment.

The abolition of so much of the handicap which is the lot of the town-dweller in attaining and retaining health is a great triumph of humanitarianism and of applied science. In securing it many can share the credit. A large part of the credit must be given to the work of engineers, architects, and sanitary inspectors. The general medical practitioner has borne a part, and medical officers of health, backed by efficient public health organisations, can claim to have played a very important role. But to be fair we must give to voluntary and official hospitals, to their staff, and to the committees responsible for their organisation, a high place in our meed of appreciation and praise.

CONTRIBUTION

The Vital Statistics of Peabody Buildings and other Artisans' and Labourers' Block Dwellings (*Journal of the Royal Statistical Society*, March 1891).

CHAPTER XXXVI

EXCURSIONS IN STATISTICS

MORTALITY FROM CANCER

Need for standardisation of statistics—Possible lines of preventive action—Has cancer increased?—Alcohol and cancer—Postscript

CANCER mortality has been the subject of multitudinous studies during the last fifty years. In this period, the registered death-rate from cancer has steadily increased. In England and Wales the average annual death-rate from cancer registered in 1851–60 was 207 per million living (standardised population) among males and 440 among females. In 1901–10 these rates had increased respectively to 784 and 942, and in 1916–20 to 957 and 996. In the year 1931 cancer headed the list of single causes of death in England and Wales (59,346 deaths), tuberculosis coming next (35,818 deaths).

In earlier years tuberculosis was Captain of the Hosts of Death. I remember Osler's remark at a Tuberculosis Congress to the effect that tuberculosis had been Captain of the Hosts of Death; it had now only the rank of a lieutenant. It would shortly become a private soldier, and there was reasonable hope that eventually it would be drummed out of the army. Now cancer has taken the place of tuberculosis. An oft-repeated but erroneous statement is made that the increased death-rate from cancer is due to the larger number of survivals to the higher ages at which cancer claims nearly all its victims, a statement only true if one carelessly gives "crude" death-rates. This cause of incomparability between earlier and later statistics can be entirely eliminated. The Registrar-General now publishes cancer death-rates for standardised populations, i.e. populations in which correction is made for varying proportions of the total population at successive ages; and Mr.

George King and I as early as 1893, when employing corrected death-rates for the first time in the investigation of cancer, showed how this standardisation for cancer statistics changed the comparative position of various communities.

The absence of standardisation has made much of the writing on cancer statistics untrustworthy. The one thing certain in cancer statistics is that, whether the death-rate from this disease has or has not increased, cancer at the present time is the greatest enemy to normal duration of life, if we omit the risks of infancy. The difference between the age-incidence of deaths from tuberculosis and from cancer is seen in the diagram on page 308, copied from a contribution of mine to the *Lancet*. Its first half shows for 100 deaths of each of these diseases the number that die in each successive age-period 0–5, 20–25 . . . 75–85.

The second half shows the deaths at each age-period *plus* all the deaths from the same cause at all lower ages.

It will be noted that by the time the age of fifty-five is reached, tuberculosis has disposed of 88·6 per cent of its victims, cancer of only 29·8 per cent of those who eventually die of this disease. The proportion of deaths from each of them which occur at the working years of life 15–65 are tuberculosis 64·6, cancer 58·6 per cent. Both diseases strike very heavily at these most useful years of life, tuberculosis especially when promise has not yet been fully redeemed in accomplishment, and cancer in maturer years when accomplishment is curtailed and we are deprived of much of the invaluable contribution to social welfare and sound judgment which persons at and beyond middle life can make.

I was a member of the Statistical Committee, and then of the Executive Committee, of the Imperial Cancer Research Fund from its initiation in 1904 until 1931, and have watched its experimental research work during these years with profound interest. This work has cleared up doubtful points in the causation of cancer and disproved many plausible but erroneous hypotheses that were advanced as explanations; and although the genesis of cancer is still mysterious, the work done by the Fund, and to some extent by other organisations, has cleared the way for the solution of the problem for which we all look with a hope that may not be unmixed with anxiety.

We know that cancerous growths occur in all vertebrate

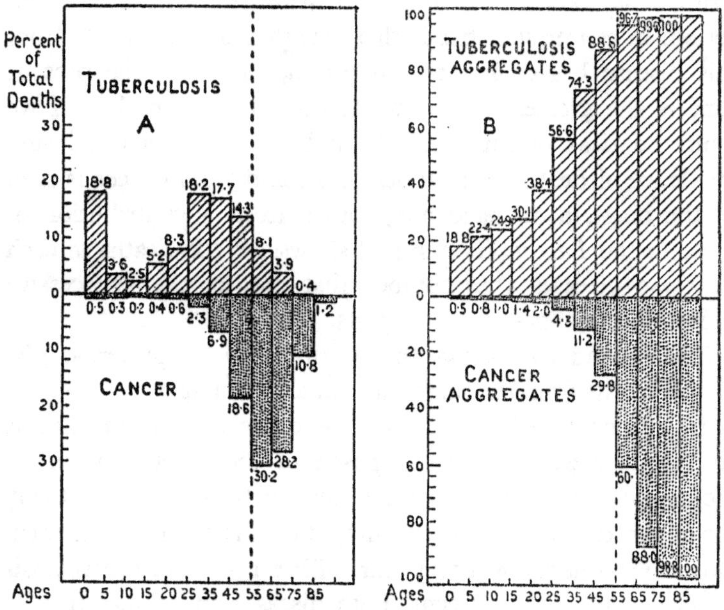

Diagram 8

England and Wales, 1901–10. A. *Percentage of Total Male Deaths at each Age-period from Tuberculosis and Cancer which occur at each Age-period.* B. *The same at each Age-period along with the Deaths at all lower Ages.*

animals. They occur in cold-blooded animals such as fish, in vegetarian animals as the cow, and in the uncivilised races of mankind. It may be said that cancer is rare among these, but among all these animals, and in savage man, death from "natural causes" in the more mature years of life in which cancer chiefly prevails is exceptional, and who will venture on guesses when there are no comparable statistics? The age-incidence of cancer is the key to open the door of all statistical problems concerning it. In abattoirs to which aged cows are still sent cancer is not uncommon, though rare in other cattle. The special conditions of civilised life, notwithstanding frequent representations to the contrary, must occupy a much less important place in the causation of cancer than has been ascribed to them, except the one factor of survival to more mature ages. On this I may quote a personal letter from the late Sir William Gairdner dated February 22, 1901, concerning an investigation made at his suggestion by Dr. Howden in 1893. I cannot find space for the whole of Sir William's letter; but the following extract gives the gist of Dr. Howden's contribution to this problem:

> At the time when the "increase of cancer" scare got into the newspapers in 1890, I suggested to Dr. Howden that without *arrière-pensée* he might go over his Index-Catalogue for thirty years, giving the facts as to cancer from his exceptionally detailed autopsies of patients in the Montrose Asylum during that period. He did this and found that there was absolutely no appreciable difference between the first half and the last half of the same series as to the proportional occurrence of cancer.

We know that various forms of local irritation favour the occurrence of cancer. The fissured tongue produced by syphilis is not infrequently followed by cancer, and the irritation of soot in chimney-sweeps and of paraffin in paraffin-workers when continued over prolonged periods may be followed by cancer. Cancer can be experimentally produced in animals by means of paraffin. Thus chronic irritation of a mucous membrane, or of the skin, is an important element in the production of cancer.

In an address given in 1923 (*Journal Royal Sanitary Institute*, Vol. XLIV, No. I (1923), I summarised the present possibility of preventive measures against cancer as follows:

> At no time has the prospect of success in tracing this disease to its initial faults been so bright as now. Meanwhile two lines of action are practicable as aids to the diminution of this disease; first, education of the public in the early symptoms of the disease, with the

object of securing the early treatment which offers the best prospect of cure; and secondly, the realisation by the public of the established fact that protracted local irritation is a chief provocative agent in causing cancer.

The Central Midwives Board have done good work in instructing midwives in the early symptoms of uterine cancer. Similar instruction of other special groups will be useful; but it is doubtful whether wide publication of information as to the early symptoms of cancer will achieve the end in view. Much more hopeful is dissemination of information as to the need for avoiding local injury of tissues and especially of prolonged local irritation. Cancer is known to be especially common in workers in petroleum and tar engaged in these occupations over many years, in the olden times in chimney sweeps, and in recent years, before necessary precautions were known, in workers with X-rays. These are exceptional provocatives of cancer; but what irritations are responsible, for instance, for cancer of the tongue, lip, and œsophagus, which in men in this country cause nearly 14 per cent of all registered deaths from cancer? Scalding hot drinks may be suggested as a possible agent; and I am informed on high authority that among Chinese women œsophageal cancer is almost unknown, but common in Chinamen; also that the Chinese wife eats her dinner of cooked rice after her husband has satisfied his hunger! In England at various ages œsophageal cancer is $2\frac{1}{2}$ to $4\frac{1}{2}$ times as common a cause of death in men as in women; and probably both indulge fairly equally in hot food and drinks. For cancer of the tongue the excess mortality in males is terribly great, varying from 11 to 27 times the death-rate in females at successive age-periods from 45 onwards. Evidently here we must assume some special source of injury especially involving men, and probably, to a less extent, this is true also for œsophageal cancer. Sir D'Arcy Power (Bradshaw Lecture, 1918) has collected evidence pointing to a close association between syphilis and cancer of the tongue; and in view of this probable inference, the thorough and systematic treatment of syphilis in its initial stages and still more the prevention of syphilis must be regarded as important measures for preventing the subsequent development of cancer.

HAS CANCER INCREASED?

Much interest attaches to the disputed question as to whether cancer mortality has increased, or whether the apparent increase is the result of improved medical diagnosis and certification. It is agreed by all that some of the increase is only apparent, but most writers on the subject consider that this explanation explains only a relatively small portion of the registered increase of cancer mortality. The Frankfort figures cited hereafter and the figures of life insurance societies, however, indicate that a much larger share of the apparent increase is thus explicable.

An initial doubt arises from the steadily improving accuracy of death certification by doctors. An early experience of mine in family practice illustrates this. I was called to see a city man aged fifty-six, who had been brought home profoundly anæmic after vomiting of "coffee-ground" matter. I had no difficulty in diagnosing cancer of the stomach. A distinguished physician saw the patient in consultation. He remonstrated with me as to the unwisdom of committing myself to a definite diagnosis of cancer; and some months later the patient's death-certificate was signed without any mention of cancer. At that time relatives objected to the word "cancer" or "malignant disease" on the certificate.

But there has also been a great increase in the treatment of serious disease in hospitals with autopsies in fatal cases; and this also must have led to increase in the cancer returns. In his Second Annual Report to the Imperial Cancer Research Fund, its director, the late Dr. E. F. Bashford, after a careful study of hospital statistics, concluded that even for hospital patients only those in which microscopical examinations had been carefully recorded were strictly comparable. Erroneous diagnoses were common on the negative as well as on the positive side.

But not merely improved diagnosis is concerned. Certification of the cause of death, although obligatory on the doctor in attendance, is necessarily unchecked in its accuracy, and many doctors prefer to give vague returns. This number is steadily decreasing; and a comparison of the number of deaths now ascribed to ill-defined diseases and old age, with the much larger number thus ascribed in earlier years, illustrates the great extent to which cancer may have replaced earlier indefinite returns.

It was such considerations as these which were in the minds of Mr. King and myself in 1892–93, when we investigated the official cancer returns. Our first task—never previously undertaken—was to make the national cancer death-rates strictly comparable from year to year. This was done by taking a common standard of age distribution (see the original paper in *Proceedings of the Royal Society*, Vol. 54, 1893). Then, after having calculated the national death-rate at each age-period from cancer, this rate was applied to the selected standard population at different ages, and thus we obtained the number of deaths from cancer per annum among a million persons in a standard population aged twenty-five and upwards. This was done for several successive periods of years and for each country in the United Kingdom, and by this means one could ascertain the true changes in the death-rate in each country. The corrections thus made greatly changed the picture given by the crude figures. This is shown by comparison of the crude and corrected figures for England and Ireland:

	Not Corrected		Corrected	
	England	Ireland	England	Ireland
1860–66	498	553	625	614
1888–90	1,091	894	1,393	912

Ireland by uncorrected statistics in the earlier years had a higher cancer death-rate than England, but the corrected death-rate was rather lower; while in the last period correction made the more favourable statistical position of Ireland very great indeed.

With the national figures for the three parts of the United Kingdom were compared the figures of the Scottish Widows' Fund Life Assurance Society. These related to persons insured for rather large sums, in whose cases certification would be likely to be exceptionally accurate, even after allowing for objections of relatives to "cancer" in a death-certificate. The annual curve for this Fund began higher and its increase was slower than that of the national curves.

Figures were also analysed from Frankfort-on-the-Main, which had exceptionally accurate records of deaths from cancer arranged according to the parts of the body primarily affected. By classifying these deaths into "accessible" and "inaccessible" cancer we were able to compare death-rates under each heading for a series of years, and showed that "accessible" cancers had increased. These results have not been supported by Dr. Stevenson's official statistics for England (see p. 492 of my *Elements of Vital Statistics*, 1923), but they have been remarkably confirmed by Professor W. F. Willcox in a contribution on "The Alleged Increase of Cancer" (*Journal of Cancer Research*, Vol. II, July 1917). In this paper Professor Willcox brought the statistics of Frankfort given in our paper (1860–89) up to the year 1913, and showed that up to that year the accessible cancers continued on the same level, while non-accessible cancers continued to increase (see diagram on p. 491 of *Elements of Vital Statistics*). Those interested in this subject should refer to a paper by Mr. R. Teece, F.I.A., on "The Increase of Cancer" in the *Journal of the Institute of Actuaries*, July 1901, and to the discussion on this paper, in which Messrs. King and Newsholme, Dr. J. F. Payne, Sir Thomas Smith, and Mr. Manly took part.

It cannot be said that we have reached the maximum registered total death-rates from cancer in England. Thus in Frankfort-on-the-Main in 1888–89 the standardised death-rate from cancer was 2,318 per million males aged twenty-five years and over as compared with 1,370 in England and Wales at the same ages. Either, then, there were causes of cancer mortality operating to an enormously greater extent in Frankfort than in England as a whole, or the Frankfort figures overstated its cancer mortality, or the real mortality from cancer in England was higher than the death-returns indicated. Probably the last-named explanation is nearest the truth.

There remains the possibility that, as my old teacher Dr. J. F. Payne always maintained, cancer of some parts of the body has increased, of others not. He specially instanced the registered increase of cancer of the alimentary system. There is a more recent example bearing on the same point. The Registrar-General's figures for England have shown that coincident with the fall in the birth-rate, the death-rate from cancer of the uterus, which is excessive in married women, has ceased to increase. Another interesting fact is that mammary cancer causes a higher death-rate in unmarried than in married women. The last named of these two facts may possibly indicate lines of preventive action, and the first points to the need for better midwifery and for stricter post-partum medical care.

ALCOHOL AND CANCER

The consecutive decennial supplements to the Registrar-General's reports give the average annual death-rates from cancer in persons engaged in a number of different occupations; and commenting on these statistics giving the experience of 1881–90, I drew attention (*Practitioner*, 1899) to the low "relative mortality figure" for cancer among coal-miners (38) as compared with coal-heavers (56). I then commented as follows:

> Can any reasonable hypothesis be framed to explain why the manipulation of coal underground should be so much less irritating than its manipulation overground?
>
> Can it be that we have to look to intemperate habits as being a main factor at work rather than the particular occupation?

I added that the high cancer mortality among commercial travellers, brewers, innkeepers, and butchers pointed to this conclusion.

This led to my obtaining figures from the United Kingdom Temperance and General Provident Institution to check this tentative suggestion. This is an insurance society with two divisions of insured persons, total abstainers from alcohol and others. I must refer to the paper named at the end of this chapter for information as to the reality of the comparability between the two groups. The same method of securing arithmetical comparability between the two groups was followed as in the joint paper by Mr. King and myself (p. 312). The broad results were as follows:

The death-rate from all causes in three years was 17·03 among the abstainers and 23·52 per 1,000 lives at risk among the non-abstainers, while the death-rate from malignant disease was 0·95 among the former and 1·34 per 1,000 among the latter. Thus the death-rate from cancer was 41 per cent higher among the non-abstainers than among the abstainers.

Unfortunately I was unable in this investigation to ascertain the site of the malignant disease, but I note that in the *Annals of Eugenics*, 1933, Parts III and IV, Dr. P. Stocks and Mary N. Karn have investigated a number of cases of cancer along with controls which show a positive association between daily beer-drinking in men and the location of cancer on lips, in mouth, pharynx, and œsophagus, but not in the stomach or elsewhere.

POSTSCRIPT

Since writing this chapter I have found several contributions written by me for medical journals, from which I make the following extracts:

CANCER HOUSES

The circumstantial evidence as to "cancer houses" sometimes appears convincing: but this may mean only a series of coincidences.

The late Professor de Morgan showed that if a sufficient number of persons were set to work at the tossing of pennies, it would eventually occur that one of these would, if he continued the process a sufficiently long time, turn up "heads" for a thousand times in succession without a single interval of "tails." . . .

It is plain that the fact that several successive families living in a house have each had members suffering in this house from malignant disease does not necessarily prove a causal relationship between the condition of the house or of the soil on which it is built and the origin of the disease. Nor does it necessitate the presumption that cancerous infection has clung to the house or any of its contents.

It was further pointed out that a succession of deaths from cancer in a given house or street might merely indicate that successive persons living in the house or street were of the ages at which cancer is a large cause of mortality.

In another investigation the tentative conclusion had been reached that cancer was specially endemic in certain cities, which were usually low-lying or flat, or bordering on streams, and it was regarded as "almost certain that there is a direct connection between the presence of subsoil water within a certain distance of the surface and the prevalence of malignant disease." This conclusion was not unlike an earlier conclusion of Haviland: but it is fairly clear that it had not been possible to exclude the fallacy that towns commonly are situate in or near valleys, and that their hospitals attract patients from distant areas. This case reminds one of the remark of a mythical Bishop, that the passage of rivers through or alongside of great towns was evidence of providential care for its inhabitants!

I may quote from one further article, illustrating the need for that standardisation of death-rates which has been already emphasised. After quoting figures from the city of Chicago, which misused the increased age at death as an explanation of the increased cancer death-rate, I added:

The fallacy of accepting the mean age at death as a test of duration of life has been repeatedly exposed in textbooks on hygiene and vital statistics; and it cannot now be rehabilitated for the purpose of showing that cancer mortality has not increased. The above is simply a variant of the fallacy involved in not carefully distinguishing between the death-rate from cancer per 1,000 living at all ages, and the death-rate from cancer at a particular age-group per 1,000 living at that particular age-group. Thus, Dr. Vivian Poore stated in a discussion on this subject (*Proc. Life Ass. Medical Officers' Association*,

May 1897): "The cause of the increase of cancer seems to me to arise from the fact that there is a great saving of life in the early periods of life and more people live to what one may call the cancerous age." Dr. Woods Hutchinson, in an article in the *Contemporary Review*, expresses the same erroneous idea in the following words: "To use a Hibernicism, cancer is increasing because more people are living long enough to die of it. . . . Cancer is the price paid for longer life."

In an article in the *British Medical Journal*, 1988, Vol. I, p. 74, I showed that the increased number of survivors to higher ages as compared with earlier years "only accounted for a small proportion of the total increase in registered mortality from cancer," and that the main statistical problem was to decide whether improved diagnosis and improved certification of deaths entirely or only partially accounted for this increase.

It is quite possible that cancer has become more frequent in certain parts of the body and less frequent in others. This point was urged by the late Dr. J. F. Payne, who showed from the statistics in St. Thomas's Hospital reports that the proportion of cancer of the digestive organs to total cancer had increased, and inferred that cancer of the digestive organs had increased. This may be true, though it cannot be said that the statistical evidence advanced in its favour is satisfactory.

CONTRIBUTIONS

On the Alleged Increase of Cancer, by George King, F.I.A., and Arthur Newsholme, M.D. (Read before the Royal Society, May 1893, republished in *Journal of the Institute of Actuaries*, Vol. XXXVI, p. 120).

The Statistics of Cancer (*Practitioner*, April 1899).

The Possible Association of the Consumption of Alcohol with Excessive Mortality from Cancer (*British Medical Journal*, December 12, 1903; reprinted in *Journal of the Institute of Actuaries*, Vol. XXXVII, April 1904).

PART VI

THE SAFEGUARDING OF DEVELOPMENT AND GROWTH

CHAPTER XXXVII

THE CARE OF INFANCY AND CHILDHOOD

Child welfare work not entirely recent—Illustrations of earlier work—Why did reduced death-rate 1–5 precede that at the age 0–1?—Birth-rate and infant mortality—Improved care of infants—Early specialised care of infants—Glasgow and Manchester—Huddersfield and Bristol—Foreign child welfare work

In writing on maternity and child welfare work, as on tuberculosis in preceding chapters, it must be remembered that I write from the personal angle of my own recollections; and that, although at various points I recall the work of others, I am obliged to write chiefly on those parts of maternity and child welfare work with which I have been most intimately associated.

I use the current phrase "maternity and child welfare work," but, in fact, I propose to postpone discussion of care of the mother, as new work specially intended to increase her welfare has been more pronounced after 1908.

The stages of development of *specialised* maternity and child welfare work illustrate how illogically British practical reform, in health as in other matters, arises and progresses. In Chapter XLI, it will be seen what a potent factor was anxiety as to national inferiority and perhaps deterioration in expediting the introduction of a school medical service. The defects discovered in school children gave added impetus to work, general or special, which would improve the health of the infant and the pre-school child or toddler, but it was not until 1914 that this work received monetary grants from the central government, grants in aid of maternity work being given at the same time. Of course, the health of the mother is the initial and always the chief means of ensuring that of the child, aided by hygienic and medical help for her children.

But although special organisations for reducing illness and

death in young children and their mothers began after 1900, it is a mistake to assume that anxiety about, and considerable effort to reduce, infant and child mortality is a recent development. The writings of Farr and Simon bearing on excessive infant mortality, if quoted, would fill many pages; and in the reports of medical officers of health from 1855 onwards similar anxiety has almost continuously been expressed. Much was written on the ignorance of hygiene and neglect of its practice, including the improper feeding of infants, excessive infant mortality having been usually attributed to these causes. A few quotations bearing on this subject are given on pp. 139–141 and more will be given in this chapter.

In earlier years efforts directed towards combating excessive infant mortality were chiefly those of general sanitation, as illustrated in the next chapter. Printed circulars were distributed on the prevention of diarrhœa, and of measles, and whooping-cough, three of the chief banes of infancy and childhood. Some authorities in the summer months distributed bottles of diarrhœa mixtures to all applicants, for the empirical treatment of this illness. This was an early instance of therapeutics as a public health measure. In Brighton in June of each year some 10,000 circulars, giving advice as to the prevention of diarrhœa were distributed house to house. These circulars laid special emphasis on the grave risk to the infant incurred when the mother ceased breast-feeding during the summer months.

In my report for 1894 I emphasised the unfavourable social conditions favouring diarrhœa, among which "the worst are probably artificial feeding by bottle and 'nursing out.' The mothers are frequently engaged as charwomen or laundresses, while their infants are left in the charge of neighbours or children."

At the same time I deplored that:

> Our educational work shows but little immediate results. There is a strong wall of prejudice, ignorance, and carelessness, through which it is difficult to break. There are, however, indications that some good is being done. One of the most hopeful features is the teaching

of the elements of domestic economy in the elementary day schools for girls in the town;

and I added:

> Much good might be done by simple instruction on the subject at Mothers' Meetings, by district visitors, and others; and I am glad to note the increasing attention which is being paid to this branch of parochial and voluntary church work.

In the same report it was stated that in 72 per cent of the houses visited because of deaths from diarrhœa, no defects were found justifying the issue of sanitary notices by the inspector; and I went on to moralise:

> The many items which conduce to produce a state of cleanliness sufficient to prevent the poisoning of infants' food cannot come within the scope of official action (for the removal of nuisances, etc.). . . . The chief means of preventing diarrhœa will remain with the householder, and they comprise the minutiæ of domestic cleanliness, care in the preparation of infants' food, avoidance of stale food, extreme cleanliness of bottles, etc.

In my annual report for 1896, after emphasising the rarity of diarrhœa in breast-fed infants, I added that for hand-fed children:

> It would be a great boon if sterilised whole milk in small bottles, each sufficing for one meal, were available by purchase for infants, and were to come into general use for infants during the summer months. This plan is now generally adopted in some countries, and I trust that in Brighton the want will soon be supplied by private enterprise.

In my annual report for 1902, sensational facts were adduced:

> Only those who frequently visit the homes of the poor in summer will realise that food can scarcely escape massive fœcal contamination. There are no pantries; food is stored in a cupboard in a living-room or bedroom. The sugar used in sweetening milk is often black with flies, which may have come from a neighbouring dustbin or manure heap, or from the liquid stools of a diarrhœal patient in a neighbouring house. Flies have to be picked out of the half-empty

can of condensed milk before its remaining contents can be used for the infant's next meal. While agreeing with Professor Delepine's conclusion that fœcal contamination of food is responsible for most of our epidemic diarrhœa, it appears to me that the swallowing of fœcal dust apart from food is responsible for a not inconsiderable amount of this disease, and that the infection more commonly has a domestic than a bucolic origin. . . . We cannot afford to neglect either of these possibilities, but . . . in this disease, as in tuberculosis, our chief enemy is in our own and in neighbouring households. . . . When we remember that some mothers prepare their infants' food with unwashed hands, the swallowing of virulent coli bacilli of human origin with this food ceases to be a matter of surprise.

In 1905 in a circular distributed widely, and particularly through registrars of births, the following advice was given in special leaded type:

Do not be persuaded to give up nursing your own baby, unless this is specially ordered by a doctor—a very rare event.

The best food for the baby is mother's breast milk without any other food whatever. It is especially dangerous to wean your baby during the summer months of June, July, August, and September.

These extracts relate chiefly to the contents of Chapter XXXVIII; but I wish here to emphasise the fact that prior to the earlier years of special infant welfare work, efforts were being made by most medical officers of health to reduce infant mortality, especially that caused by epidemic diarrhœa, while some attempt was also being made to increase maternal care, especially when young children had measles or whooping-cough.

I note that in my circulars to the public the statement that deficiency of cream causes rickets repeatedly occurs. I was, I confess, greatly dissatisfied with the relative lack of success of these efforts in my own experience; and Dr. G. F. McCleary in his admirable book on *The Early History of the Infant Welfare Movement* (H. K. Lewis, 1933) quotes the late Dr. J. F. J. Sykes, M.O.H. of St. Pancras, as finding that circulars of advice were apt to be misunderstood, the directions as to methods of feeding infants, when artificial feeding became necessary, having been even regarded as recommendations of artificial in lieu of breast-feeding. This led to the pioneer work done in the St. Pancras School for Mothers, initiated in 1907, which meant the replacement of printed by personal counsel, in which the value of personality was added to that of the written word.

In my Brighton annual report for the year 1904, I recorded an infant death-rate of 133 per 1,000 births, as compared with an average of 156 in the ten years 1894–1903, and added:

> We have no right to be contented until the infant mortality is less than one-tenth of the births.

But in 1932, the infant death-rate in Brighton had become 41, one twenty-fourth of the births, and the rate for the whole country in 1930 was only 60 per 1,000 births. Progress had exceeded a reasonable forecast. What has produced this marvellous change?

Various explanations are given, and one point is clear: no one factor is responsible for this great change, but a number of influences have co-operated in effecting it. And why had it not occurred earlier, for in the next four annual age-periods succeeding infancy marked reduction of mortality had been occurring for more than twenty years before 1901? We will consider this point first.

THE ANTECEDENT REDUCTION OF DEATH-RATE AT AGES 1–5

This was discussed by me in various reports to the Local Government Board, and to these I must refer for discussion of reasons why infancy had not in years before 1901 shared the benefit experienced at the ages 1–5.

The following remarks are drawn chiefly from my *Report on Child Mortality at ages 0–5 in England and Wales* (Cd. 8496). In this report I compared the English experience 1871–75 with 1911–15, which is near enough to our time-limit of 1908 to be utilised here. Between these two periods:

Death-rate under one year had declined			29 per cent
” at ages 1–2		”	41 ”
”	” 2–3	”	50 ”
”	” 3–4	”	53 ”
”	” 4–5	”	50 ”

I then noted that infantile mortality had declined to a less extent and that the decline had begun later (not until 1901) than the decline at ages 1–5, at which ages a declining death-rate is shown from 1871–75 onwards. I enunciated what are probably the reasons for this difference in date and amount of lowered death-rate. Congenital causes of mortality had not been attacked with great success; and "*the preservation of life in infancy is more closely a question of intimate personal hygiene than in the next years of life.*" I then continued as follows:

> The influence of improved personal hygiene is seen in the decreasing infantile death-rate in the last ten years (i.e. since 1904), and it is reasonable to expect that the increasing attention now being paid to the hygiene of pregnancy, of parturition, and of the post-parturition period in the mother will ere long result in a closer approximation of the degree of decline of infant mortality to that attained for the four following years of life.

The accompanying diagram shows the course of events in successive quinquennial periods since 1871–75.

This diagram is drawn from death-rates given in a table on page 12 of Cd. 8496, and it will be remembered that *actual* death-rates at the ages 1–5 are very low as compared with death-rates 0–1. A diagram on page 13 of that report shows relative death-rates for each of the first five years of life. In Diagram 9, in view of the fact that the course of events is practically identical in each of the ages 3–5, I have given the average relative rates for this age period instead of the fuller details in the original report.

I have not given actual death-rates for each age-period, but—in order to make the curves easily comparable—have in each instance stated the death-rate in 1871–75 at ages 0–1, 1–2, and 3–5 respectively, as 100, and all subsequent rates in proportions to this fixed point. By this means the differing course of the three curves becomes easily visible. The infant

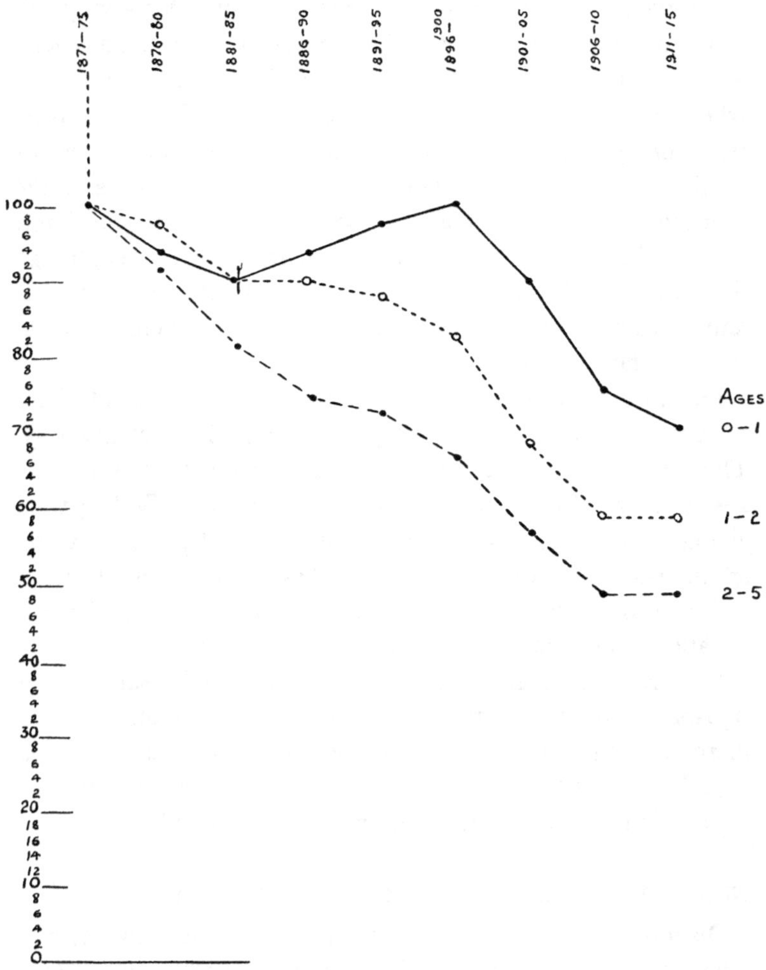

Diagram 9

Relative Mortality Figures in quinquennial periods 1871–75 to 1911–15 at Ages 0–1, 1–2, and 2–5, the death-rate at each age in 1871–75 being given as 100

death-rate has not consistently declined, and has in fact shown no continuous change until after 1900; while from 1880 onwards (even earlier it may be added) the curves for 1–2 and 3–5 have shown consistent and marked diminution—especially the curve for 3–5. We may well repeat our question—why this procrastination in decline of infant mortality? And the answer I give is that italicised on page 326. It is a true answer; but whether it is a complete answer I cannot say. To give a fully trustworthy answer a more compete analysis of causes of death at each age period will be needed. A large share of the reduced infant mortality after 1900 has been in diarrhœa, and this fits in with my italicised statement, though it is strange that educational influences should then have led to so precipitate a change. There is still room for a more complete historical study of the national mortality at ages 0–5.

(As an opportunity to write it may not recur, I add here a further reference to my Report on Child Mortality 0–5. This report set out fully the variations in death-rates at ages 1–5 in every chief sanitary area in England and Wales; thus giving—and this I have often said is the chief practical value of vital statistics—valuable "pointers" as to where investigation and reform are most urgently needed. The discovery of these variations was in fact the chief aim of the report.)

We have then not discovered a completely satisfactory explanation of the failure prior to 1901 of infant mortality to share the improvement already seen for many years at ages 1–5; but the italicised statement comes nearest to such an explanation, and fits in with the factors mentioned below.

INFLUENCE OF BIRTH-RATE ON INFANT MORTALITY

Diagram 10 shows the historical course of these two events —births[1] and infant deaths—during the years 1871–1930. Here again I have not given actual rates, but have stated the birth-rate and the infant death-rate of England and Wales in 1871 as equalling 100, and each subsequent rate in proportion to this.

[1] On page 115 of my *Elements of Vital Statistics*, ed. 1923, is given a similar diagram, showing birth-rates in proportion to the number of married women of child-bearing ages.

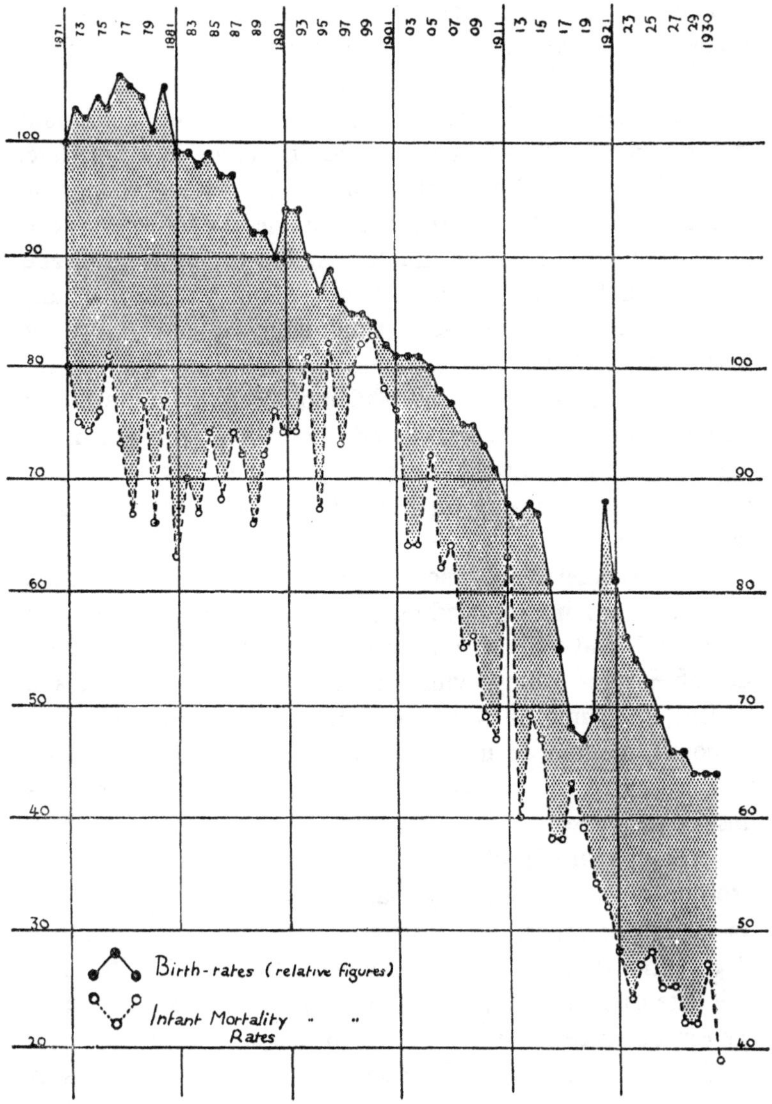

Diagram 10

England and Wales.—Curves of yearly Birth-rate and Infant Mortality rate 1871–1930 (Relative Figures)

Note.—Point 100 *for infant mortality begins at point which* = 80 *for birth-rate.*

The curves demonstrate that the course of the national birth-rate has not consistently corresponded with that of the death-rate of infants under one year per 1,000 births.

The English birth-rate gives no indication of continuous decline prior to 1876–80, and after that it declined at a rapid rate. By 1908, the latest year concerning us at present, that is, in about twenty-eight years, the birth-rate had fallen 27 per cent. A lower birth-rate means smaller families on an average, and the smaller families, although they are found more generally in the relatively well-to-do than among wage-earners, are found in the latter also on an increasing scale. In fact the change in birth-rate between 1876 and 1908 was so great, that smaller families limited to the relatively small number of families who are not in the wage-earning classes could not have produced the great change in the national birth-rate shown in the diagram.

Now a smaller family means, for the working-class mother, more time and an improved exchequer to devote to the care of each child, and it is reasonable to believe that here is a considerable factor in improving each infant's prospect of life and health. The family in which there is only one or two children is, however, often an unsatisfactory nursery of character, and such a family, by cultivating indulgence and bad habits, is mischievous also on the physical side of life. But we may reasonably regard families, say of four or five children, as more likely to be reared healthily than families in which there are seven or eight children. This statement is subject to a multitude of exceptions; and I have no doubt that a large family, when adequate care can be given, will be reared as successfully as—even more successfully on the side of character—than a small family in circumstances otherwise equal. Occasionally one sees statistics of the infant death-rate in families classified according to the number of births in each family, the small families always showing in the aggregate more favourable results. The statistics thus collected, so far as I have seen them, are not trustworthy, for the reason that the small families on an average have a better social position and a higher standard of hygiene than the poorer and large families which furnish the relatively high infant death-rates. *Non ceteris paribus.* Elsewhere I have discussed this subject more fully (see for instance, p. 117 of my *Elements of Vital Statistics*, 1923 edition, and my reports on Infant Mortality to the Local Government Board, 1910–16[1]), and have shown that many districts with a high birth-rate have a low infant death-rate, and that the converse position also often appears. But one may accept the probability that, *ceteris paribus*, the successive infants in a small family of the wage-earning class are more likely to receive adequate care than those in a large family.

That smaller families have not been a chief factor in reducing infant mortality is made clear by the curves on page 329, which show that between 1880 and 1901 the average rate of infant mortality remained almost stationary, or increased, while the birth-rate in the same period declined 20 per cent: in later years with a birth-rate which has continued to decline even more, a striking and almost continuous reduction of the infant mortality rate has occurred, which is out of proportion to the decline in the birth-rate.

We must seek for other reasons than smaller families for the factors which have been especially responsible for the reduction of infant mortality shown in Diagram 10. We may at once give first place to the dramatic improvement in the care of infant life since the beginning of the twentieth century. It should be remembered that preventive work for infants would bear fruit more quickly than preventive work directed, for instance, against tuberculosis, as the former is concerned with a single year of life only, and the lives at risk rapidly pass out of the statistical period concerned, to be replaced by an ever-flowing tide of infants. An important place must be accorded also to improved social and economic conditions. Sickness and unemployment insurance payments have contributed to this; and so, especially has the improvement in the drinking

[1] For reference see page 371.

habits of parents (p. 374). Sanitary improvements, including better methods of supplying and storing milk, have taken a large part. These factors overlap, and give mutual support. They have all been made more effective by the work of health visitors and of child welfare centres, although the main effect of their special work is to be seen chiefly in the years following 1905 or even 1908.

I have not separately particularised the reduction in the infectious diseases of infancy. Both at ages 0–1 and 1–5, this reduction has been experienced; especially of diarrhœa, but also of measles, whooping-cough, and pneumonia. But it was not until 1901 that effective attacks on diarrhœa may be said to date, and one must associate this with the italicised sentence on page 326.

THE RAPIDLY IMPROVED CARE OF INFANTS

To the influences producing better care of infants must be attributed the main share in securing the reduced infant mortality shown in the diagram on page 329. This was so, even in the years preceding 1909, with which in this volume we are concerned. In the period now under review this increased and improved care was only partly due to the work of special agencies (health visitors and infant welfare centres); it was even more the result *in this earlier period* of ameliorative measures undertaken by parents on their own initiative, and of the activities of voluntary and local governing bodies, apart from *specific* child welfare work.

Among these influences and measures first place must be given to the dual effect of domestic sanitation and of elementary education. On sanitation I write more fully in the next chapter. Elementary education became compulsory for all children between the ages of five and fourteen in the year 1870. It meant for the next generation an almost universal habit of reading, and with it some elementary acquaintance with rules of health (see Chapter XLI). This universally more instructed outlook on life was additional to the teaching of the elements of health to the extent to which it has, directly and indirectly, been embodied in actual instruction during school life. The late Dr. Wheatley, M.O.H. of Shropshire, drew marked attention to this factor in an address to the Society of Medical Officers of Health. Scholars must have exerted on mothers, and through them on infants, a great pressure in favour of cleanliness; for there has been in school-life a constant stimulus of emulation towards tidiness and cleanliness; and the scholars may almost be said to have been actively concerned in coercing their mothers to enable them to arrive in school in a creditable condition. The marvellous reduction of uncleanliness and of infestation with head and body lice which has been experienced under the pressure of the school nurse's work, has been a powerful factor in the same direction (p. 382). The medical inspection of school children, aided by the valuable work of school nurses, if it had secured nothing beyond this, would have greatly improved national health, not only of school children, but also of infants and pre-school toddlers. The discovery of malnutrition, with its multiform causation, and of actual disease in scholars has in addition led to home visits, and to remedial action which has been valuable to the infant as well as to the older children. School medical inspection on a national scale only dated back to 1907–8; but, before that year, elementary education was already of high hygienic value for the future. The girls in school in 1870–80 are the mothers of the infants in the years 1900–8, and their school work and their subsequent reading of newspapers and miscellaneous reading matter must have influenced for good, to an incalculable extent, their babies in the early years of the present century. The earlier part of the dramatic fall of infant mortality since 1900 owes much to this cause, and it must have been still more effective in the years since 1908.

This general influence received additional impetus from the work done by health visitors in their domiciliary visits, and by school nurses, and by them and by the medical officers at child welfare centres and at school clinics.

Their efforts have helped to reduce the amount of infectious disease; quasi-medical care, with expert consultations when needed, has been given to the mothers of multitudes of infants previously lacking this help; and instruction as to sunlight, fresh air, ventilation, personal cleanliness, clothing, and especially dietetics, has been popularised and disseminated. In the main, it is through their activities that this knowledge has now become the common possession of a great majority of the working-class mothers in the land. So much is this so that, in various towns, the mother in the classes which can afford to pay moderate medical fees, are now pressing for infant consultations for their children; and there can be little doubt that, where private medical practitioners do not train themselves for this hygienic work and organise it, such officially arranged consultations will become general.

If I were to state what, in my view, have been the greatest gains from general and special health work for infants and pre-school children, I would cite first the all-round improvement in the care of infants and young children, including the formation of good habits and orderliness of life; and next to this the special enlightenment which has secured the changes in infantile hygiene responsible for the reduction of rickets. This is perhaps the greatest of the enemies of healthy childhood; and in women it is a chief cause of difficult child-bearing. In its more serious forms, as shown by bone deformities, it is rapidly decreasing in prevalence, the administration of cod liver oil in infancy, or its equivalent in vitamin content, preferably as part of the infant's regular food, having become general in child management.

RELATIVE VALUE OF GENERAL AND SPECIAL WORK

It is not easy to determine the relative share of *general* and of *specialised* child welfare work in producing the rapid reduction of infant mortality between 1901 and 1906. For many years general measures aiming at this result had produced no patent effect on the national infant death-rate, but towards the end of last century better educated women were becoming mothers and by 1905 not a few health visitors were already at work. Their number did not suffice to enable personal contacts to be made with more than a relatively small minority of the mothers in the land; though we know that the influence of health education is never confined to those directly receiving it. We must divide the credit for the new steady reduction of infant mortality in the first five years of the present century between the relatively small amount of specialised child welfare work and the general enlightenment of the population, the work done in sanitary administration in educating the public mind and conscience, and the improvement in domestic sanitation and personal hygiene resulting from these more general sources of enlightenment and reform.

EARLY SPECIALISED CHILD WELFARE WORK

Some of the early developments in special child welfare work prior to 1908, so far as I can recall them, are given in the following paragraphs. Beginning with my local experience in my Annual Report for 1894 I noted success in obtaining one "female sanitary visitor." The number of births in that year was 3,055. The following comment was made:

> The next generation of mothers, especially if practical domestic economy is inculcated in the elementary day schools, will be better prepared to fight this almost entirely preventible cause of death (diarrhœa). In the meantime the female sanitary visitor and the sanitary inspectors visit the houses in which such cases are apt to occur (especially houses in which a birth has been registered during the last six or eight months), and distribute circulars setting forth simple precautionary measures.

We evidently had not "got far."

This solitary nurse gave weekly "talks" to all parish mothers' meetings who would receive her. She visited cases of measles and whooping-cough (sanitary inspectors also did this) which had been notified by school teachers, and she also undertook anti-diarrhœal work.

In 1906 the nurse and I started a school clinic, to which teachers sent boys and especially girls suffering from pediculosis, eczema, impetigo, and ringworm, and much useful work was thus accomplished.

GLASGOW AND MANCHESTER

I have before me a report written by me in 1892 in which the appointment of a female health visitor was urged. It set out her potential value in the above directions, and in advising as to nursing and thus reducing the number of deaths when young children are attacked by infectious diseases. In support of my application I quoted letters from Dr. J. B. Russell, M.O.H. of Glasgow, and from Dr. J. F. W. Tatham, M.O.H. of Manchester, showing what was already being done in these cities.

Dr. Russell said that in Glasgow they had five female inspectors who devoted special attention to domestic cleanliness, and made some 20,000 visits and 30,000 re-visits per annum. They also reported any nuisances found where they visited, and helped in prosecutions where these were necessary.

Dr. Tatham, after alluding to the existence of female visitors for many years under the auspices of a voluntary association, stated that since April 1892 the salaries of four to six of these visitors were being paid by the City Council, while their work was still carried on, like that of the many voluntary health visitors under the supervision of the ladies' branch of the Manchester and Salford Sanitary Association.

This, I believe, was the first instance of the payment of female sanitary and health visitors by a local authority. It is typical of what has happened so often in public health work, especially on its personal side. The work is initiated by voluntary workers, and then gradually, as it proves its utility, is taken over, partially or entirely, by the Sanitary Authority. Voluntary organisers have a freer hand to begin and carry on work on experimental lines than the representatives of the ratepayers, and to voluntary pioneers public health has been and continues to be indebted in planning out promising new work, while also giving most valuable help within the setting of official work.

The duty of each district visitor in Manchester was as follows:

> To visit from house to house in her district, and to carry with her carbolic powder, carbolic soap, etc., and to explain to the recipients the methods of using these disinfectants.

Dr. Tatham added:

> The visitors are instructed to direct attention to the evils of bad smells, want of ventilation, and filth of all kinds, and to give homely advice to mothers on the feeding, clothing, and nursing of their children, to report all cases of sickness immediately to the M.O.H., and to endeavour to promote the comfort of the sick or to arrange for their removal to the hospital. They are especially enjoined to urge the importance of cleanliness, thrift, and temperance on all possible occasions, and to endeavour to teach the mothers of families how to provide wholesome and economical food for their households.

They were also expected to observe the sanitary condition of the houses visited, and especially to report "concerning the method adopted in each case for the feeding of children, especially of infants under two years of age."

Dr. Tatham gave his opinion that "these services are a great boon to the sick, the suffering, and the helpless residents of the poorer districts of the city"; and he stated that the unpaid services rendered by the lady superintendents of these district visitors "can only be described as invaluable."

This ladies' branch of the Manchester and Salford Association started in 1862. The actual home visitors were paid from voluntary funds until 1892, when this burden began to be transferred to the common funds of the city. Dr. McCleary, in a fuller account of this organization (*op. cit.*, p. 87), states that in 1905 the city had become divided into sixteen districts for Manchester and Salford, each with its own visitor.

FURTHER HEALTH VISITORS

In various parts of England and Scotland it had become partially realised that sanitary authorities must concern themselves not only with nuisances, defective drains, and overcrowding, but also with infant hygiene and with the care of the sick. Action in the new direction started many years before it began to show its benefit in reduced national infant mortality, as was bound to be the case in view of its small extent when related to needs. McCleary states (*op. cit.*, p. 89) that in 1905 there were some fifty towns in which the local authority utilised the services of female health visitors. The work had begun on an exiguous scale, but it had begun. The name "health visitor" had not been standardised, and the newer name adopted in United States of America of "public health nurse" had not yet emerged.

These official visitors were additional to the voluntary visitors organised by health societies. Sheffield, Birmingham, Chesterfield, and Glasgow were among the early workers in this field.

Work of this kind was gradually improved as well as extended, and in some areas the adoption and enforcement of the compulsory notification of births to the M.O.H. made it possible to give prompt advice to the mother before wrong methods of feeding, etc., for her infant had been initiated. I do not propose to consider in this volume the gradually increasing value of midwives in the same field. To the extent to which they have been rightly trained they are the most valuable of all agents in the promotion of infant hygiene at a time when it is most needed and advice concerning it is most sympathetically received; and the passing of the Midwives Act in 1902 rendered possible the gradual abolition of unqualified midwives and the improved training of all future midwives. The practical value of the co-operation in infant health work between midwives and mothers will be seen best in considering events after 1908.

HUDDERSFIELD

The Huddersfield Corporation, led by Dr. S. Moore, their M.O.H., and with the very effective co-operation of Mr. Alderman Benjamin Broadbent, in 1906 secured from

Parliament local powers which enabled the M.O.H. to learn of all births in Huddersfield within thirty-six hours of their occurrence. Similar powers were soon given to other towns, and in 1907 the central government adopted a Bill introduced by Lord Robert Cecil, now Lord Cecil of Chelwood, for the notification of births, which enabled any local authority to secure these powers without special legislation. In 1915 the Notification of Births (Extension) Act made early notification of births universal, and empowered each local authority to exercise their existing general powers "for the purpose of the care of expectant mothers, nursing mothers, and young children."

Mr. Benjamin Broadbent took an important part during many years in promoting child welfare work. Wide publicity was given to his scheme for Longwood, a special district of Huddersfield in which he himself was born.

In 1904–5, when he was Mayor of Huddersfield, he announced that every infant born in Longwood would receive a present of £1 on completing its first year of life, and a promissory note payable on the child's first birthday was handed to the mother when she was first visited by the assistant medical officer, who acted as health visitor. This was accompanied by appropriate advice, repeated in periodical visits during the year. This was excellent "publicity," and all over the country the scheme was described.

Thus every district benefited indirectly. In speeches made by Mr. Broadbent, I have heard him emphasise the great moral value attaching to the interest taken in mothers and their infants, irrespective of the above scheme. He did not pass a perambulator without entering into conversation with the mother or nurse; and the human interest displayed, and the mother's realisation that her baby was a subject of communal as well as of parental anxiety must have been a valuable aid in increasing the efficiency of parental care. The good effect of this scheme and of the system of medical health visitors inaugurated in Huddersfield about the same time must be looked for chiefly after 1908, the time limit of the present volume, and it is necessary to note that in Huddersfield, as in the rest of England, much decline in infant mortality had occurred before Huddersfield's machinery for improved direct specific work became fully effective.

A few notes are added as to infant welfare work in this and other countries in this earlier period. Nathan Straus initiated the provision of pasteurised milk in New York in 1893, and in 1902 his organisation was supplying nearly a quarter of a million bottles of milk monthly. Dr. H. L. Coit in 1892 worked out a plan for the supply of good milk. He coined the phrase "certified milk" and he worked out in detail the procedure of certification of milk. Dr. Pierre Budin's first "Consultation de Nourrissons" was initiated in 1892.

In 1895 Budin organised his second Consultation de Nourrissons at the Maternity Hospital, Paris.

In 1894 Dr. Leon Dufour started the first Goutte de Lait, to supply milk which was modified and sterilised.

The number of infant consultations and milk depots rapidly increased in France towards the end of the century.

In 1899 Dr. Drew Harris, M.O.H. of St. Helens, Lancashire, initiated a Municipal Milk Depot in that town. At the end of the first year 140 infants were being fed on milk from the depot.

In 1901 Liverpool established two Municipal Milk Depots on the advice of Dr. E. W. Hope, M.O.H.

Some twelve municipalities followed in 1901–7, the Battersea depot being opened in 1902. These depots supplied sterilised milk specially modified for infants. Whatever may be said against these milk depots as possibly inclining mothers away from breast feeding, there is no doubt that they greatly influenced public opinion in favour of improved infantile hygiene.

Dr. McCleary in November 1905 began to hold consultations for the infants fed at the Battersea Municipal Milk Depot. A similar consultation was started by Dr. Chalmers in Glasgow in 1906. In the same year Dr. Pritchard started his Infant Consultation in Marylebone.

In 1905 the first International Congress of Gouttes de Lait was held in Paris.

In 1906 the first National Conference on Infant Mortality was held in London. At this Congress, the Right Hon. John Burns, the President of the Local Government Board, presided, and gave an important address, which is happily preserved for us in McCleary's *Early History of the Infant Welfare Movement* (Lewis, 1933). This address gave a great impetus to child welfare work all over the country.

In 1904 the late Dr. J. F. J. Sykes, M.O.H. of St. Pancras, in an official report, drew marked attention to the importance of pre-natal conditions, and concluded that "efforts should first be exhausted upon the mother before confining attention to the infant." If special emphasis be laid on the word "confining," this dictum enunciates a principle of fundamental importance.

In July 1907 the St. Pancras School for Mothers was opened, the work of which was concentrated in the main on efforts to aid the *nursing* mother. No special pre-natal consultations were held.

The Midwives Act came into operation in April 1902, and from April 1905 it became illegal for an uncertified woman to call herself a midwife. From April 1910 the practice of midwifery by unqualified women became illegal.

This is not a complete statement of the various special agencies for the welfare of infants which functioned during the whole or part of the period 1901–8. There are omissions on the official side, and more on the side of voluntary organisations. The sketch, however, suffices, I think, to enable one to form an approximate conclusion as to the part which these special agencies played in securing the marked and rapid decline in the English rate of infant mortality between 1900 and 1908.

The next chapters may be regarded as restating with some additions the substance of this chapter. The chief addition is a discussion of the great influence of alcoholic drinking on poverty and of poverty on alcoholism, and of these on infant mortality. It should always be remembered that public health efforts (including special child welfare work) are not carried out *in vacuo*. They influence and are even more widely influenced by contemporary social changes, of which the most important are named in the following chapters.

ILLUSTRATIONS OF DIFFICULTY IN STATISTICAL ASSESSMENTS OF PUBLIC HEALTH WORK

Public health workers are beset with demands to show results of their work—to "produce the goods" to use a common phrase. Sometimes in public health work this can be done, more often not. Infant mortality provides a happy hunting-ground for such (usually amateur) statisticians.

It must have been in connection with some such criticism that in November 1917 I wrote the following statement for the then president of the Local Government Board, which, I think, sets out the chief principles involved:

> Infant mortality has declined rapidly since more active measures for the protection of child life have been taken. The decline has taken place under the influence of a number of co-operative circumstances, including better houses, improvement of the milk supply, better scavenging and sanitation generally, and the special measures taken as the result of the Notification of Births Act. These have included advice and medical assistance for mothers and their infants, home visits by health visitors giving hygienic advice and assisting in the removal of influences, whether of habits or home circumstances, which are unfavourable to the health of the mother or child.
>
> The causes of excessive infant mortality being complex, it is impossible statistically to measure the influence of any one factor, such as the action taken as the result of the notification of births. To attempt this is to assume that results in human hygiene can be checked in the same way as experiments in a physical or chemical laboratory.
>
> There is a flagrant illustration of this absurd attempt in a recent official report issued at the cost of the Government, in which it is stated that:

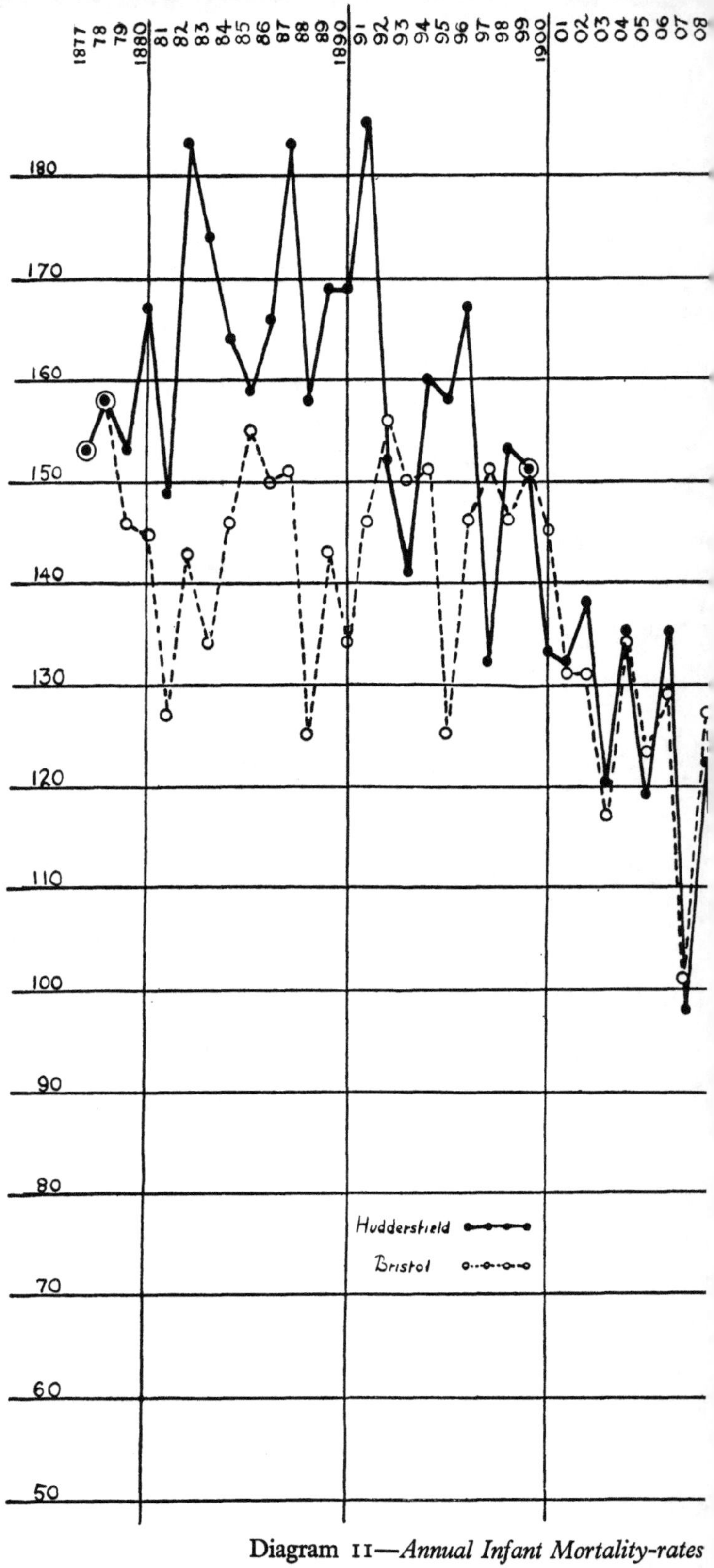

Diagram 11—*Annual Infant Mortality-rates*

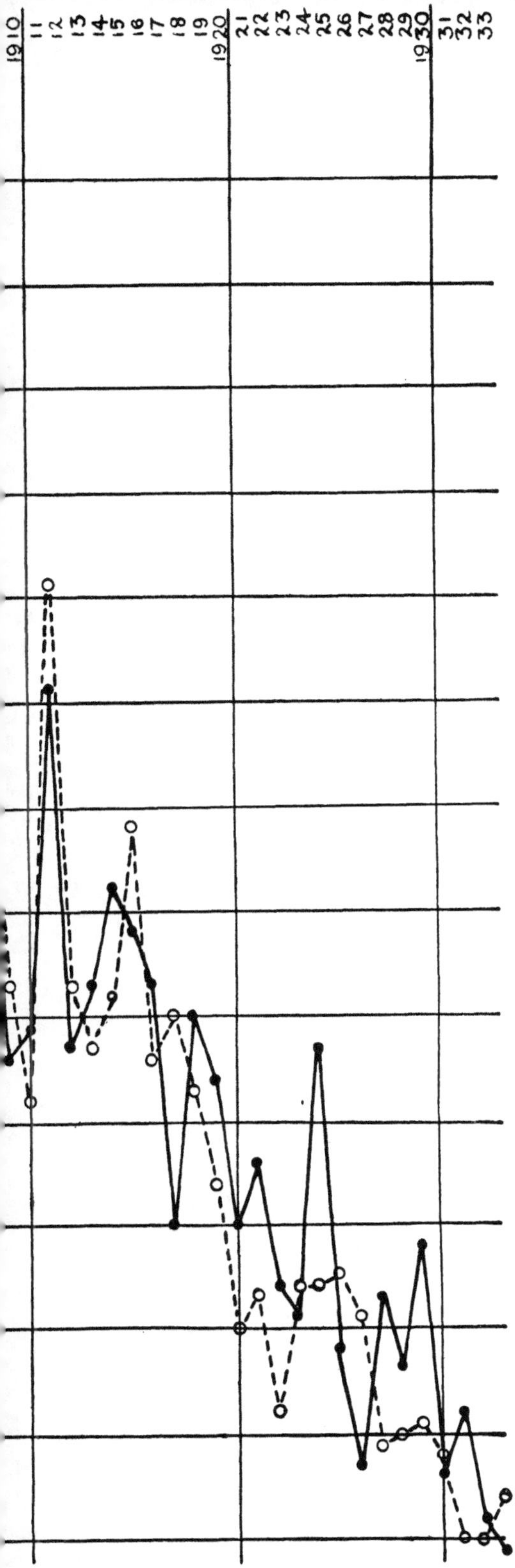

per 1,000 Births (1877–1933)

"A study of the infantile death-rates in towns where such measures (i.e. milk depots, infant clinics, etc.) have been adopted—Liverpool, Bradford, Poplar, Glasgow—does not support the contention that these methods are of much value in seriously decreasing the evil."

The statement here quoted is misleading because:

(1) As indicated above, it assumes that only one cause of change in the death-rate has been operating, viz. infant clinics, etc. Or

(2) That the other causes of change in the infant death-rate have been operating equally in every town.

(3) It assumes that the measures taken as the result of notification of births, including infant clinics and health visiting, have been operating for a sufficiently long time to enable the result to be statistically stated. This is not so, and attempts in this direction are comparable to the action of the small boy who week by week examines the seeds which he has planted to ascertain whether they are growing.

It cannot be too constantly borne in mind that, when complex causes are in operation, to attempt by statistics to prove the influence of one of these is likely to lead to serious errors. A much safer line is to argue on well-established general principles. It is certain that knowledge is better than ignorance: it is certain that a mother who receives the best counsel as to her own health and the health of her infant is in a better position for securing health than a mother who does not receive this counsel: it is certain that a mother who is helped by medical treatment or by the provision of a nurse or mother's help when required, is enabled to safeguard her own health and that of her child better than the mother who does not receive such assistance. These are obvious general principles and action in practical life must be taken on these lines.

HUDDERSFIELD AND BRISTOL

A further example is furnished by a comparison of total infant mortality rates in Huddersfield and Bristol during a long period.

The data on which the earlier part of this diagram (1877–1907) has been constructed are copied from the Annual Report for 1907 of the late Dr. D. S. Davies, the M.O.H. of Bristol. By kindness of Dr. Parry, now M.O.H. of Bristol, I am able to continue the diagram up to 1933. First, I will give Dr. Davies' remarks in his 1907 report on the two curves for Huddersfield and Bristol respectively, which in his report were given on opposite pages. In my diagram the same curves are superimposed. In commenting on his two diagrams Dr. Davies manifested the philosophical detachment of mind, and that determination not to be contented with less than scientific demonstration which characterised him throughout life, and which fitted in with his familiar name of "Doggie" Davies when we were fellow-students at St. Thomas's Hospital. He expressed his "sympathy with any work undertaken for the control of excessive infant mortality" and hoped that "the appointment of special health visitors will enable me shortly to undertake in Bristol some useful work to this end." But he warned the Town Council that "we must be careful in our use of statistical methods, lest too much be claimed and disappointment result." And he then pointed out that the great improvement in Huddersfield, "claimed as due to the special measures taken there," had been associated with "a practically identical improvement during the same years in Bristol without special measures to this end having been taken." The possible slightly greater improvement shown in the Huddersfield figures "may be due to the special measures adopted there . . . but there is no advantage in deceiving ourselves as to the extent of the improvement to be expected."

On a further page Dr. Davies summarised the comparative experience of the two towns as follows:

In the ten years 1897–1906, the rate of infant mortality was 135 in both towns, while it was 117 in Huddersfield in the three years 1905–6–7, and 117·3 in Bristol. Huddersfield had more industrially employed women aged 20–25 (21 per cent as against 15 per cent in Bristol of married or widowed women), but the proportion of employed women at ages 25–35 was equal in the two towns, and at ages 35–45 was greater in Bristol.

Mr. Broadbent interviewed me in 1918, when this comparison had been again brought forward, and after examining the experience of these two and of other towns I gave my conclusion that comparisons of results of child welfare work in terms of total infant mortality necessarily gave inconclusive results.

Writing on June 9, 1918, Mr. Broadbent suggested that "all the years before 1905 should be eliminated, because no direct efforts were being made before then"; but this did not remove the fact, as I said, that prior to 1905 some decline of mortality occurred and the subsequent course of the curves for Huddersfield and Bristol did not differ greatly, although Bristol had no health visitors before 1912. My own comment was:

> The course of infant mortality is almost identical in each town. This is an illustration of the *non ceteris paribus* . . . the causes of variation between different districts are so numerous that other causes are liable to conceal the important influence of child welfare work, and especially of home visiting.

In further correspondence Mr. Broadbent agreed as to the presence of other causes of difference such as housing, industrial occupations, and sanitary arrangements, especially the persistence in Huddersfield of pail closets and middens, and I confirmed this in the following comment:

> If one could subject communities to the rigidly controlled and simplified experimentation possible in chemistry, it would be easy to reach final conclusions on social problems; but unfortunately good work in one direction may be largely counteracted by bad influences in the same community. One does good service by displaying existent differences in infant mortality, and by emphasising that this is a complex social and sanitary problem, and that there is no one remedy for it any more than there is one pill or any pill to cure an earthquake.

I confirmed Mr. Broadbent as to the value of the Huddersfield work, even though Bristol's infant death-rate showed an equal decline, for the influence of the special educational efforts at Huddersfield and elsewhere was not limited to the towns where it began. Modern daily journals happily prevented this. And apart from cheap newspapers accessible to all, the "schoolmaster was abroad." Furthermore one had to bear other considerations in mind. Reduction of total infant mortality was an extremely crude measure of the value of special efforts. After all, there were non-preventible or partially non-preventible causes of death, which made the deaths in the first four weeks of life after birth responsible for nearly half the total deaths in the first twelve months. A dispassionate study of the history of infant mortality in these two towns from 1877 to 1934 demonstrates, I think, the folly of attributing to one factor what undoubtedly has resulted from many changes in sanitation, family hygiene, and social life, the share of each of which scarcely admits of statement by elementary methods of statistics, while the data for more elaborate statistical analysis are defective.

CHAPTER XXXVIII

ENEMIES OF CHILD LIFE

SUMMER DIARRHŒA

THIS subject must be discussed, as it has filled a very considerable place in the history of public health and in my personal epidemiological work in the last half-century. From 1912 onwards there has been a marvellous reduction in the toll levied by diarrhœa on infantile life, a change which is almost as striking as the reduction of typhoid fever. The reduction in the prevalence of diarrhœa lagged behind that of typhoid, suggesting at once in retrospect a difference in the causation of the two diseases.

In writing of diarrhœa in these pages, I concern myself only with epidemic enteritis which is chiefly fatal to infants in their first year of life. In the past dysentery and typhoid fever of an anomalous type have sometimes been veiled under the name diarrhœa, but for the present broad outline of the causes of the decline and fall of diarrhœa, this may be ignored. So also may changes in nomenclature in death registration, though it will be understood that the comparative figures here given show the direction and trend of events, perhaps not the exact prevalence of diarrhœa in any given year.

The magnitude of the change in the experience of Brighton is shown by the fact that in none of the three quinquennia, ending with 1900, did its average diarrhœal death-rate in Brighton fall below 23·7, while in the quinquennium 1927–32, it averaged only 8·0 per 1,000 births. In the decade 1901–10 there was some little improvement, though not enough to overcome the maleficent influence of hot summers. The last year in which an excessively hot summer succeeded in overcoming the inhibitory measures operating against diarrhœa was in 1911. Since then the peaks of excessive prevalence of diarrhœa in years of high summer temperature have remained relatively low. Similar remarks apply to the experience of England as a whole during the same period, the highest national death-rate from diarrhœal diseases of children under one year of age per 1,000 births being 31 in 1896–1900.

There was no considerable improvement until after the terrible outburst in 1911, though there were great variations from year to year. Perhaps some improvement is evident in the years 1902–10. But in more recent years a marked change appears; and it has become clear that infants are now no longer the helpless victims of epidemic diarrhœa even in hot summers, for hot summers have recurred, with relatively little excess of diarrhœa.

Typhoid fever, unlike epidemic diarrhœa, showed a continuous decline during several decades in the nineteenth century. In 1891, the death-rate from it was less than half of the rate in 1871; and in 1931 it had become only one-sixtieth of the rate in 1871. There is thus a marked difference in the national experience of these two intestinal diseases; and as we now conclude that defects of domestic sanitation and lack of cleanliness in methods of infantile feeding are chiefly responsible for the belated improvement in the diarrhœal rate, we may next examine experience in earlier years. Brighton may be taken as fairly typical of other districts.

From 1869 to 1874, after which year Dr. Taaffe, the first M.O.H. of Brighton, took over the work, Mr. Noel Humphreys wrote quarterly reports on the health and vital statistics of Brighton, which were printed and circulated. Mr. Noel Humphreys was Dr. Farr's colleague at the General Register Office, Somerset House (p. 274), and his remarks on infant mortality may, I think, be regarded as reflecting the views of his distinguished chief.

Reviewing the figures for the third quarter of 1870, a hot and dry season, with an excessive loss of infant life from infantile diarrhœa, he considers that this "may to a great extent be traced to the neglect and ignorance of parents," and recommends that, pending the effect which general elementary education is likely to have:

> in the meantime a good deal might be done by turning our almost universal system of parochial visiting to account for the purpose of impressing . . . the vital importance of simple sanitary precautions as to cleanliness in person and food and ventilation.

Commenting on the statistics for the third quarter of 1871, Mr. Humphreys says, "its low temperature had the effect of retarding the usual summer epidemic of diarrhœa." As is well known, experience until recent years had invariably shown that epidemic diarrhœa is most prevalent and fatal to infants and children under two years of age, that it is a disease chiefly of the summer months, the number of deaths varying with the summer heat; and that in this country it prevails excessively in towns, as compared with rural districts.

A further extract from Mr. Humphreys' 1871 report shows that he was imbued with the missionary spirit of William Farr. He states:

> In assuaging the severity of recurring epidemics invaluable assistance might be rendered by sanitary associations of ladies, who, having educated themselves in these matters, would devote a portion of their energy in parochial duties to bringing a knowledge of their importance into the homes of the poor.

And again in 1872 he remarks:

> The working classes . . . are evidently sadly in want of some knowledge of the elements of physical and sanitary science; to this ignorance may in great measure be attributed a large proportion of the preventible mortality which is continually occurring around us.

Dr. Taaffe, M.O.H., in 1874, emphasises the same point. "My own experience," he says, "is that numbers of infants are literally killed by improper feeding."

My own comments on the same subject (p. 323) show similarly that the neglect of infant hygiene was occupying the minds of sanitarians; and the extracts given above could doubtless, with variations, be indefinitely multiplied if one searched the reports of medical officers of health throughout England.

But as already stated, marked decline of diarrhœal mortality did not show itself until the second decade of the present century, when the numerous circulars of advice and warning which medical officers of health distributed in profusion were beginning to be supplemented by personal visits made by sympathetic and competent health visitors to the homes of the people, and the good effect of more widely distributed factors, including general education, began to emerge (p. 333).

In reviewing my annual reports from 1887 to 1908 I find that each year epidemic diarrhœa occupied considerable space, and my uncertainty as to its exact causation and prevention is indicated by the following extract from page 206 of the 1899 edition of my *Vital Statistics*:

> The prevalence of diarrhœa is a matter of great importance, and ought to receive further elaborate and combined investigation by skilled observers.

This was followed by the preparation and publication (*Public Health*, December 1899) of my individual contribution to this end, in an elaborate paper entitled, "A Contribution to the Study of Epidemic Diarrhœa," in which I gave the results of a detailed statistical investigation of the incidence of diarrhœa in the English great towns. This took the form of a Presidential Address given to the Society of Medical Officers of Health on my election, November 1899, as President of the Society. In it I attempted to weigh all available evidence on the subject, and set out some general conclusions.

Other studies of the subject had already been made. G. B. Longstaff (*Society of Medical Officers of Health Transactions*, 1880–81) arrived at the conclusion that:

> Summer diarrhœa is caused by the pollution of air, water, and food with some product or products of the decomposition of organic matter during very hot weather.

This broad statement would describe the inexact state of our knowledge to-day, except that we should lay less stress on air and water.

Dr. Hope (Liverpool) had also shown the close relationship of diarrhœa to infant feeding, and Dr. Spottiswoode Cameron (Leeds) had told how in an experimental area, a lower death-rate from diarrhœa followed special scavenging and swilling of backyards, unshared by other areas of the town in which these special measures had not been adopted.

In 1888 an exhaustive report on the subject had been published by the Local Government Board, written by the late Dr. Edward Ballard. This is mentioned later in this chapter.

My contribution consisted of a study of the death-rates from diarrhœa in the twenty-eight large towns of England, in each of the seventeen years 1892–98, and of their relation to conditions of soil, temperature, rainfall, sanitary circumstances, and social position. The differences shown in twenty-eight diagrams and in a detailed comparison of these towns are most striking. This is indicated in the following instances of death-rates from diarrhœa under one year of age per 1,000 births (average of seventeen years):

Four lowest	London	23·3
	Halifax	12·4
	Birkenhead	23·2
	Huddersfield	15·7
Four intermediate ..	Brighton	27·6
	Portsmouth	31·4
	Sunderland	31·7
	Norwich	32·7
Four highest	Blackburn	41·3
	Bolton	42·0
	Leicester	48·4
	Preston	60·4

In the following diagrams reproduced from the original address the extreme contrasts are displayed. (The vertical

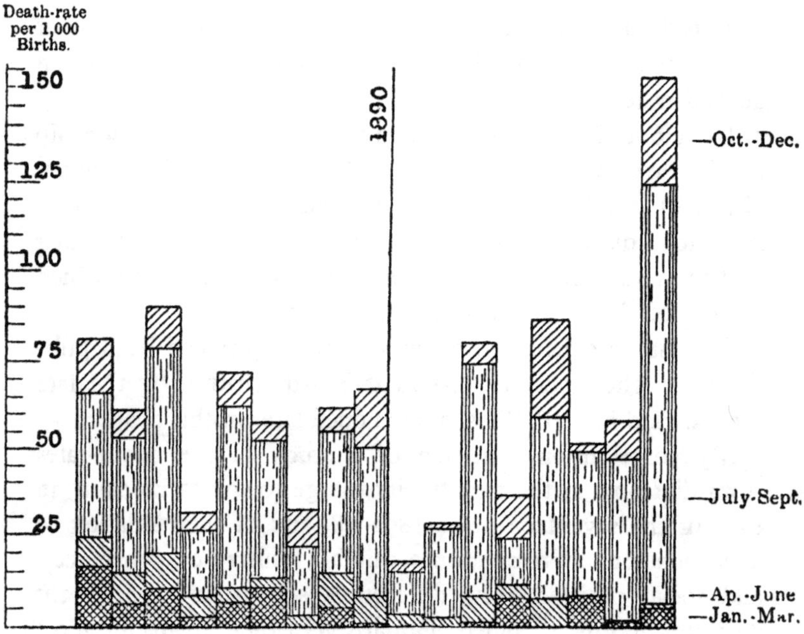

HUDDERSFIELD (1882–98).
Estimated population 1898 = 102,454.

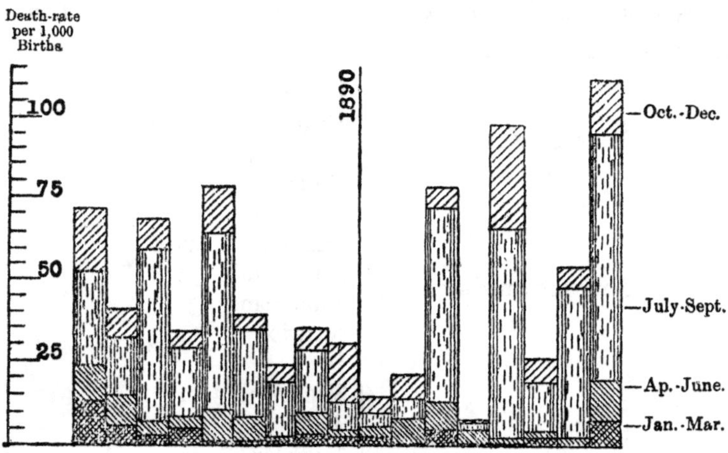

HALIFAX (1882-98).

Population estimated 1882 = 74,713.
„ „ 1898 = 96,729.

Diagram 12

Huddersfield and Halifax

columns are divided into four parts, giving the death-rate from diarrhœa in each successive quarter of the year.) Each diagram states the death-rate from diarrhœa in infants under one year of age per 1,000 births.

Huddersfield and Halifax during the years investigated (1892–98) had the lowest death-rate from infantile diarrhœa, while Preston, Lancashire, had the highest, Leicester coming next to it in height.

Briefly stated, the following conclusions were derived from this statistical study.

1. Epidemic diarrhœa in England is chiefly a disease of urban life, but no exact relationship to density of population or overcrowding is visible.

2. To a preponderant extent epidemic diarrhœa affects the wage-earning and especially the labouring classes.

3. Towns with the water-carriage system of sewerage, as a rule, have much less diarrhœa than those retaining "conservancy systems" (pails, privies).

But the last rule was not universally true; for some towns still having chiefly pail-closets, as Halifax, Huddersfield, and Oldham, had a remarkably low death-rate from diarrhœa.

Similar inconsistencies appeared in respect to scavenging, and it seemed that the efficiency of methods adopted was not easily capable of statistical statement. Furthermore, hilly towns with little sunshine and warmth in summer had relatively little epidemic diarrhœa. This explains the favourable position of towns like Huddersfield and Halifax in years before special child welfare work had begun, and while their house-sanitation was still unsatisfactory.

A good illustration of the importance of domestic sanitation in diminishing diarrhœa is given by contrasting Nottingham and Leicester, two Midland industrial towns, whose circumstances appear to be fairly equal in the years contrasted, except in regard to domestic sanitation. This illustration is given at this point, though it relates in part to years subsequent to my presidential address. In the following table taken from my

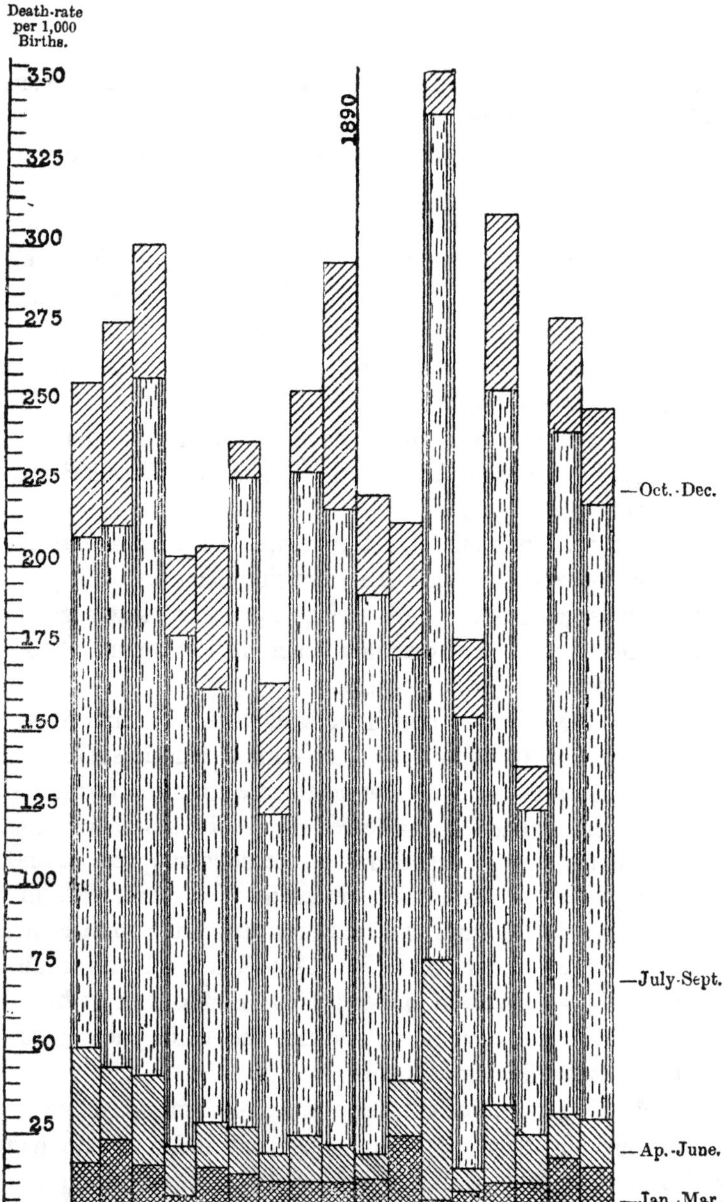

PRESTON (1882-98).

Population estimated 1882= 97,656.
,, ,, 1898=116,356.

Diagram 13

Preston

annual report to the Local Government Board for 1909, the diarrhœal mortality in each town in each period is given as proportional to that of 1889–93 stated as 100.

	1889–93	1894–98	1899–1903	1904–0	1909
Nottingham ..	100	139	145	119	96
Leicester ..	100	115	89	78	48

Leicester greatly improved its position, as regards diarrhœa, Nottingham scarcely at all, and this is coincident with the fact that half the houses in Nottingham continued to have pail-closets, while during the period under consideration, Leicester had entirely replaced these by water-closets (see also p. 204).

While hygienic excremental disposal was an important factor in diminishing the infection to which epidemic diarrhœa presumably is due, one could conclude that there are other concurrent factors which may reduce the evil influence of domestic insanitation.

4. Among these factors, the condition of the soil comes first to be mentioned. In the well-known report of Ballard, emphasis was laid on the relatively low mortality from diarrhœa in towns built on solid rock, even though other conditions were unsatisfactory, and the experience of the Lancashire towns, and of Huddersfield and Halifax confirms this conclusion. In my address I emphasised the influence of gradient as well as of soil as a factor in self-cleansing.

The discrepancies of experience already indicated are further explained in part by:

5. Local difference in temperature and rainfall in the summer months. I stated this dogmatically as follows, after a careful examination of local experiences:

> Given two towns equally placed as regards social and sanitary conditions, their relative diarrhœal mortality is proportional to the height of the temperature and the deficiency of rainfall of each town, particularly the temperature and the rainfall of the third quarter of the year.

I must refer readers to the original study for further details. Referring to earlier investigations of mine on rheumatic fever (p. 224) and diphtheria (p. 194) it was clear that whereas in these two diseases more than a single year's prevalence of the favouring climatic conditions is required for the production of a major epidemic, "epidemic diarrhœa becomes epidemically prevalent after a few weeks' persistence of the favouring climatic conditions."

At this point a suggestion made by me should be mentioned. It may have been inspired by similar suggestions made by Farr as regards cholera and density of population (pp. 100 and 302). In both of these instances Farr, many years ago, proposed a possible factor of correction for altitude above river level (for cholera prevalence) and for density of population (for the general death-rate), which should be applied before statistical comparisons of insalubrity were made. Similarly I suggested that "a series of meteorological factors of correction might be devised" in contrasting, for public health purposes, the position of towns as regards epidemic diarrhœa. I added, however, that:

> This is an unnecessary refinement, and is only mentioned as indicating the need for allowance for meteorological conditions in determining the merits of the relative position of towns in respect of diarrhœa.

In all these three instances the suggested arithmetical correction failed to give a satisfactory analysis of the factors concerned, and subsequent experience has shown their superfluity. It has, for instance, become clear that diarrhœa is controllable in the hottest years by measures of personal and domestic hygiene. The suggested factor for cholera had an erroneous basis; as to that for density of population, see page 302.

Special significance was attached by Ballard to the fact that the rise of diarrhœal mortality does not begin in England until the mean temperature recorded by the 4-foot earth temperature has attained about 56° F; but this is almost the same as stating that the mean weekly air temperature has reached 63° F. Both indicate the cumulative effect of the sun's heat on changes of decomposition in the soil and in food, and presumably on some micro-organism to which we may assume epidemic diarrhœa to be due. My final conclusion was that:

> The fundamental condition favouring epidemic diarrhœa is an unclean soil, the particulate poison from which infects the air, and is swallowed, most commonly with food, especially milk.

I should now attach special importance to contact infection, from uncleanly handling of the infant's food, though the close association of reduced diarrhœa and improved scavenging, substitution of water-closets for pails and privies, and the reduction in horse manure, point to the importance of dried dust and of flies in conveying the infection of epidemic diarrhœa.

I am not now certain that so much importance should be attached to "soil" except when it is impregnated with fœcal matter, and there occurs direct infection from a mother's fingers, or from flies carrying organic filth.

Like other observers I pointed to milk, the chief food of infants, as the usual vehicle of infection, while maintaining that in epidemiology there is usually a composition of causes, and that there must be no neglect of satisfactory sanitary arrangements, good scavenging, etc. It was necessary also that milk and other foods should be kept very cool.

The late Dr. James Niven, basing his conclusion on a weekly fly census in the summer months of several years, regarded flies as the common vectors of infection and the number of flies as a better index of the prevalence of epidemic diarrhœa than either temperature or rainfall in the summer months.

Similarly Dr. F. J. Waldo in his Milroy Lectures (1900), stressed the importance of horse manure as provoking epidemic diarrhœa, and this view is compatible with the remarkable decrease of the disease since motor- replaced horse-traction in towns.

Perhaps none of us emphasised adequately the risks of personal infection from the mother or nurse in charge of the infant, or of other domestic sources of infection; and this brings me to the last stage of this prolonged, though still incomplete, study of epidemic diarrhœa. All hygienists agreed in regarding milk and perhaps still more farinaceous foods as responsible for each summer's outbreak of epidemic diarrhœa, and this view appeared to lean to the conclusion that infection was of domestic origin.

But it was also commonly believed that the farm was the chief source of diarrhœal infection. We are indebted to Professor S. Delepine for a contribution to the *Epidemiological Society's Transactions* (Vol. XXII, 1902–3) which, with the discussion on it, has clarified this problem. He described an epidemic of diarrhœa affecting simultaneously a large number of people. This was traced to milk from a particular farm, and might have been due to the horribly insanitary conditions there prevalent, or to the milk from a particular cow on the farm which had a diseased udder. Delepine proved the presence of fœcal pollution in the milk; and inferred that there may be "a more intimate connection than has been generally recognised between epidemic diarrhœa and fœcal contamination of milk."

In his paper, which embodied valuable data as to the milk of farms, and the influence of temperature on the bacteriological contents of milk, he noted that while (in my address already summarised) I had agreed as to milk being the vehicle of infection, I had not attached so much importance as he (Professor Delepine) did to infection in the cowshed. His results, he added, while not excluding infection in transit or in the home of the consumer, indicated that infection at the farm "must be of paramount importance." He suggested that enteritis in the cow may be the source from which virulent bacilli are derived. He also regarded temperature as a more important factor in producing diarrhœa than deficiency of rainfall, on which point one may still remain uncertain. There is in summer a direct inverse relationship between temperature and rainfall.

In the discussion on Professor Delepine's paper I brought forward figures from experience in Brighton which were expanded each year until 1907, when my last local report was written. I may therefore use these more complete figures as bearing on domestic *v.* farm infection. In the years 1903–7 there were 202 deaths in Brighton from infantile diarrhœa, and it was possible to state exactly the method of feeding in each case. The method of feeding of 2,045 infants during the same period was ascertained. These lived in houses inspected house-to-house in the routine work of the sanitary inspectors, and they constituted a fair sample population. The detailed figures showed that breast-fed babies had only one-tenth, that babies fed on cow's milk had one-fourth, and that babies fed on condensed milk had seven times as many deaths from diarrhœa as would fall to their share were the deaths from diarrhœa evenly distributed among all the babies. This meant that condensed milk in this experience was especially dangerous, and that milk derived directly from a farm was much less dangerous. Some of the ways in which condensed milk may become infected are stated on page 323. Further details are given in a contribution to the *Journal of Hygiene* (Vol. VI, April 1906).

Dr. Meredith Richards in Croydon obtained results confirming the experience of Brighton.

My medical assistant, Dr. T. B. Heggs, examined specimens of condensed milk and found that in the process of condensation and preservation of milk the B. Coli had usually been killed off.[1] It is possible that the use of condensed milk may have formed an important pre-condition of diarrhœa by producing malnutrition, with a semi-scorbutic condition or preliminary catarrh of the digestive tract. And here we pass

[1] In 1911 Dr. F. J. H. Coutts, of the medical staff of the Local Government Board, made an exhaustive inquiry into Condensed Milks (*Food Reports No. 15*). Living bacteria were found in samples of condensed milk; but Dr. Coutts states, "it appears probable that coli bacilli of intestinal origin present in the original milk are as a rule destroyed in the manufacturing processes. Most tubercle bacilli are also destroyed."

indistinctly from the standpoint of direct infection to that of previous conditions favouring infection. It is in this borderland that the best work in infant hygiene has been done.

But the main conclusion established by the varying experience of breast-fed infants, of infants fed on fresh cows' milk, and of infants fed on condensed milk, was that the infection of diarrhœa is domestic in origin. This conclusion is now, I believe, generally accepted. The relative share in carrying infection of flies, of domestic dust, or unsterilised feeding bottles, and of the nurse's unwashed hands, must be conjectural, and obviously all these possible vehicles of infection must be guarded against.

CONTRIBUTIONS

A Contribution to the Study of Epidemic Diarrhœa. Presidential Address before the Society of Medical Officers of Health, November 1899 (*Public Health*, December 1899).

The Public Health Aspects of Summer Diarrhœa (*Practitioner*, August 1902).

Remarks on the Causation of Epidemic Diarrhœa in the Discussion on Professor Delepine's Paper (*Transactions Epidemiological Society*, 1903).

Domestic Infection in Relation to Epidemic Diarrhœa (*Journal of Hygiene*, Vol. VI, April 1906).

CHAPTER XXXIX

RICKETS, MEASLES, AND WHOOPING-COUGH

MEASLES IN WAR-TIME

I HAVE devoted a long chapter to Epidemic Diarrhœa for several reasons.

(1) It was by attack on this disease that the first step in the modern infant welfare movement was taken; attempts to diminish mortality from measles and whooping-cough playing a considerable though minor part in this earlier work.

(2) Diarrhœa is a good instance of the value of public health effort even when only an incomplete knowledge of causation is possessed. We have now no reasonable doubt that epidemic diarrhœa is caused by infection or by some toxic agent produced by a specific contagium. And we cannot doubt that the measures of municipal and domestic hygiene, which have been followed by the rapid decline of this infantile scourge, have included the direct prevention of this contagion.

(3) In the prevention of diarrhœa an improved dietary for healthy infants played an important part, and by this gateway the physiological side of hygiene found an entry into public health practice. This entrance of physiology into public health showed itself especially in the discouragement of the advice to wean their infants often given to mothers for inadequate reasons; and such artificial feeding as was inevitable became more satisfactory and especially more aseptic than in the past. Among the various improvements in artificial infant feeding, perhaps the most influential for good among the very poor has been the increasing substitution of dried for other forms of milk, with some fruit juice added as a precaution against scurvy. Mention has already been made of the mischief, apart from diarrhœa, often caused by sweetened condensed milk and farinaceous foods given during the first nine months after birth.

RICKETS

The great diminution of rickets in recent years is an outstanding feature of the child welfare movement; and this has resulted from the improved feeding of infants and the correlative general hygienic improvements, especially the increased appreciation of fresh air and sunshine. This reduction in rickets has meant a lowered death-rate from bronchopneumonia and therefore from measles and whooping-cough. The reduction in the death-rate from the last-named diseases must be ascribed in part to reduction in the prevalence of rickets.

One cannot fail to be struck with the parallelism between the decline in the prevalence of epidemic diarrhœa and of rickets; and as rickets is a disease of malnutrition, it is certain that the reduction of rickets has been largely due to the reduction of diarrhœa, with its immense drain on nutrition and the occurrence of prolonged "marasmus," which in the past has figured so largely in the list of causes of death in infancy. Alongside of these diseases must be remembered the large number of puny, rachitic survivors after attacks of diarrhœa.

Quite apart from intercurrent diarrhœa, rickets had been the chief of the enemies of child health in multifarious ways, and most visibly by delaying and diminishing growth, by making it deformed, and thus becoming responsible for the greater part of the crippledom of the young. Rickets and tuberculosis have been the twin enemies of child health and development, both of them happily now in process of extinction as the direct result of the application of modern hygiene. The history of crippledom in this country during the last thirty years is a typical example of the way in which with improvement of medical and surgical skill deformities are successfully corrected. Then follow efforts to prevent the need for surgical skill.

HISTORY OF CRIPPLEDOM

This history is embodied in the science and art of orthopædics, an account of which is given in the *Life of Sir Robert*

Jones (Hodder & Stoughton, 1934). He was chief among the leaders in this work. Orthopædics is a branch of pædiatrics, and as neither word has become so familiar in this country as in America it may not be superfluous to state that the root of the word pædiatrics is derived not from the Latin "pes" (a foot), but from the Greek *παις παιδος* (a child). Thus orthopædics is concerned with correcting and with preventing deformities of any part of the body or limbs in children.

When I was a medical student frequent operations were undertaken to correct knocked-knee by operation on the internal condyle of the femur, and to straighten extreme bow-legs by fracturing the bones and resetting them in a less crooked position. These deformities were then terribly prevalent. There is a story in the biography just mentioned of a father who brought his son for treatment—"but there must be no breaking of bones." "But," said R. Jones, "you would not object to fracturing," and the father responded, "No, of course not," and so the child was cured.

A reference bearing on the question of school hygiene (Chapter XLI) is worthy of continued publicity. In 1888 R. Jones gave an address on the "Hygiene of School Children" in which he dealt with the question of physical training, and inveighed against the artificial deportment imposed on girls in boarding schools.

> Many of us have sent daughters or sisters to schools spirited and healthy, and have lived to see them return round-shouldered, deformed, martyrs to headaches . . . threatening their whole future happiness.

And he concluded by forecasting:

> We ought soon to eradicate rickets, and with it, at one stroke, the pitiful deformities, which follow in its path. . . .
>
> All this cannot be now far off, and when it comes we poor physicians and surgeons, many of us at least, may be relegated to the ranks of the unemployed.

The vast improvement that has occurred since the above words were written was happily seen in large part by Sir

Robert Jones before his death in 1933. He had done invaluable work in fulfilling his own forecast. In 1895 he quickly seized the importance of Roentgen's discovery, and with Dr. Holland was the first in England to apply it in the discovery of a small bullet embedded in a boy's waist.

During the Great War the orthopædic hospitals established on his initiation by the War Office secured skilled specialist treatment to soldiers, justifying Lord Moyniham in bracketing R. Jones with Almroth Wright (in the prophylaxis of enteric fever) as two of the greatest benefactors during the war. I can only mention R. Jones's later work in initiating a network of large country hospitals for crippled children, served by after-care clinics, and directly related to public health administration in every county in England. There was created an admirable co-operative system in which voluntary officials and workers combined for the benefit of crippled children. Others were at work with the same object, but to Robert Jones must be given the honour of training a multitude of skilled workers in this speciality, and thus rendering possible the success of the present advanced and successful methods of treatment of cripples.

On one aspect of anti-tuberculosis work on which I have laid special stress in Chapter XXX he was especially emphatic:

> There can be no policy more obstructive to the objects we have in view than that advanced and incurable cases (of tuberculosis) should be sent back from sanatoria and other institutions to their houses, and so expose to infection their children . . . at the very period when the danger is greatest. The human bacillus could be largely eliminated if the authorities insisted on the proper care and isolation of the consumptive.

MEASLES AND WHOOPING-COUGH

Over 90 per cent of the total deaths from measles and whooping-cough occur at ages under five; and with the decline in the birth-rate the proportion of the total population chiefly at risk—children under five—has also decreased. In comparing successive periods, therefore, the death-rate from these diseases must either be stated in terms of the child population, or death-rates for all ages together must be standardised to eliminate this source of arithmetical error. Whichever of these two methods of statement is adopted it is found that the death-rate from both diseases has declined materially. Inasmuch as measures of isolation, disinfection, or other public health measures have not been practised or have proved largely ineffective, this reduction is reasonably attributable to better nursing, to improved hygiene in the homes of the poor, and especially to the reduction of rickets, rendering broncho-pneumonia less fatal when it complicates these two diseases. The greater fall in whooping-cough than in measles supports the important role I have ascribed to rickets in infant mortality. Some idea of the lower death-rate from measles and whooping-cough and from diarrhœa may be gathered from the following table:

England and Wales. Standardised Death-rate at all Ages

	Measles	Whooping-cough	Diarrhœal Diseases
1861–70	377	450	974
1901–10	318	286	874

These figures are remarkable. They show that at this earlier period, when special national child welfare work was small in amount, the improvement as concerns measles and whooping-cough was far greater than that for diarrhœa. Reduction in the death-rate from measles and whooping-cough was being earnestly sought by medical officers of health, who were especially active in educational propaganda. Already rickets was declining in prevalence, and must have exerted much influence in the same direction. But it gives one pause to remember that improvement in infant feeding, as judged by diarrhœal mortality, was secured more slowly than improvements in other branches of hygiene.

The almost routine recurrence of measles every second year is well known; but the occurrence of major epidemics at longer intervals, described by Whitelegge and others, is not so generally recognised. Both major and minor epidemics appear to be almost unavoidable, and in towns it is rare for a child to escape in one or other of two successive epidemics. The main object in present circumstances is to secure that the attack shall be postponed until the child is over four years old, after which age an attack is much less likely to prove fatal. In years which come after the limit of this volume, successful results have been obtained from treatment by the serum of convalescent patients, or, less satisfactorily, by serum obtained from adults who have had measles in childhood. Much saving of life may be expected on these lines.

Measles patients when placed in a hospital ward do not do well unless careful bed-isolation and free aeration are secured. When measles breaks out in an institution for infants and young children, the first duty of those in charge, after removing patients already attacked, is to break up those remaining in the institution into smaller groups, as for instance by distributing them in wards for adults. They should be widely spaced, and each patient screened from other measles patients, and nursed under strictest aseptic precautions.

Measles in adults unprotected by an attack in childhood may be terribly severe, and in the Great War I saw lamentable illustrations of this among Highland soldiers at the Bedford camps, and in the camps on Salisbury Plain to which New Zealand recruits, suffering from measles acquired in crowded quarters while coming from that distant land, arrived to join as combatants. War has the capacity—whether through over-crowding or otherwise—to intensify the measles virus. This was strikingly illustrated also in America in the North *v.* South war. A further illustration is given as an appendix to this chapter.

In describing a Brighton epidemic of measles in 1904 I drew attention to the fugitive vitality of the infection of influenza, and remarked that "for several years it has appeared to me that the same must be true in regard to measles." I gave reasons why disinfection after a portion of the cases (as there was no compulsory notification of this disease) was unlikely to do good, and that even were it otherwise the rush of patients would, if disinfection were attempted in all known cases, overwhelm our administrative machinery. In order to test whether in fact the absence of disinfection means retained infection, my staff undertook a special investigation. We knew of 625 houses recently invaded by measles. In 534 of these the occupants were the same a few weeks later as on the first visit, and no further children had been attacked by measles, although terminal disinfection had been abandoned. In 66 houses new families were living in the houses recently invaded by measles or new babies had been born. Altogether there were 86 "new" children in these presumably infected houses which had not been disinfected after the recent epidemic cases. Of the 86 new children, 59 were said to have had measles previously, leaving only 27 unprotected and possibly exposed to infection. No cases had occurred among these. Further details are given in my Annual Report, Brighton 1904. Although these data are scanty, they led to my permanently abandoning disinfection after measles. Dr. C. V. Chapin of Providence, U.S.A., led the way in abandonment of terminal disinfection after scarlet fever and diphtheria; and in this country Dr. Duncan Forbes, my successor in Brighton, similarly was a pioneer in abandoning disinfection after these diseases. Such disinfection can now be regarded as futile when it goes beyond what can be effected by domestic cleaning and washing.

MEASLES IN WAR-TIME

Although the problem is one of adult as well as child welfare, I may insert here an illustration of the terrible danger involved in the close aggregation of infants and children if measles gains an entrance, and if, as is generally the case, there occurs, along with measles, attack by additional catarrhal infections. In such circumstances a most virulent symbiotic infection is produced, with terrible loss of life.

At the time of the South African or Boer War (1900–1) I wrote several editorial articles for the *British Medical Journal.* The first of these was entitled "The Waste of Life and Efficiency in South Africa" (*British Medical Journal,* January 1901) and two later articles in the same journal on "The Mortality in the Concentration Camps in South Africa" (*British Medical Journal,* November 9, 1901). In these camps military and in part humane considerations had led to the aggregation of Boer women and children in concentration camps. After a full analysis of the number of persons thus aggregated, and their death-rates, my article stated:

> We have no sympathy with those who would make political capital out of the high death-rate in the concentration camps. The camps appeared to be a military necessity, and it was doubtless regarded as more humane thus to mass the women and children than to leave them to starve on their half-ruined homesteads. The results, however, have been calamitous.

I need not recall the figures which showed a terribly high death-rate from measles and broncho-pneumonia. While agreeing that the "habits of the Boers probably made matters worse" it was added:

> This is simply a further reason for not permitting the continuance of aggregation under such unsatisfactory conditions. . . . We have serious doubts as to the efficiency of the sanitary control of the camps. It is due to inefficient sanitary control that a large share of the dysentery and enteric fever in the military camps has occurred, and the statistics give ground for suspecting that similar inefficiency has characterised the control of the concentration camps.

A practical remedy was proposed:

> The one essential thing is to split up the camps into a number of much smaller camps on new and unpolluted soils. Large numbers of cases of measles cannot safely be treated together unless under the most favourable hygienic conditions. Failing these conditions,

the aggregation of patients must be stopped. The conscience of the public is very properly touched on this subject . . . and it may be hoped that prompt measures will be taken in the direction indicated.

The editor of the *British Medical Journal* Dr. (afterwards Sir) Dawson Williams, writing to me on December 16, 1901, said:

You will see that the suggestion that the camps should be thinned out and broken up has been to some extent at least adopted. . . . I think we are entitled to claim credit for the action of the *Journal*; it is at least a curious coincidence that Mr. Joseph Chamberlain (then Colonial Secretary) telegraphed at 4.25 p.m. on Friday, November 8th, to Lord Milner asking whether aggregation of large numbers would not involve excessive mortality; and on November 9th, at 1.10 p.m., requesting (as had been urged in the editorial articles) that the statistics of child mortality in the camps should be placed on the basis of definite classification by ages. Your article was published in the *Journal* dated Saturday, November 9th, but could be obtained in London on the morning of Friday, November 8th, and you will remember that it was freely quoted in the daily papers of November 8th. A copy of the *Journal* was also sent on Friday, November 8th, to the Secretary of State for War. . . . Apparently the responsible people have accepted advice and are prepared to do what is practicable.

CHAPTER XL

SOME SOCIAL ASPECTS OF THE HEALTH OF THE CHILD

Poverty and health—Maternal ignorance—Social disabilities —Fecklessness of mothers—Alcoholic indulgence

In preceding chapters I have described some aspects of child hygiene as seen in my life-time, and have discussed not only the sanitary circumstances which influence the health of the child but also the supremely important factor of improved parental care. But further remarks as to the economic and ethical aspects of family life are needed if I am to convey my convictions resulting from long-continued study of this subject.

POVERTY AND HEALTH

These remarks bear chiefly on the intermingled influence of poverty and of the character of the parents on the health of their infant. In continuing in this chapter the study of preventive medicine as applied to the infant, I propose to distinguish between the poverty which is unavoidable by parents and the poverty which may not unfairly be regarded as at least partially self-inflicted. It is a subject on which I have frequently written. The statements set out here are more fully given in a series of Reports on Maternal and on Infant and Child Mortality to the Local Government Board published in 1908–16.[1]

We must accept it as axiomatic that increase of family

[1] *Report on Infant and Child Mortality* (Cd. 5263), pages 142, issued 1910. *Second Report on Infant and Child Mortality* (Cd. 6909), pages 411, issued 1913. *Third Report on Infant Mortality in Lancashire* (Cd. 7511), pages 204, issued 1914 (contains contributions by Drs. S. M. Copeman, Farrar, Lane-Claypon, and Manby). *Report on Maternal Mortality in Childbearing* (Cd. 8085), pages 140, issued 1915. (contains contributions by Drs. Lane-Claypon and I. Cameron).

income makes it easier to ensure the health of children. A steady improvement in the average economic status of the community has occurred during the present century, notwithstanding the Great War and the increase of unemployment. Insurance funds have done much to counterbalance the privations and dangers of unemployment, and it is clear that the children of wage-earners even in 1934 *on the average* are better clothed and better fed than they were in the nineteenth century. This does not mean that the position is altogether satisfactory, only that it is less unsatisfactory than it was. For poverty, even when only partial, is seriously detrimental to the children affected by it.

We have already seen that diarrhœal mortality is much heavier among the poor than the well-to-do. This statement holds equally true for such diseases as measles and for total infant mortality. The best figures as to the social incidence of total infant mortality are those prepared by the late Dr. T. H. C. Stevenson for the Registrar-General's Annual Report, 1911. In that year the deaths of infants per 1,000 births were 77 in the upper and middle class, 133 in the wage-earning class, 133 for skilled and 152 for unskilled labour, and 97 for agricultural labourers, as against 148 for textile operatives and 160 for miners.

To what extent is poverty itself responsible for these differences? Figures given in my Report on Mortality at ages 0–5 (Cd. 6909) go far to justify the statement that to blame poverty *per se* is a first-class error. Ireland and Norway are both poorer countries than England and Wales; but in 1906–10 England's infant death-rate was 117, that of Ireland was 94, and that of Norway (in 1909), 72. The rural circumstances of the last two countries more than offset the preponderance of town life in England. The comparison of infant mortality given above between agricultural labourers (very poor) and skilled labourers illustrates the same point. We need to analyse the circumstances of poverty more closely. To quote my above-mentioned Report:

In this connection it is significant that prior to 1900 the average infant mortality in England and Wales failed to decline, notwithstanding steady improvement in the average economic condition of wage-earners during this earlier period. Improvement in the average condition of wage-earners as a whole is, of course, not inconsistent with the continuance of extreme poverty in a considerable proportion of the total population; and such poverty is injurious to both mother and infant, diminishing the immediate prospect of life and deteriorating the physique and health of the infants who survive an ill-nourished childhood. But the fact of an average improvement in respect of poverty (in this earlier period) remains. Evidently, then, in recent years some further influences, beyond the beneficent effect of reduction of poverty in proportion to total population, have come into action.

MATERNAL IGNORANCE

That maternal ignorance is a chief factor in the causation of excessive child mortality is, I have said elsewhere, "comfortable doctrine for the well-to-do person to adopt." It embodies an important aspect of truth, but it is mischievous when it leads to the notion that what is chiefly required is the distribution of leaflets of advice, or the giving of theoretical instruction in personal hygiene.

There is little reason for thinking that the average ignorance in matters of health of the working-class mother is much greater than that of mothers in other classes of society. Furthermore, it would appear that working-class mothers give their infants the supremely important initial start of breast-feeding in a larger proportion of cases than do the mothers in other stations of life.

The mothers in all classes may be ignorant; in both there has been deficient training in habits of observation, especially as to the beginnings of illness and the formation of good habits; but the mother in comfortable circumstances is able to ensure for her infant certain advantages which the infant of the poorer mother often cannot obtain. Among these are the following:

(1) The well-to-do mother is commonly able to devote herself to her infant and have assistance in this duty; the working-class mother is single-handed, and has also to perform

unaided all the duties of her household, including the washing and cooking for the family.

(2) The well-to-do mother is commonly able to ensure that the milk for her infant is purchased under the best circumstances, is stored in a satisfactory pantry, and is prepared in a cleanly manner. The working-class mother often is supplied with stale, impoverished milk, may have no pantry, and except when suckling her infant is handicapped at every stage in the cleanly preparation of her infant's food.

(3) If the well-to-do mother is ill, adequate medical and nursing assistance is at once available, and the child's welfare can be safeguarded; if the working-class mother is ill, the child must often suffer with its mother.

(4) If the child of the well-to-do mother falls ill, everything that good nursing and medical attendance can furnish is commonly at once available; for the child of the working-class mother the state of matters is remote from this ideal, for facilities for medical attendance and nursing vary greatly in different districts in the extent to which they are available for the poor.

(5) Infants and nursing mothers are both quickly affected by their environment. This environment is complex. The mother forms the chief environment of the infant. If she is overworked and suffering from chronic fatigue her infant must suffer; directly, because the mother's milk under these circumstances is liable to be impoverished or otherwise unwholesome; or indirectly, owing to insufficient attention to the infant. The infant of the well-to-do mother is less likely to suffer in either of these ways.

(6) Not only are the milk supply and the storage and preparation of artificial food important parts of the environment of the infant, but so also are the housing conditions of the family, and the sanitary conditions of the back-yard and of the street in which the house is situate. The superiority in these respects of the circumstances of the one mother and infant over those of the other is obvious.

Both mothers in the past have commonly been ignorant. But the *ignorance* of the working-class mother is more dangerous, because *associated with relative social helplessness.* To remedy this the environment of the infant of the poor in essentials needs to be levelled up towards that of the infant of the well-to-do, and medical advice and nursing assistance needs to be made available for the poor as promptly as it is for persons of higher social status.

I have already emphasised the removal of ignorance and the specific instruction of mothers in child hygiene as responsible in large measure for the reduced infant mortality since 1901. But this is only successful when the disabilities of the mother in the poor family mentioned above are removed or reduced.

FECKLESSNESS OF MOTHERS

Probably more important than actual ignorance is carelessness or fecklessness of mothers. In the essential duty of breast-feeding the infants of the poor are better served than those of the well-to-do; but, for the reasons just set out, maternal carelessness among the poor in other respects is fraught with much greater risk to the infant than corresponding carelessness among the well-to-do.

This carelessness is being diminished under the pressure of public opinion and of the example of other mothers. A child welfare centre in this way is a great influence for good. Not only is the mother influenced by the medical advice given, but she is subjected to the stimulus of comparison of her child with the children of other mothers, and to the valuable influence resulting from the evidence of active interest in her child. The effect of these influences is confirmed by the systematic visits of a tactful and judicious health visitor.

INTEMPERANCE

Alcoholic indulgence of parents is a major cause of excessive infant mortality in a proportion of total families, which still remains higher than would be inferred if we trusted the too optimistic impressions on this point now current. It is at this point especially that we reach the special region of voluntary or self-imposed poverty. Alcoholism is not the sole cause of self-imposed poverty. Gambling is another road to this goal, and poverty may also arise from extravagance or carelessness apart from these two great vices.

Short of drunkenness the systematic indulgence in drink of one or both parents, i.e. indulgence which involves the diversion of a considerable proportion of the family income to drink, necessarily implies that an available margin of wages is being spent, which, more wisely expended, would have served to pay the additional rental needed for satisfactory housing, and still more to supply the children with more milk or a more satisfactory total dietary than is now given them. The immediate physical gain obtainable from an increased ration of milk in children of school and pre-school ages has been abundantly demonstrated. It is in large measure a question as to whether the parents shall have their beer or the children shall be more satisfactorily nourished and cared for. The question is not, however, merely or chiefly one of diversion of limited funds from a useless and often harmful luxury to important necessaries. It is much more than this.

As regards experience before the Great War let me quote from the annual reports of two distinguished health officers, Drs. Hope and Niven, giving their experience in Liverpool and Manchester respectively.

Dr. Hope (Annual Report, 1907) gives the history of 874 families taken consecutively, because in each of them an infant had died. In these families 3,801 infants had been born and 1,895 had perished, nearly all in their first year; while

> side by side with this, other parents under similar conditions, with the same income, following the same occupations, the same hard struggle against poverty, had reared all or nearly all of their children. The question arises, To what is this remarkable difference due?

The answer in Dr. Hope's words is as follows:

Long series of cases of this description are recorded, in which obvious drunkenness in an extreme degree is the pre-eminent feature associated with the loss of the infant, the money wasted, the parent drink-sodden, and every feature of intelligent attention to the infant wanting. With these there comes the long string of examples in which the alternations between the gaol and the workhouse are factors, which make it abundantly plain that the children of the family have had no proper maternal solicitude bestowed upon them and have perished in consequence.

Dr. Hope goes on to contrast these conditions with those of poor Jewish families among whom "thriftiness and sobriety were universal; no drunkenness," and great care was taken by the mother as to the children's food. Among them infant mortality was low.

Similarly, Dr. Niven states that the infant mortality in the Cheetham District of Manchester in 1894–1903 was 115, as compared with 184 for the whole city. He explains that Cheetham is a very poor and crowded district, and adds:

The quarter is inhabited by Jews. It is the custom among these Jews for married women to stay at home. . . . There is practically no drunkenness, and these poor people are in consequence comparatively well-nourished. They are not very clean.

He further animadverts on "the squalid destitution in towns which accompanies drink and pawning facilities." (See also Dr. Niven's more recent comment on p. 168.)

Since the writing of the Reports just quoted there has been much improvement in alcoholic habits; but the amount still spent on alcoholic drinks remains almost incredibly high. The exceptionally trustworthy estimate of Mr. G. R. Wilson, B.A., based on official records, is that in Britain in the year 1933, £4 19s. 4d. was spent per head of population, or £7 10s. for every person aged twenty and over. Total abstainers are necessarily included in this average. Of the total alcoholic expenditure, some 80 per cent is spent on beer.

All alcoholic drinks are now much more highly taxed than

in the past, and comparing pre-war with post-war experience it may approximately be said that the nation drinks half as much as it formerly drank, and pays twice as much for it. According to Sir Josiah Stamp's recent estimate, working-class families spend from 13 to 17 per cent of their weekly earnings in drink. He regards it as a justifiable estimate also that over 20 per cent of our national poverty (in the sense, I presume, of privation of some element necessary for well-being) is "directly attributable to drink."

The reduction in total consumption on beer and other alcoholic drinks has been so great as to render it difficult to realise that any mischief still ascribable to drink is as great as may be inferred from these estimates. An authentic fact will enable one to visualise their truth. Although in 1928 convictions for drunkenness only numbered 58,000 in England and Wales as compared with 189,000 in 1913, yet in 1928 they were about 13 per 10,000 of the total population, including women and children.

In the same year over sixteen standard gallons of beer *per capita* were consumed. This implies a very much heavier annual consumption of beer than sixteen gallons per individual by a portion of the adult population; and social and health workers will have no difficulty in agreeing with a statement made by me in 1916 that if abstinence from alcoholic drinks could be ensured in our crowded industrial towns there would be rapid reduction in their infantile mortality. Alcoholic abstinence would do more to secure this improvement than any other single social reform.

The evils generated by alcoholic indulgence are well known. This indulgence is a chief impediment to healthy housing, for it has robbed the family of money which should have been spent on the family's rental. It is also a chief cause of the many accidents in child life. It destroys the efficiency of home life. It leads to neglect, carelessness and dirtiness in feeding, and generally it means badly nourished infancy and childhood. It is, furthermore, a provocative—by removing or lowering self-restraint—of the venereal diseases which still play havoc with child life.

When we recall these and many allied evils for which alcoholic indulgence is responsible, we can have no hesitation in concluding that reduction in alcoholism has been an important factor in producing the lowered infant mortality of the present day.

This conclusion, based on the general considerations set out here and more fully in the official reports referred to above, confirms the inference suggested by Fig. 11, p. 80, of my *Second Report on Infant and Child Mortality* to the Local Government Board, 1913 (Cd. 6909) which shows the close correlation between the curves from 1890 to 1912 of (*a*) the infant death-rate, (*b*) the *per capita* consumption of beer and spirits, and (*c*) the annual proceedings for drunkenness. The curves, reproduced in the accompanying diagram,[1] have an almost irrisistible suggestiveness. Of course, correspondence does not necessarily imply causation. The falling infant death-rate is also a sequence of other social changes not directly related to alcoholic habits, which need to be considered. For, as I have pointed out,

> Intemperance is a symptom of social evil as well as its cause. It not only results from example and habit acting on an individual of feeble will power, but it is also a common sequel of the toxæmia of over-fatigue, the habit of excessive drinking being acquired in the foolish attempt to counteract fatigue by this means. Excessive drinking is a product of uninteresting surroundings, and more particularly of bad housing and of domestic discomfort. The consideration of intemperance, therefore, cannot be separated from that of housing conditions, and in the search for the easiest point at which to break the vicious circle of influences dragging parents and children down, there is need in some instances for direct attack on intemperance, and in others for equally vigorous attention to the avoidance of chronic over-fatigue, to improvements in housing, and to the provision of wholesome means of recreation.

---

[1] Reproduced by permission of H.M. Comptroller of the Stationery Office.

England and Wales:—*Curves of Infant Mortality, of per capita consumption of beer and spirits*, 1890–1912 *inclusive, and of proceedings for drunkenness in terms of population*, 1890–1911. (In each curve the figure for 1890, or in the case of spirits for 1891, is stated as 100, other years being stated in proportion to this).

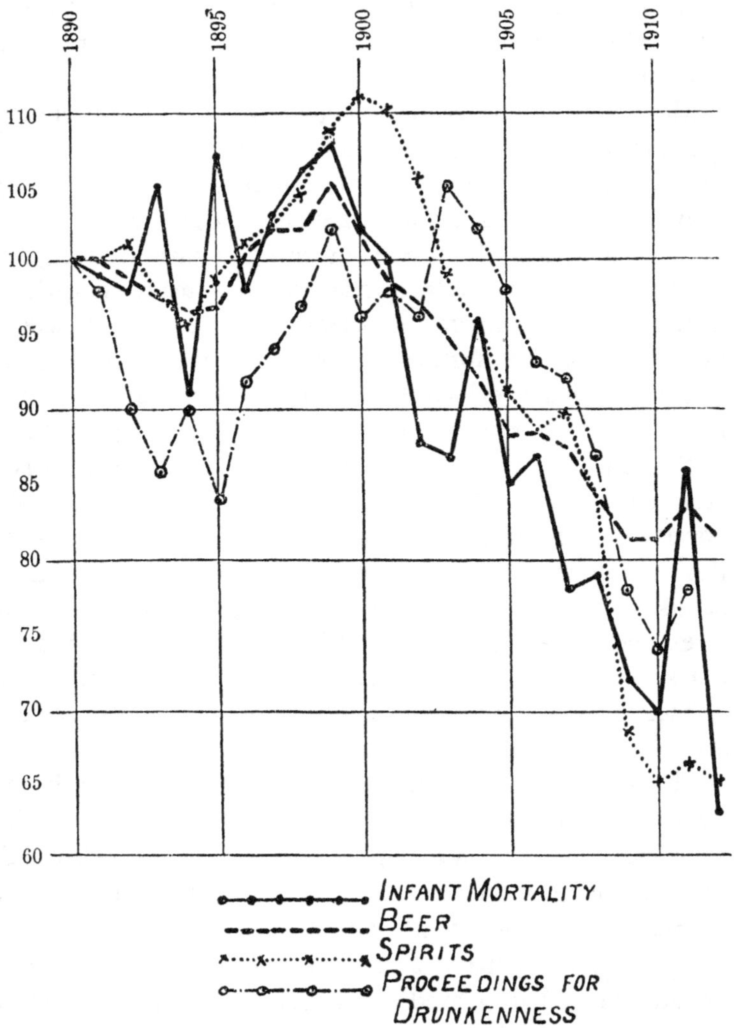

Diagram 14

Clearly, intemperance, like poverty, of which it is often the creator, is a complex phenomenon, in the reduction of which many factors are involved. I need not stress its religious aspect. We have all seen instances of the changed character and conduct, and almost immediate improvement in family comfort and health, when men and women are brought under religious influence.

Many social influences have helped to reduce drunkenness. The increase of cycling and motoring has done much; and the money spent in picture-shows once or twice a week, often by whole families, has doubtless helped to depopulate the public-houses and reduce the torrent of beer-drinking. And beyond all these in importance there has been the steady educational work of various temperance societies, which has so influenced public opinion that abstinence day by day from alcohol is no longer regarded as evidence of crankiness, but has become the normal practice of a high proportion of the total population.

To sum up: poverty in the extreme sense of the word is a great enemy of child-life. It is especially injurious when the poverty is self-imposed, partially or entirely, especially when this self-imposed poverty results from parental alcoholic habits. For in this instance there is not merely serious diversion of expenditure from the needs of healthy life for the children, but superadded to this are the more serious moral effects of alcoholism—carelessness and indifference, with actual neglect, sometimes culminating in protracted cruelty.

The reduction of alcoholism has meant improved health for a vast number of infants, and the possibilities of preventive medicine under this heading are far from being exhausted; and we must give the reduction of poverty and increased care of infants and young children produced thereby its meed of importance, while maintaining that health visitors and child welfare centres have played a great part in producing the more rapid decline in infant mortality which has occurred in recent years.

CHAPTER XLI

HEALTH AT SCHOOL

No sudden change from environmental to personal hygiene—Infection and contagion the first and continuous urgent school problem—Prophylaxis in growth—Medical diagnosis for school absentees—The feeding of school children—Lower age limit for school attendance—Nursery schools—Steps towards a school medical service—Illustration of divergent views—The value of enlightened public opinion—The scholastic side of school hygiene

THE history of the evolution of the British School Medical Service presents many points of interest, but I necessarily confine my description chiefly to the points which have impinged on my personal experience. The scattered work of local medical officers of health and others, and investigations on special problems of school hygiene, have now widened into a national school medical service, which legislatively and largely in practice is an essential part of the Public Health Service in England.

Long before its official organisation, the hygiene of school life was the subject of study and care on the part of many medical officers of health, teachers, and other social workers. The extracts given on page 146 show how this work appealed to me as a young M.O.H. I devoted time and study to it. My knowledge crystallised in a manual of *School Hygiene: The Laws of Health in Relation to School Life*, which was published in 1887. Many editions followed, the last of these under my own hand (the 8th) in 1902. In subsequent editions Dr. James Kerr was the chief author, and I took but little part. Altogether sixteen editions had been published by 1924.

Recalling my personal experiences, in 1899 at a Sessional Meeting of the Sanitary Institute, I read a paper introducing a discussion on "The Health of Scholars, with special reference to the Education Code of the Board of Education." This paper discussed some of the chief problems then occupying the minds of social workers. I began by enunciating the practical opinion that:

> To secure the greatest economy of effort and the maximum result, measures for the promotion of the national health should be in the directions in which there is the greatest scope for their operation;

and that efforts to secure a high standard of health among those under fifteen, and more particularly among those under ten years of age were of supreme importance.

But from the same utilitarian standpoint, I pointed out the importance of remembering that a larger share of each day is spent under the conditions of home life, than under the conditions of school life.

I criticised the allowance of floor space prescribed by the Education Department (afterwards the Board of Education), and the ventilation of schools.

I characterised "cleanliness of the schoolroom as the most indispensable physical condition, next to its lighting and ventilation." I described a scheme for the Brighton Schools for excluding from school children with chronic contagious complaints like impetigo, ringworm, and lousiness, the M.O.H. giving the certificates needed to claim, in respect of these children, the average monetary grant from the Education Department, which was dependent on such certification. The scheme also included use of the inspectors of the Society for the Prevention of Cruelty to Children, who brought pressure to bear on neglectful parents, to secure the care needed for each scholar. This programme may have been suggested by the pioneer work of Dr. James Kerr, then school medical officer in Bradford. From 1902 onwards he developed this work in London, rapidly and successfully, and the example of London was followed throughout the country. His work in promoting the personal hygiene of school children deserves to be told in detail. The cutaneous contagious ailments, then very prevalent, have become relatively uncommon. Pediculosis, whether of the scalp or the body, and other parasitic conditions are now exceptional. The school nurses first appointed were chiefly engaged in the detection and then in the guidance and supervision of the necessary work of personal cleansing at the school and in the homes of the children, and one cannot easily exaggerate the influence on health of the vastly improved cleanliness of school children throughout the whole of Britain which followed on the school medical work before and after it was nationally organised in 1908.

I give here a few particulars of Dr. Kerr's earlier work.

Dr. James Kerr was born in 1862, practised as a physician in Bradford 1893–97, and from 1897–1902 as a specialist in eye and ear diseases. His persistent representations as to defective children to the Bradford School Board led to his being appointed part-time medical superintendent to the Board, and he began a series of investigations of various problems in school life, the aim being prophylaxis in growth. This led to his receiving in 1896 the Howard Medal of the Statistical Society for an essay on School Hygiene. I had the good fortune to be the adjudicator of the Society for this essay, and thus first became acquainted with the extent and originality of this Bradford work. It comprised inquiries into the visual acuity of 9,000 children, the senses, speech, and mental condition of 1,222 retarded children, standards of hearing, mouth-breathing, and some other subjects.

In 1902 Kerr was appointed medical officer to the School Board for London, and he was the chief organiser of the Second International Congress on School Hygiene, held in London in 1907.

I have already noted the invaluable work in cleanliness of scholars initiated by him and carried through with great success in London, thereafter followed all over the country. In his first annual report to the London School Board he wrote:

¶ The detection of children whose efficiency in school is damaged by dirt, parasites, chronic diseases of the ears, or impaired visual acuity, is just beginning. The treatment of all these matters has to be thorough, but is a routine of the most monotonous and uninteresting description. The burden at present falls on the hospitals, and they have not yet adapted themselves to it. Whether even with time they ever can efficiently discharge this public duty is at least doubtful.

In 1906 Kerr was emphasising the need for treatment, medical inspection not being an end in itself. There was required:

Public provision of treatment for certain common conditions, in order to free hospital authorities from crowds of common cases, which at present they cannot manage to their own satisfaction.

In 1907, pursuing the same subject, he wrote:

A point has now been reached to decide whether the greater part of medical inspection shall remain fruitless, or whether the Council will take steps which will justify their later interference to see that younger dependents have a fair chance of properly benefiting by the education offered. Treatment as a public concern will have to be considered in respect to certain educational matters, such as visual troubles, discharging ears, ringworm, and the care of the teeth, in which neither the private practitioner nor the hospitals can give any hope of either sufficient or satisfactory treatment.

Like other towns Brighton adopted a system of notification by school teachers of absentees who were suspected to be suffering from an infectious disease. (This local arrangement is described in the *British Medical Journal*, September 2, 1899.) I regarded it as necessary that the Sanitary Authority should develop a system of medical inspection and inquiry into the history of *all* temporary absentees before they were allowed to resume school attendance; and while expressing the opinion I then held that the School Board should "not usurp the place of the parent or of the Board of Guardians in providing food for the underfed scholar," I added that it would be "no additional interference with the sense of independence of parents to provide free medical diagnosis for poor children who are suffering from slight ailments, for which the parent cannot afford to call in a doctor." And I suggested further that:

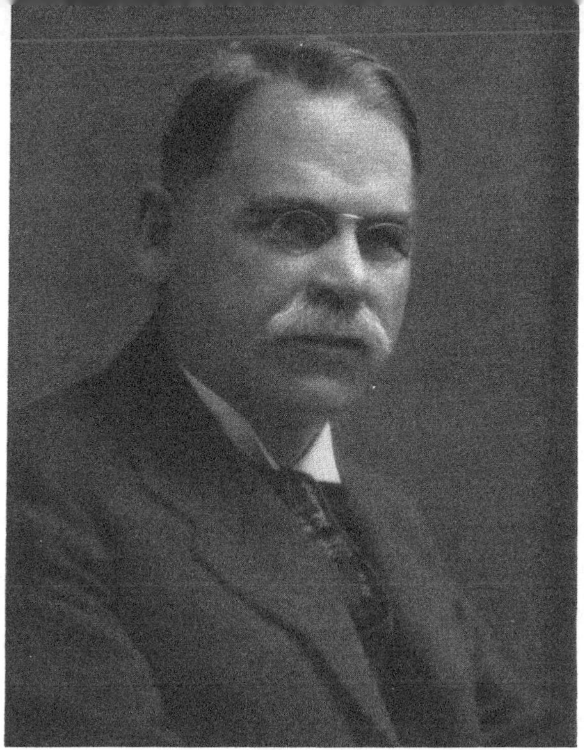

[*Elliot & Fry*

DR. JAMES KERR

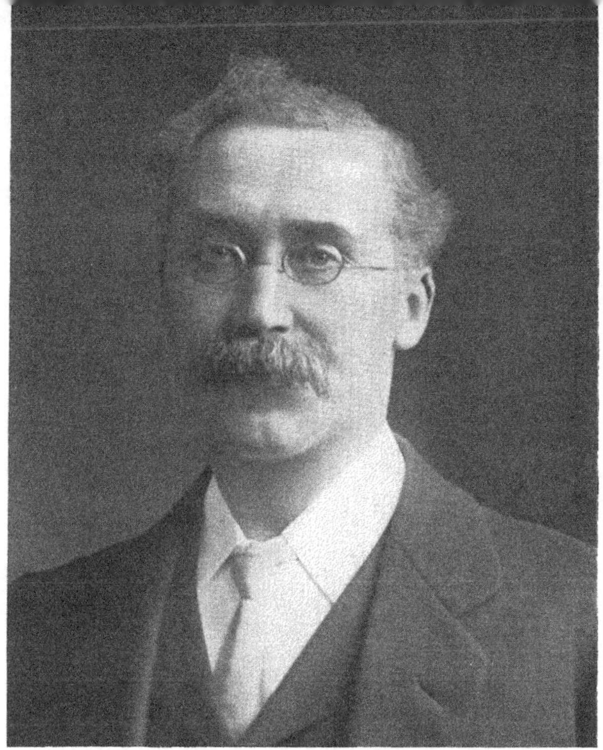

SIR LESLIE MACKENZIE

The largely increased use of hospitals and dispensaries, without any sense of pauperisation, appears to point in the direction of the provision of State doctors for each district, just as there are now State teachers. If such State doctors could be provided for school children, and their services were freely available for the labouring classes, there would be a great diminution in the incidence of infectious diseases in connection with school life.

Evidently I was more sanguine in 1899 than I am now as to the extent to which such a system, or any system, would prevent the spread of measles, whooping-cough, and diphtheria by personal infection. More mature experience has shown that as regards two of these diseases our chief hope lies in immunisation against attack. Difficulties of diagnosis, even when a doctor sees a pupil, as well as failure to obtain medical advice, mean that many infectious cases almost inevitably are overlooked.

I have quoted the above paragraph in full, as showing that somewhat early in my work I had come to the conclusion that for the poor State aid was needed for a better medical service. More on this hereafter.

The feeding of badly nourished school children was also discussed by me in the same paper. In 1899 voluntary workers in Brighton had collected funds for free breakfasts for children recommended by the school teacher. Each of the families concerned was made the subject of a social inquiry by the sanitary inspectors in my department, and these reports were approved by me as a condition of continuance of the free breakfasts. A frequent difficulty, alas! was how to deal with the families in which the father was at work, but his earnings went to the public house. Attempts were made to coerce him by threats of legal action for cruelty, but they failed because the wife would not bear witness; and in the end the voluntary Committee very properly gave the breakfast, even though the strict economist might, and sometimes did, accuse us of subsidising drunkenness. I doubt if at the present day such cases can be satisfactorily dealt with, while ensuring that the child is adequately fed.

The problem of feeding school children is still with us; but happily in this year (1934) there is a reasonable prospect that very many children at school will receive daily a glass of pasteurised milk. The great improvement in vigour and growth which follows this practice has been demonstrated in large-scale experiments in schools both in England and Scotland. Of course, this is only an interim reform. It should be associated with persistent teaching as to what constitutes a complete dietary in children for whom no special ration of milk is called for.

In 1884 there was an agitation against "over-pressure" of children in elementary schools (p. 401), and this may have helped to direct attention to the real problem of under-feeding. Voluntary efforts to improve nutrition were started in many districts, and the evidence of physical defects discovered during the Boer War (1899–1900) led to further action. In 1905 an Inter-Departmental Committee sat on the Medical Inspection and Feeding of Children attending Elementary Schools. They found that a considerable number of local authorities had established some measure of school medical inspection. In 1906 the Foreign Office collected and published information as to school-feeding in other countries, and then a permissive Act (Elementary Education (Provision of Meals) Act) was passed, authorising education authorities to open canteens at a cost not exceeding a halfpenny rate. This meant the introduction of a new policy for education authorities. They were made to step into the region of the work of Guardians of the Poor. Further extensions of the responsibilities of Education Authorities occurred in provision for the care of blind and deaf and of epileptic children; and finally, after the period dealt with in this volume, there was imposed upon them in 1921 the duty of treating sick or defective scholars not otherwise provided for. It is only since the medical activities of the Education Committee, of the Public Health Committee, and of the Committee which took over the former medical work of Board of Guardians of the

Poor, came under a single large Local Authority, that satisfactory co-operation between the various branches of medical work undertaken at the expense of public money, has been rendered fully practicable.

THE LOWER AGE LIMIT FOR SCHOOL ATTENDANCE

In work as M.O.H. I had forced on my attention the recurrent devastating spread of infectious diseases among children in infants' schools. In March 1902 I read a paper to the Childhood Society entitled, "A Plea for the Exclusion of Children under Five Years of Age from Public Elementary Schools," which was widely discussed. It fitted in with a period of financial stringency in the country, and was widely acted on by local Education authorities. It should be explained that in England compulsory attendance for children begins at the age of five years, but at the time when the above paper was read, 10·2 per cent of the total scholars in elementary schools in England were under that age. In a later paper on the same subject I claimed the support of Mr. (later Sir Robert) Morant, quoting the following remarks from his official Memorandum to the Education Code or 1905:

> Children under 5 years of age are not required by law to attend school, and there is reason for believing that the attendance of such children is often accompanied by danger to health.

Mr. Morant went on to state that evidence pointed to the conclusion that children not coming to school until they were six years old or more "in general compared favourably at a later age with children whose attendance began at an earlier age." This statement was quoted in a paper contributed by me to the Proceedings of the Second International Congress on School Hygiene, London, 1907, which led to a "full-dress" discussion of both sides of this problem of the lower age-limit. In this paper I elaborated the financial, the economic, and the health aspects of the question, stressing under the last-named heading the general effects of breathing polluted air as well as the spreading of infectious diseases.

It was pointed out that the aggregation in schools necessarily meant much pollution of the air, and that in large rooms the evils of aggregation were exceptionally great. The need for greater movement of air increases with the size of the room. Children and their clothes are now much cleaner than at that time, but it still remains true that in a private family the dangers of close aggregation are less than when the children of many families are collected in a single larger room. This is especially so in the spread of infection like that of measles. I did not anticipate that exclusion of the younger children from school would entirely prevent the spread of measles, for older children brought infection home, where its fatality was terrible among infants and pre-school children.

The problem is modified now that artificial immunisation against measles has become practicable, though not yet generally practised; and in respect of this disease—the chief offender—the discussion can now be limited to educational considerations.

On this side of the problem the quotation from Mr. Morant's memorandum in 1905 and other quotations were utilised by me to justify my statement in 1907 that "the educational uselessness of school attendance under five years of age may be regarded as officially confirmed." But this does not necessarily condemn attendance of children under five at school; it may indicate that the conditions of school life at this age need to be fundamentally changed. Dr. Kerr, in a report to the London County Council, 1905, urged that the curriculum for these children had been lacking in intelligence, and that what was needed was not withdrawal of these children from school, but an improved kind of education and the appropriate training of teachers; for, as he urged, children "learn more in the years from three to five than they will learn in the same period at any time subsequently." The school he advocated is rather a nursery with specially trained attendants. For "in the infant department the child has chiefly to grow. Nutrition and sleep are its chief functions." The process of education is extremely active in these early years; but the teaching required is teaching in social adaptation. This means the acquisition of habits of cleanliness and of discipline, as well as the ability to walk and run. Dr. Kerr laid it down that pencils, paper, needles, and pins should not be handled by children below six, though free-arm drawing is valuable. My comment on this programme was that in my view

> the school is not the best place for such training as is desirable at these ages. It is most naturally and effectively acquired at home (when the home is satisfactory), and in healthy play with other children; or in crèches in charge of a nurse rather than a teacher, when the mother cannot give the requisite attention.

Present arrangements in nursery schools are now more in accord with the above-stated principles; and I appreciate the extreme importance of early formation of habits of self-control and social conduct, as these largely determine physical health and mental and moral welfare in adult life. This side of child welfare work is being increasingly stressed in the teaching given by doctors and nurses at child welfare centres, and it is among the most important spheres of growing social work. The work is being continued in nursery schools. These are still relatively few in number.

STEPS TOWARDS A SCHOOL MEDICAL SERVICE

Many events converged to the establishment of this service.

The Education Act of 1870 appointing School Boards, followed in 1876 by the imposition of an obligation on all parents to cause their children to receive elementary instruction during the ages five to fourteen, was supplemented in 1880 by making school attendance compulsory, and in 1887 by the abolition of payment of school fees by parents. A great State responsibility for the welfare of all school children was thus created; and the transfer of the powers of School Boards in 1902 to Local Education Authorities, who were County Councils and County Borough Councils along with some smaller Sanitary Authorities, meant that these authorities, who dealt with the problems of health and local government, are now called on to concern themselves with the education and health of the children placed under their care in schools.

Meanwhile a double current in favour of greater attention to school hygiene was increasing in volume and force.

Social enthusiasts and medical officers of health were largely responsible for this pressure, which led to the appointment of the official committees mentioned in the following paragraphs. The urge in this direction was increased by the recruiting statistics, revealing the physical unfitness of many soldiers in the Boer War, 1899–1900.

Dr. Frederick Warner's examination of over 50,000 school children in and about 1892 aroused general attention. School Boards began to appoint medical advisers. In London Dr. (later Sir William R.) Smith was appointed in this capacity by the London School Board in 1891, and in 1893 Dr. Kerr in Bradford. A chief duty of these new officers was to control medical certificates of absentees, and to examine pupil teachers, etc.

In 1893 the Elementary Education (Blind and Deaf Children) Act imposed on Education Authorities the duty of appointing medical officers for the purposes of the Act, and in 1899 there followed the medical provisions under the Defective and Epileptic Children Act. The introduction of medical supervision in school work was thus started.

In 1903 a Royal Commission on Physical Training in Scotland was appointed, and in England an Inter-Departmental Committee on Physical Deterioration in 1904. Drs. Leslie Mackenzie and Matthew Hay in Scotland published figures showing great variations in the physical conditions of Scottish children in various social strata, and the Inter-Department Committee enlarged the scope of similar data, and discussed in some detail the questions of school feeding and of medical inspection of scholars. The Society of Medical Officers of Health, after hearing a paper read by Dr. Meredith Richards (*Public Health*, Vol. XV, p. 128), passed resolutions, which were forwarded to the Board of Education and the Local Government Board, advocating *inter alia* that "the hygienic control of public elementary and of other public schools should devolve on the medical officer of health of the district"; and that "the medical officer of health should be required to record the action taken by his department in regard to schools, and to forward annually to the Board of Education such portions of his report as relate to this subject."

The appointment by the Board of Education of a skilled medical adviser in school hygiene was urged in a further resolution.

From an editorial article on "The Organisation of the Medical Inspection of Schools," which I wrote in 1903 (*British Medical Journal*, November 14, 1903), I take the following paragraph in further illustration of the early stages of advocacy of medical inspection in England. I began by referring to methods of school hygiene in foreign countries, described by me on another page of the *Journal*, and emphasised the need for different beginnings in England.

> In Belgium and France general sanitary administration is . . . almost embryonic. In England, on the other hand, general sanitary administration is elaborate and complex, and in a large proportion of its sanitary districts is efficiently carried out. . . .

I then stated that although the control of sanitation of schools and of infectious diseases on the whole was more efficiently carried out in England, there was much less work done than "in certain German schools over such matters of personal hygiene as eyesight, adenoids, deafness, and so on." Reference was then made to

> the excellent work done by Dr. Kerr as Medical Officer to the Bradford School Board, and the similar work in relation to the special problems of school hygiene which is now being done by him and his medical assistants under the London School Board.

Referring to the London work I said:

The work is one of the best instances that could be adduced of the further possibilities of valuable medical work in school hygiene. Each scholar represents a certain social value, capable of being increased by attention to his physical, intellectual, and moral culture. This value will be diminished or lost if through neglect of early treatment of disease or of hygienic precautions the scholar suffers in health. Hence medical inspection of scholars as well as of schools is imperatively demanded in the interest of the community. It is this personal aspect of school hygiene which, except in a comparatively small number of districts, has been neglected in this country.

This article, written in 1903, from which I have already freely quoted, went on to detail the extensive duties which should be entrusted to the proposed school medical inspectors. They should have final control, not only over questions of ventilation, cleansing, arrangements of desks, etc., but also regulate the programme of physical exercises, and give "clear instruction to the older scholars in the laws of health." They should, most important of all, make

periodical medical examinations of each child, if possible at least once a year, a dossier being kept for each child, so that progress may be noted as to weight, height, eyesight, hearing, etc. . . . Such a record would speedily lead to further investigation in the case of those children who were being neglected in their homes.

At this early stage I emphasised and entered into some detail as to the need that

if efficiency is to be secured and overlapping to be avoided, the medical inspectors must act in collaboration with the M.O.H. of each country or borough.

The British Medical Association was active in forcing the hands of the Board of Education; and in Scotland much pioneer work in expediting the medical inspection of school and scholars was accomplished. Dr. (now Sir Leslie) Mackenzie's book on *Medical Inspection of Schools* (published in 1904) embodied the results of much personal investigation, and was an almost complete guide to the future medical inspectors of schools.

AN ILLUSTRATION OF DIVERGENT VIEWS

As I write I have before me a copy of a petition in 1907 to Mr. R. McKenna, then President of the Board of Education, and of the correspondence on this petition in which I took part, signed by distinguished physicians and surgeons, and endorsed by the British Medical Association.

The object of the petition, as originally drafted, was to secure adequate teaching of hygiene and temperance in all schools and training colleges; but there had been introduced into the petition a paragraph in favour of "the establishment of a Medical Bureau in the Education Department," with some recommendations as to its relation to general public health work. Voicing the attitude of many medical officers of health, I took strong objection, as a member of a prospective deputation, to the last paragraph of the petition, which affirmed that:

> It is impossible for all these duties (anthropometrical records and records of the health-condition of each child) to be performed by either the Department or by the personnel of the Public Health Medical Service of the country. Their fulfilment constitutes a considerable development of work special to the Education Department, and therefore should be controlled by the Board of Education.

On receiving a copy of this petition I at once wrote stating that health administrators, including, I believed, the majority of medical officers of health, could not accept this statement, and I resigned my position on the Committee which had dealt with the educational side of the petition, as a protest against introducing at a late stage this "foreign" question as to who were the appropriate authorities to carry on the local work of medical inspection of scholars. The late Sir Lauder Brunton wrote begging me "not to upset the apple-cart": and in answer I indicated the difficulties involved in introducing into the petition "the entirely separate question of the mechanism" of school medical inspection, including a recommendation for the adoption of a method which "would secure the least result and involve the most expense." I added that this new school medical work was essential in "the evolution of the work of the M.O.H., which remains incomplete until it embraces the medical work proposed in the petition to be done in an independent department."

The late Sir Victor Horsley, F.R.S., then wrote to protest against my comments. In answering I wrote with the frankness which Horsley always displayed in controversy, "the fact is you (the petitioners) are all almost without exception amateurs in respect of practical administration." The administrative scheme outlined by him was described by me "an admirable example of prospective local inco-ordination." In a further letter I summed up the methods proposed by him as follows:

> To attempt now to set up independent school doctors, unco-ordinated to a chief executive medical officer (for all health work), means . . . giving us probably for another thirty years inefficiency in school medical work like that of a large number of districts in which there are still part-time medical officers of health.

Brunton and Horsley and their co-petitioners were actuated by burning social zeal, and they furthermore represented many educationists who desired to keep the proposed new school medical service separate from the public health service.

At that time public health work in many districts admittedly was inadequate and unsatisfactory. The petitioners failed to appreciate that the addition of school medical inspection to other sanitary duties would make it practicable to employ full-time medical officers more generally; and that in towns in which an efficient sanitary service already existed, full access to schools and scholars immensely increased the possibility of complete public health work.

A later incident in my Brighton experience illustrated these two schools of thought. When "the duty to provide for the medical inspection of children" was enacted by the Education (Administrative Provisions) Act, 1907, it became necessary for the Brighton Town Council and its Education Committee to consider action. The Town Council passed a resolution asking the Education Committee to consider the subject and report on it, after consultation with the M.O.H. I received notice of the meeting of the Committee to be held for this purpose, and was asked to be in waiting. After a long time I was called, and was forthwith informed courteously by the Chairman of the Committeee that they had considered the matter and proposed to appoint a special school medical officer who would not be related to public health administration. I at once explained that my instructions had been to consult with them, which did not mean simply hearing their decision; adding that all I could now do was to report to the Town Council that I had been unable to consult as instructed by them. The Committee evidently appreciated the difficulty. I ceased to be M.O.H. of Brighton in February 1908 and my successor as M.O.H. became also School Medical Officer, with a staff of school doctors and of school nurses under his general control.

The adoption of a general system of school medical inspection became law in 1907 by the inclusion in the Education (Administrative Provisions) Bill of that year of a private member's clause, which put upon all Education Committees the duty to provide for systematic medical inspection of all scholars, and gave them powers to make provision for their health and physical condition.

The central control of school hygiene was placed in the hands of the Board of Education; and under the leadership and driving power of its Secretary (Sir Robert Morant) and its newly appointed chief medical officer, Dr. (afterwards Sir George) Newman, who had hitherto been the M.O.H. for the metropolitan borough of Finsbury, the new service soon expanded and became a potent factor in revealing physical defects in children and thereby impelling remedial and preventive action.

The first "Memorandum on Medical Inspection of Children in Elementary Schools," issued in November 1907, set out the intentions of the Board of Education that the administration of the Education (Administrative Provisions) Act "should rest upon a broad basis of public health," and that it should also "use to the utmost extent the existing machinery of medical and sanitary administration, developing and supplementing it as required, rather than supplanting it by bringing into existence new agencies, partially redundant and possibly competing."

The memorandum added that the Board of Education view the whole subject of school hygiene not as a speciality or as a group of specialities existing by and of themselves but "as an integral factor in the health of the nation. The application of this principle requires that the work of medical inspection should be carried out in intimate conjunction with the Public Health Authorities and under the direct supervision of the medical officer of health."

This quotation shows that in its initiation the Board of Education endorsed the principles on which the school medical service should be conducted, for which many members of the public health medical service had strenuously contended.

The new service was not established without much controversy with medical practitioners and with their Association. Those wishing to learn more of these earlier difficulties may refer to page 367 of my *International Studies on the Relation between the Private and Official Practice of Medicine* (Vol. III, England and Wales, Allen & Unwin, 1931), in which Brighton once more illustrates difficulties encountered. In this instance the British Medical Association attempted to prevent the appointment of full-time school doctors and to boycott them when appointed by the Brighton Education Committee. Happily the policy of the Association is now consistent with the public interests.

THE DUAL ASPECT OF SCHOOL MEDICAL WORK

I am tempted to add comments which may serve to bring into relief the dual aspect of school medico-hygienic work. It is an educational as well as a medical problem. A main object of medicine is to anticipate, and often to prevent, the onset of disorder or disease of any part of human personality. At first the chief and most urgent task of school medicine was to detect physical defects and to secure their treatment. This at the present day is still the most urgent daily work of the school doctor and of the school nurses who help him; and it will continue to be so for many years, perhaps always. It will become less preponderant in school medical work when the admirable work already done at child welfare centres—institutions of the general public health service—has been more fully developed, and when the care given to infants has become equally general for pre-school children, for the "toddlers" in whom between the ages of two and five much disease develops, seriously handicapping subsequent school life.

Thus on its purely medical side closer and more complete co-operation between scholastic and non-scholastic official medical care of children is needed. The two services should indeed be one; and there can be no future separation of the two without serious injury to the public health.

But there remain the problems of physical, mental, and moral culture—all of them needing fuller application in practice if health in its fullest sense is to be secured; and with these problems the teacher, the physiologist, and the psychologist are concerned as well as the physician and hygienist. Much has already been done in these branches of school hygiene; the physical training in elementary schools is admirable. The fact that in some medico-hygienic respects school medical work forms an integral part of satisfactory school education explains the opposition of some experts in school hygiene to the combination of school with general public health work. Dr. Kerr expressed this view in his Annual Report to the London County Council for 1908:

> The whole State provision for aiding the growth and development of the child from the time it ceases to be entirely dependent upon its parents until it attains puberty now constitutes this formal education. The only scientific doctrine to follow as a guide for legislation is that any public supervision of, or provision for, the growth and development, that is for the general care, of children should be under

the education authority. The recognition of this unifying principle will simplify laws and avoid endless overlapping and complications in practice.

Happily now every Education Committee throughout England is an integral, though largely autonomous, part of the County Council or Sanitary Authority of its area of work, and the dual responsibility can be met. There is much hope of as rapid progress on this physiological and psychological side of educational life as on its medical or clinical side. Nor is this triple path of progress confined to school life. The same impetus is being appreciated in the work of child welfare centres, in which training of conduct and in good habits forms as important a subject as correct methods of feeding and clothing and general hygiene.

The initiation of the school medical service illustrates the importance of public pressure in securing reform. Not five years before the new service started, the Board of Education's attitude to the medical supervision and care of children had been one of passive opposition. Similarly influential opinion on the London County Council then regarded such a service as foreign to the work of the Council, and belonging to poor law and sanitary authorities. But politicians, like Government Departments—who are their executive—have their ears open; and "public opinion," that persuasive and irresistible force when right is on its side, brings mental and moral coercion to those whose eyes have hitherto been shut. The schoolmaster, the hygienist, and the "uplifters," anxious for health and fitness, and regarding its attainment as a religious end, were indeed abroad.

CONTRIBUTIONS

School Hygiene: The Laws of Health in Relation to School Life, published in 1887. Eighth Edition 1902, Sixteenth Edition 1924 (rewritten by Dr. James Kerr).

The Health of Scholars. An Address at the Sessional Meeting of the Sanitary Institute, December 1899 (*Journal of the Sanitary Institute*, Vol. XXI, Part II).

The Lower Limit of Age for School Attendance. A Plea for the Exclusion of Children under Five Years of Age from Public Elementary Schools (Childhood Society, *Public Health*, July 1902).

The Lower Limit of Age for School Attendance (*Proceedings of the Second International Congress on School Hygiene*, August 1907, and *Practitioner*, November 1907).

For references as to chronicity of infection in scarlet fever and diphtheria, see page 185.

CHAPTER XLII

CASSANDRAS

Fears of decadence in every generation—Over-pressure or under-feeding—Evidence of national deterioration unsatisfactory—Explanation of increased sickness certification—Dubious evidence of inherited inferiority—Post-bellum evidence of physical improvement

CASSANDRA'S prophecies of evil for her country though disbelieved came true; and the race of Cassandra is still widely represented, and receives much credence. Will these prophecies prove true? Is this pessimism as to the national future justified, so far as physical health is concerned? The possibilities of decadence in character are more difficult to assess.

In each succeeding decade of my long experience as a physician, statements have been made that the standard of health and sanity of the community must necessarily be lowered by modern medical care, whether it be concerned with prevention or repair, and that a like statement applies largely to the non-medical care which accompanies—or should accompany—medico-hygienic treatment.

I have been comforted by an ineradicable belief that what is socially desirable or in accord with Christian principles cannot be injurious to the welfare of oncoming generations; and this chapter attempts to give reasons for thinking that there is no substantial evidence of widespread physical decadence, or support for the view that the maintenance and extension of sanitary and sanatory work is incompatible with man's well-being.

I may recall some of my former protests against certain Cassandra-like utterances of the past, extending in part beyond the range of medicine. In an address as President of a Brighton scientific society in 1893, on "Civilisation and the Survival of the Fittest," I concluded as follows:

Unfavourable forecasts however plausible they may appear, we will not believe. There are many instances, in which prophecies have been falsified by events, which make us distrustful of "long views." The Duke of Wellington in 1832 said that "few people would be sanguine enough to imagine that we shall ever again be as prosperous as we have been." Since that time the wealth of this country has advanced by leaps and bounds. The break-up of the Turkish empire in Europe has been foretold for centuries. Malthus foresaw impending bankruptcy, unless population was restrained. We are further removed from bankruptcy than in his time, although the population has trebled. The coal measures of England may some day be exhausted, but not one of us will stay his hand from the coal scuttle on a cold winter's day on this account.

Even earlier than this I had upheld an optimistic view. In an article in a weekly journal written in 1885, I doubted the general occurrence of "Over-pressure" in schools concerning which there was then much agitation. I recalled that this was no new cry, for Charles Dickens had already caricatured it when he described Dr. Blimber's private school as a mental hothouse in which "mental green peas were produced at Christmas, and intellectual asparagus all the year round," and that following on this "over-pressure," it was sadly true that "young Toots, when he began to have whiskers, left off having brains."

Elementary education had become compulsory in 1880, and this meant, I added, that:

there had been forced into the schools the weakly and underfed wastrels of our crowded cities;

with the collateral consequence in the opinion of a distinguished alienist that

to educate a half-starved child at all is to overpress it.

I contended that:

A child, though half-starved, is better, from a sanitary standpoint, in a well-warmed and well-ventilated schoolroom, than wandering in the streets. The brain-work involved in school life will burn up less of his scanty food than would be required to keep up his temperature in resisting the external cold.

It is only fair to add that I went on to advocate dinners for all poorer scholars, and that then we should not be exposed to the risks which in Sir James Crichton Browne's eloquent words meant:

> The children want blood, and we offer them a little brain-polish; they ask for bread and receive a problem; for milk, and the Tonic Sol-fa system is introduced to them.

I may illustrate my obstinate disbelief in decadence by recalling that after reading a paper at the Jubilee Meeting of the Manchester and Salford Sanitary Association, April 24, 1902, I was asked to sign a petition to the Board of Education in favour of improved physical education in schools, but was obliged to decline, because by doing so I should have been committed to assertions in the petition of race degeneration, based on figures as to recruits, which had failed to convince my judgment.

The figures of rejected recruits at the time of the Boer War in 1899 aroused the public conscience, and led to various investigations.

In contributing in 1903 to a symposium on National Physical Deterioration which appeared in the *Manchester Guardian*, I challenged the premises on which several distinguished contributors had already discussed this question. The following extract from my contribution may be quoted from a reprint of the contributions to the symposium in a volume entitled *National Physical Training: An Open Debate*, ed. by J. B. Atkins, London 1904.

> The number of recent rejections of recruits is stated to have been exceptionally high, and particularly so in our great manufacturing centres. To argue from this increase that the average physical status of the population has declined is most fallacious. To begin with, there has not been in the last half-century a period at which so many recruits have been required in so short a time as since the commencement of the Boer War.

I pointed out that the greater demands had necessitated accepting recruits of inferior physique, and I urged the need for comparable data in comparing successive periods. In this connection the efforts of the British Association between 1878 and 1883 to obtain data on the physical examination of Britons at various ages may be mentioned.

Prior to 1904 the Director General of the Medical Department of the Army, citing increase in rejection of recruits, had, in the words of my contribution to the afore-mentioned symposium:

> Expressed the opinion that the increase in the rejections could be explained in one way only—"the masses from whom the Army recruits are chiefly taken are of an inferior physique to what they were twenty-five years ago." Further inquiries, however, showed that a large proportion, and probably the whole, of the excess of rejections at the later period was due to improvements in the returns, to more rigid enforcement of standards of height, girth, etc., and to other similar causes.

I then commented as follows on some figures published in the Report of the recent Royal Commission on Physical Training (Scotland):

> The figures of height and weight of school children in Edinburgh and Aberdeen show marked inferiority in the Edinburgh children; and the earlier statistics show similar differences in different social strata. Do these figures, however, justify the remark in the Report of the Royal Commission (p. 25) that "there exists in Scotland an undeniable degeneration of individuals of the classes where food and environment are defective?" Degeneration from what? For our present purpose the quoted statement is beside the mark. If it implies that the Edinburgh children have degenerated as compared with a past generation of Edinburgh children of the same social stratum the statement is unsubstantiated, and this is the point with which we are concerned. To say that the poor are punier, smaller chested, and thinner than the well-to-do is to state a sad commonplace, but it does not help us in determining whether there has been any "degeneration," as compared with the past. We are driven back upon our main question. What evidence is there that the mass of the population—i.e. the artisan and labouring classes—have degenerated as compared with the mass of the last or previous generations?

Mr. J. B. Atkins gave evidence before the Departmental Committee on Physical Deterioration, quoting my contribution to his symposium, and I may give here a paragraph from the Report of the Committee as follows:

> The Committee hope that the facts and opinions they have collected will have some effect in allaying the apprehensions of those who, as it appears on insufficient grounds, have made up their minds that progressive deterioration is to be found among the people generally.

I need not give the well-known facts showing that the average span of life from birth onwards has lengthened, and that this is true for each age above sixty, as well as in the earlier part of life, though the higher ages have gained much less than the young.

It is conceivable, of course—and is widely believed—that although the average duration of life has been marvellously prolonged (*a*) its quality has, and it is alleged must have, deteriorated in view of the saving of weakly lives by modern medicine and surgery, and especially in view of the saving of delicate infants and of consumptive patients from death.

(*b*) It has been assumed without proof that some deterioration of the quality of average human life must have occurred as a result of the fact that the birth-rate has remained relatively high[1] among the financially poor, while among the well-to-do it has greatly declined.

(*a*) It is true that multitudes are now alive who, had the conditions of the eighteenth and of the first half of the nineteenth century continued, would be in their graves. This has been brought about by improved social conditions, including better sanitation, housing, and more abundant food, and modern medicine and surgery. But it is also true that many of those who in the past would have been maimed by the evil factors in life, are now less exposed to these, and under improved medical treatment and better general conditions of life are in excellent

[1] This in 1934 is much less the case.

health. Who shall strike a just balance between these forces? Varicose veins and hernia, for instance, need no longer be causes of industrial inefficiency; and appendicitis has ceased to be dangerous or disabling when properly treated.

Infant mortality, as we know, has been halved or more than halved in the last forty years. Does not this mean a vast increase in the number of weakly survivors to higher ages? To suggest this is to ignore the fact that measures which prevent infantile deaths have also protected and improved the standard of health of all infants; and observation of modern children cannot fail to convince one that in the aggregate their health is better than that of a generation ago. It is fallacious to assume that children's epidemics exclusively or even chiefly sweep off the weakly children; but they do make very many children weakly.

The returns of Friendly Societies and of the insured under the National Insurance Acts show that the proportion of the insured who now receive sickness benefits has greatly increased. Is this not evidence of a lowered standard of health? The fact is as stated, but the inference remains unproved. In times of unemployment, claims for monetary sickness benefits increase; and apart from this factor, doctors now more fully recognise the importance of rest in the treatment of sickness, and so the certification of disabling sickness is swollen. Furthermore, under the conditions of sickness insurance in this country it is difficult for the doctor, who is always employed directly by the free choice of the patient, to refuse a certificate of disabling sickness, even though he may doubt its necessity. He, not unreasonably, gives his patient the benefit of the doubt; and this is especially so when resumption of work after illness should be contemplated.

Personally I do not regard this increased sickness-certification under our Insurance Acts, however serious it may be financially, as proving a reduced standard of health. It would not be difficult, as others like myself have suggested, to devise future benefits varying inversely with the duration of past claims. These would reveal the true inwardness of the present benefit claims. In repeating this suggestion, let me add, that no reflection on the honesty of most doctors or patients is implied. Careless certifiers are only a minority among insurance doctors.

The evidence as to the average health of the population, considered dispassionately, appears to me to show that decadence or deterioration has not occurred. It may have, and probably has, occurred among limited groups of the total population. The state of these groups calls for social and sanitary measures, not mere relief; but the general population present unmistakable evidence of an enhanced standard of health.

(*b*) There remains to be considered the effect on the nation of the reduction in the national birth-rate, which has been greatest in that section of the population most favourably placed for physical, intellectual, and general cultural development. Surely a lowering of the standard of ability in the general population, physical and mental, must follow? I have discussed this problem rather fully in my *Health Problems in Organised Society. Studies in Social Aspects of Health* (p. 250, P. S. King & Son, 1927) and on page 290; and can only briefly outline here the considerations involved.

It is necessary to distinguish sharply in one's mind between intrinsic inferiority and inferiority associated with present social circumstances. Either of these factors might produce a deterioration of health and of the mental and moral qualities which are even more desirable than physical health. Doubtless the children of the very poor are handicapped, relatively to other children, in their possibilities of accomplishment in life, whether in health or in intellectual attainment, though this handicap is being steadily reduced. But there is also, as I have written on page 241 of the above book:

> Abundant evidence that the relative (not absolute) poverty of larger families in countless families is compensated for, largely if not completely, by the care of devoted parents, and by the inestimable

value of the social training in what is best in life which a complete family affords.

Nevertheless, we have yet far to travel before the child of the poor will, in essentials of environment, including education and culture, have equal opportunities with the child of the well-to-do to realise his potentialities of growth and development in every respect. Meanwhile it is wise to be silent concerning too hastily assumed essential class inferiorities. As regards inherited inferiority I may quote here an Inaugural Address given by me on October 21, 1904 to the York Medical Society (*Lancet*, November 12, 1904). The subject of the address was "Social Evolution and Public Health."

In this address I quoted Professor Karl Pearson, who had recently expressed the extreme view that:

> We have two groups in the community—one parasitic on the other. The latter thinks of to-morrow and is childless, the former takes no thought and multiplies.

I also quoted Mr. Arthur (Lord) Balfour who, in a meeting of the British Association, September 1904, had said that inasmuch as when men win their way from lower to middle rank their progeny diminishes:

> It seems that as the State contrives education so as to allow this rising from a lower to an upper class, so much does it do something to diminish the actual quality of the breed.

Commenting on this last statement, I remarked:

> Mr. Balfour's statement seems to involve the assumption that the line of fission between the more and the less efficient members of the community lies horizontally between the various classes. There is no reason to think that this is so. *It is more probably oblique* if not vertical.

And generally while holding that there was:

> strong reason to believe that innate inferiority is the only form of inferiority which is permanently transmissible, I am satisfied that no sufficient evidence has been produced to show that there is innate inferiority in a large proportion of the wage-earning classes.

The whole problem is beset with difficulties, in particular this difficulty of distinguishing between the inextricably mingled influence of nature and nurture. Both extremes of thought present a distortion of truth; we are neither creatures of fixity of inherited characters nor are we clay in the potter's hand which is shaped by the circumstances of life. Neither view comprehends entire humanity. Biological Calvinism and environmental determinism form a double enslavement, if we accept them as compassing the circle of life. Environment, in its widest sense, mental and moral, as well as physical, is the material out of which character is formed; but man can largely vary his environment at will, and can thus in large measure determine not only his physical, but also his mental and moral well-being.

POSTSCRIPT

During the Great War infants and children in Britain were better fed, and a considerable jump in average weight and height resulted, which has not been lost. The wives of the fighting forces received pay, and but little money was wasted on alcoholic drinks.

After the Great War this improvement has continued. There is evidence of this in most parts of the country, though some exception may need to be made regarding the average physical condition of children in the "black" areas in which large-scale unemployment has been long-continued. Even in these areas there have been countervailing factors, constituted by the weekly payments under unemployment insurance, and the reduction in the wasteful spending of a large share of the family receipts on beer. The following statement made by Dr. A. S. N. MacGregor, M.O.H. of Glasgow, in his Annual Report for 1931 states the position fairly:

The boys and girls entering school from whatever social group are appreciably taller and heavier than formerly, a gain which, it is important to notice, is substantially augmented during school life. This is the general experience throughout the country. Since the war the school population has decidedly improved in physique, as measured by the heights and weights of the scholars.

Dr. Auden similarly, comparing the experience of school girls aged fourteen to eighteen in Birmingham in 1895 with that of 1925, found that the proportion of pupils whose height is above the average has improved at all these ages. It appears probable that deterioration has not been taking place, but that, owing to the rapid development of the national conscience, our biological standards in human affairs have risen considerably. Unfortunately we lack satisfactory records of standards in the past. But we know that University race crews have gone up steadily in physique in every decade of the last century.

As regards standards of intelligence we may be less certain, but, as Dr. Kerr says in his *Fundamentals of School Hygiene*, 1926:

> Intelligence is measured or expressed by mental ability. Whatever it may be in the single individual, with half a dozen of them it is proportioned to physique as shown by nutrition and bodily development. Attention to this physique is more necessary for the State than any academic education. . . . It is obvious that with such intimate mixture of races as exists in England, it is almost nonsense to regard the various social strata graded by poverty as representing mental levels of graded hereditary inferiority.

CONTRIBUTIONS

Presidential Address on Civilisation and the Survival of the Fittest (Brighton and Sussex Philosophical Society, 1893).

An Inaugural Address on Social Evolution and Public Health. York Medical Society, October 21, 1904 (*Lancet*, November 12, 1904).

INDEX OF SUBJECTS

(*See also under chapter headings*)

INDEX OF PROPER NAMES

www.ingramcontent.com/pod-product-compliance
Lightning Source LLC
LaVergne TN
LVHW011104300926
849160LV00008B/278
9781138906471